The Intentional Relationship

Occupational Therapy and Use of Self

Renée R. Taylor, PhD
Professor
Department of Occupational Therapy
University of Illinois at Chicago
Chicago, Illinois

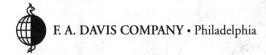
F. A. DAVIS COMPANY • Philadelphia

This book is dedicated to the exceptional therapists whose work was featured in this book. Generously, they contributed their time, personal reflections, and revealing stories of practice to serve the interest of education and knowledge development in this under-recognized area of occupational therapy.

Preface

This book emerged from an ongoing curiosity and a fair amount of frustration in trying to locate a detailed, comprehensive, and integrated textbook on therapeutic use of self specific to the field of occupational therapy. As a professor teaching in this area, my interactions with students and practicing occupational therapists inspired me to learn more about the interpersonal aspects of practice. As a practicing psychotherapist, I was also interested in learning how I might blend knowledge from the field of psychology with existing occupational therapy knowledge as it pertains to the therapeutic relationship.

I began this inquiry by conducting a nationwide survey of 568 practicing occupational therapists randomly selected from a membership database provided by the American Occupational Therapy Association (Taylor, Lee, Kielhofner, & Ketkar, 2007). The objectives of this study were to determine the degree to which occupational therapists value the client-therapist relationship, to identify variables that challenge the client-therapist relationship, and to summarize the interpersonal strategies that are currently being used to respond to such challenges. Results from this survey revealed that, across practice settings and client populations, practicing occupational therapists are frequently encountering clients who are demonstrating a wide range of emotional, behavioral, and interpersonal difficulties. Most experienced occupational therapists place a high priority on their interactions with clients but at the same time feel that their training in this area could have been more sophisticated and comprehensive. The findings from this study confirmed the need for a text addressing these issues for use by educators, students, and practitioners of occupational therapy at various levels of development.

In preparing to write this book, I first reviewed the occupational therapy literature in order to get an idea of the historical terrain of thinking about therapeutic use of self in the field. There is a rich history of thought as well as changing ideals regarding what constituted effective therapeutic use of self at various times in history. As an educator and a practitioner, I am fully aware that there often exists a gap between the ideals expressed in literature on a topic and what actually occurs in everyday therapeutic encounters. Consequently, I sought to shape the contents of this book around practitioners' expressions of the dilemmas and challenges they face in therapeutic use of self as well as their descriptions of the way they attempt to manage these circumstances. Additionally, I decided to look for instances of excellence in therapeutic use of self in occupational therapy that could be shared with practicing occupational therapists, occupational therapy assistants, educators, fieldwork supervisors, and students of occupational therapy.

This quest took me across the globe where I extensively interviewed and observed occupational therapists who were nominated by their peers as being uniquely talented in terms of their ability to relate to a wide range of clients. This journey taught me volumes about therapeutic use of self in occupational therapy, and my goal is to share what I have learned with you in this book.

Renée R. Taylor

Acknowledgments

This book would not have been possible without the ongoing support of Gary Kielhofner, who not only believed in the ideas behind the book but also provided some of the international linkages necessary to include the work of therapists from diverse nationalities and cultures. Also critical to the energy behind the production of this book were its acquisition editors, Christa Fratantoro and Margaret Biblis of F.A. Davis who inspired me to think expansively about use of self. Special thanks goes to Christa, an editor whose enduring support, creative suggestions and feedback, and ongoing belief in a novel approach kept me going. I would also like to thank Denise LeMelledo, Deborah Thorp, Carolyn O'Brien, and Berta Steiner for their time and care in producing this book. Finally, special thanks to the following occupational therapy students whose intelligent in-class questions and critical editorial feedback helped to refine the presentation of the contents of this book. In particular, I'd like to thank Emily Ashpole, Robin Black, Joel Bové, Kim Daniello, Kelly Doderman, Barbara Flood, Mark Kovic, Anne Plosjac, Abigail Tamm-Seitz, Rachel Trost, Jennifer Utz, Angie Vassiliou, and Debbie Victor.

Foreword

Literally speaking, a *foreword* heralds in other words. Dictionary definitions describe a foreword's aim as introductory. If asked to choose one word to herald in this book and introduce occupational therapists to its merits, I would choose the word *well-considered*. And because I have been asked to say more than one word, I'll elaborate on my meaning.

This book is well-considered because its focus on the therapeutic use of self is timely and crucial within health care systems struggling against pressures to compromise good intentions and relations. Taylor's model of the intentional relationship reminds practitioners that the use of self in occupational therapy needs both theoretical and practical attention. Her background as psychotherapist and her role as occupational therapy educator give her a unique vantage point for considering, creating, and proposing such a model.

Taylor's work draws both power and credibility from research that explores the stories and experiences of occupational therapists thought by their peers to possess relational artistry. From various cultures and locations, these therapists share insights into their successful interactions. In modest ways, these master therapists offer wisdom from which practitioners of all ages and career stages can benefit.

Itself well-considered, this book will foster consideration among its readers. Taylor's reflective exercises invite the development of values essential to the therapeutic use of self. We know that interpersonal skills learned in the absence of values that nurture them fall short of being therapeutic. Use of self that is *conscious* requires reflection sufficient to develop an awareness of personal traits, intentions, and actions. Use of self that is *therapeutic* presses past such awareness, asking that practitioners enact the respect and empathy that honor human dignity. Because it invites individuals to consider their interactions within the moral context of professional lives, the book is a call to mindfulness.

Although an enormous step in itself, understanding of the human need for respect and empathy is not enough. Such understanding must be paired with solid learning of effective approaches to meeting that need. This book fosters such learning through open discussions of behaviors that cause empathic breaks and through practical guidelines for meeting personal challenges found in daily practice. Because students hunger for such knowledge, this book will have educative power.

I have spent much time in thought, writing, and teaching about the therapeutic use of self. I value work on the topic that is well-considered. This book is such a work. Taylor and I share the belief that the therapeutic use of self is the essential stuff of occupational therapy rather than its "fluff." Promise and power lie within this book, and I am pleased to herald it in.

Suzanne M. Peloquin, PhD, OTR, FAOTA

Contributors

Kristin Alfredsson Ågren, MScOT, RegOT
Dagcenter Valla
Linköping, Sweden

Belinda Anderson, MEd, MS, OTR/L
Select Medical
Skokie, Illinois
Chicago Lighthouse for the Blind and Visually Impaired
Chicago Board of Education
Chicago, Illinois

René Bélanger, OTR, MBA
Hôtel-Dieu de Lévis Hospital
Laval University
Quebec City, Quebec, Canada

Carmen-Gloria de Las Heras, MS, OTR/L
Reencuentros
Santiago, Chile

Kim Eberhardt, MS, OTR/L
Rehabilitation Institute of Chicago
University of Illinois at Chicago
Chicago, Illinois

Vardit Kindler, OTR/L, MEd
Dvora Agmon Preschool, Israel Elwyn
Mish'aul – The Israeli Center for Augmentative
Communication and Assistive Devices
Jerusalem, Israel

Kathryn M. Loukas, MS, OTR/L, FAOTA
Raymond School District
Raymond, Maine
University of New England
Bitteford, Maine

Stephanie McCammon, MS, OTR/L
University of Illinois Medical Center
Chicago, Illinois

Roland Meisel, MS, OTR/L
A-Rehab, Inc.
Stockholm, Sweden

Jane Melton, MSc (Advanced OT), DipCOT (UK)
Gloucestershire Partnership
National Health Service Trust
Gloucestershire, United Kingdom

Anne Reuter, State-Approved Occupational Therapist
In Motio Outpatient Rehabilitation Center
Plauen, Germany

Michele Shapiro, OTR, Doctoral Student
Beit Issie Shapiro Community Organization
Raanana, Israel

Reviewers

Bette R. Bonder, PhD, OTR/L, FAOTA
Associate Dean
Occupational Therapy
Cleveland State University
Cleveland, Ohio

Elizabeth Cara, PhD, OTR/L, MFT
Associate Professor
Occupational Therapy
San Jose State University
San Jose, California

Mariana D'Amico, EdD, OTR/L, BCP
Assistant Professor
Occupational Therapy
Medical College of Georgia
Augusta, Georgia

Janis Davis, PhD, OTR
Assistant Professor
Occupational Therapy
Rockhurst University
Kansas City, Missouri

Christine deRenne-Stephan, MA, OTR/L
Visiting Clinical Professor
Occupational Therapy
University of Puget Sound
Tacoma, Washington

Linda S. Fazio, PhD, OTR/L, FAOTA, LPC
Associate Professor
Occupational Therapy
University of Southern California
Los Angeles, California

Terry L. Jackson, MS, OTR, LCDC
Coordinator of Education
Rehabilitation Sciences
University of Texas Medical Branch
Galveston, Texas

Barbara Kresge, MS, OTR
Lecturer and Admissions Chair
Occupational Therapy
Tufts University
Boston, Massachusetts

Jaime Munoz, PhD
Assistant Professor
Occupational Therapy
Duquesne University
Pittsburgh, Pennsylvania

Jane Clifford O'Brien, PhD
Assistant Professor
Occupational Therapy
University of New England
Biddeford, Maine

Marjorie E. Scaffa, PhD, OTR, FAOTA
Program Director
Occupational Therapy
University of South Alabama
Mobile, Alabama

Victoria P. Schindler, PhD, OTR, FAOTA
Associate Professor
Occupational Therapy
Richard Stockton College
Pomona, New Jersey

Sharan L. Schwartzberg, EdD, OTR, FAOTA
Professor and Chair
Occupational Therapy
Tufts University
Boston, Massachusetts

Janet H. Watts, PhD, OTR
Emeritus Associate Professor
Occupational Therapy
Virginia Commonwealth University
Richmond, Virginia

Contents

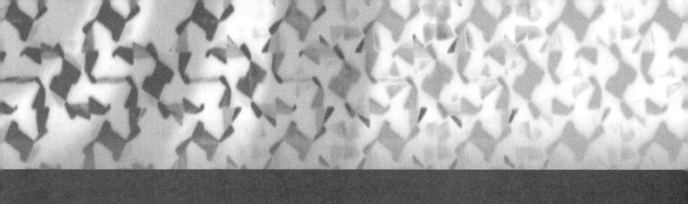

PART I

Theoretical Foundations and Guidelines for Practice

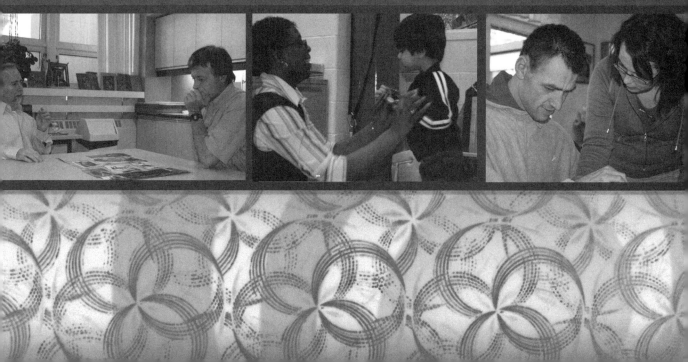

CHAPTER I

THE CHANGING LANDSCAPE OF THERAPEUTIC USE OF SELF IN OCCUPATIONAL THERAPY:
An Historical Overview

In a recent national study of 568 practicing occupational therapists in the United States, more than 80% of respondents rated therapeutic use of self as the most important determinant of the outcome of therapy (Taylor, Lee, Kielhofner, & Ketkar, 2007). However, less than half of these therapists thought they were adequately trained in use of self upon graduation. Moreover, less than one-third thought there was sufficient knowledge about use of self in occupational therapy (Taylor et al., 2007).

These therapists' perceptions of the importance of therapeutic use of self are supported by other research studies. A growing number of studies indicate that the client–therapist relationship is a key determinant of whether occupational therapy has been successful (Ayres-Rosa & Hasselkus, 1996; Cole & McLean, 2003). These findings are paralleled by extensive evidence in the field of psychology that a positive therapeutic relationship is the only variable consistently associated with successful psychotherapy outcomes (Bergin & Garfield, 1994; Orlinsky, 1994). Moreover, the demonstrated relation between a positive therapeutic relationship and good therapy outcomes is strong and consistent across highly distinct and often theoretically opposing orientations to practice (Fig. 1.1).

Additionally, the occupational therapists' opinions that their education did not adequately prepare them to manage challenging interpersonal situations in practice are also understandable. Only recently was the use of self included as one of the major categories of intervention in the occupational therapy practice framework (American

Occupational Therapy Association, 2002). Many educational programs have only just begun to consider developing required courses that focus solely on this topic, such as the one developed by Peloquin and Davidson (1993). Only 4% of the therapists who responded to the national study reported that they took a course focused only and specifically on the therapeutic use of self (Taylor et al., 2007).

Finally, the gap identified by therapists between the importance of therapeutic use of self and their field's inadequate knowledge about this area is reflected in the current literature of the profession. On one hand, the field has adopted strong values related to the importance of the use of self in practice. On the other hand, few detailed and extensive descriptions of therapeutic use of self skills for practice actually exist. Thus, the literature of the field leads one to conclude that, although therapeutic use of self is critically important, how to do it is somewhat abstract. The aim of this book is to offer a specific conceptualization of therapeutic use of self and make concrete the skills involved (Box 1.1).

History of Therapeutic Use of Self in Occupational Therapy

Although occupational therapy does not have a consistent conceptualization of therapeutic use of self, the topic has

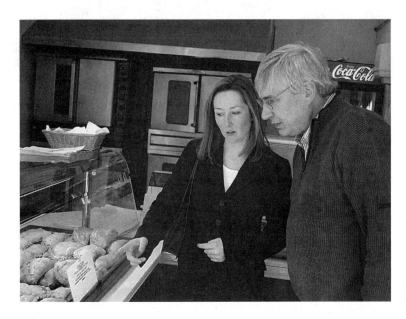

FIGURE 1.1 Jane Melton considers use of self as highly relevant to her practice

been addressed throughout the field's history. Ideas about how therapists should interact with clients have changed as the field's conceptualization of its practice has been transformed. Examining these different perspectives on therapeutic use of self provides an important backdrop for understanding where to begin when conceptualizing the use of self in contemporary occupational therapy.

Historical analysis has identified three distinct eras in occupational therapy, characterized as paradigms (Kielhofner, 2004). The earliest occupational paradigm reflected the humanistic ideas and practices of the field's founders. This paradigm built on the ideas of earlier European moral treatment. It focused on the individual's experience of doing and on his or her capacity and motivation to function during interaction with physical and social environments. This first paradigm was replaced during the mid-20th century by a paradigm of inner mechanisms that ushered in concern for addressing clients' underlying impairments. Rooted in the medical establishment, this paradigm sought to correct internal failures of body and mind. During the latter part of the 20th century a new, contemporary paradigm returned the field to its initial focus on occupation. As we will see, each of these eras had its own particular approach to the therapeutic use of self.

Moral Treatment

Nascent descriptions of therapeutic use of self were introduced in Europe in the late 1700s during the moral treat-

ment era (Bing, 1981; Bockoven, 1971). Moral treatment was a humanitarian approach that emphasized the facilitation of self-determination through engagement in everyday tasks and activities. Consideration and kindness were put forward as essential interpersonal values. Supporters of moral treatment also argued that all activity prescriptions should be based on in-depth understanding of the client's preferences and interests (Bing, 1981).

Early Occupational Era

When occupational therapy emerged during the 20th century, its leaders emphasized the humanistic approaches of moral treatment (Kielhofner, 2004; Schwartz, 2003). Central to the thinking during this era was that the therapeutic relationship served as a means by which to encourage engagement in occupation. The field's early leaders recognized that the success of therapy depended on the ability of the therapists to persuade or motivate clients (who often were in negative frames of mind) to undertake the occupations they were being offered as therapy.

One early leader, Susan Tracy, argued that the therapists should appeal to the intrinsically attractive and satisfying nature of activities. She saw the therapeutic role as one of suggesting possibilities and finding inviting ways to present opportunities for action. Tracy, along with another early founder of occupational therapy, Dunton, emphasized the importance of occupational therapists being skilled craftspeople who could serve as positive role mod-

---

Box 1.1 Definitions of the Therapeutic Use of Self

Mosey (1981, 1986) described the conscious use of self as the ability to deliberately use one's own responses to clients as part of the therapy. She characterized use of self as a "legitimate" skill across all frames of reference. To select appropriate ways to respond to a client, the therapist had to possess self-awareness, empathy, flexibility, humor, honesty, compassion, and humility.

Denton (1987) similarly described use of self as conveying an attitude of respect and acceptance to clients so self-esteem could be restored. Self-esteem could also be enhanced by the way in which a task or activity was presented to the patient. In addition, a therapist was considered effective in his or her use of self if he or she succeeded in modeling characteristics of a mature, competent, and admirable person for the client.

Schwartzberg (1993) defined therapeutic use of self as comprising understanding, empathy, and caring. Effective use of self was defined as remaining neutral but engaged, accepting the client as he or she is, being tolerant and interested in the client's painful emotions, and being able to interpret the client's expectations of therapy accurately.

Hagedorn (1995) defined therapeutic use of self as the artful, selective, or intuitive use of personal attributes to enhance therapy. Hagedorn clarified that the notion of an artful use of self should not be misconstrued as behaving in artificial or deceitful ways toward clients. Instead, artfulness referred to selecting aspects of one's own personality, attitudes, values, or responses that were predicted to be relevant or helpful in a given situation. In turn, therapists were expected to control or suppress those aspects of self that were not appropriate for the situation. According to Hagedorn, therapists were not expected to be perfect; instead, they were expected to be aware of their strengths and limitations, sensitive, honest, and genuine with clients. Therapists were also expected to manage stress effectively and to have personal integrity.

Cara and MacRae (1998) defined therapeutic use of self as developing an individual style that promotes change and growth in clients and helps furnish them with a corrective emotional experience. A corrective emotional experience is one in which a therapist's behavior toward a client during therapy contradicts the way others have behaved toward the client in the past and demonstrates to the client that he or she is worthy of caring and empathy.

Punwar and Peloquin (2000) defined the therapeutic use of self as a "practitioner's planned use of his or her personality, insights, perceptions and judgments as part of the therapeutic process" (p. 285). This definition was also used in the American Occupational Therapy Association's Occupational Therapy Practice Framework (American Occupation Therapy Association, 2002).

---

els for standards of performance and appreciation for crafts (Dunton, 1915, 1919; Tracy, 1912). Dunton (1915, 1919) and two other founders, Meyer (1922) and Slagle (1922), underscored the importance of understanding the personalities of clients so therapists would know what activities were likely to appeal to those clients.

In addition to appealing to clients' innate dispositions and using the intrinsic attraction to occupations, another approach was to appeal to the client's sense of the importance of participating in therapy. For example, Haas (1944) thought it important to instill faith in the client concerning the therapeutic process. He recommended that the physician introduce each client to the occupational therapy director to underscore the value of occupational therapy and to build the patient's confidence in the treating therapist.

At this time, the physical and social environments were also emphasized as client motivators (Bing, 1981; Kielhofner, 2004). Thus, the therapist functioned to ensure that the physical context and social milieu was attractive and inviting and that it embodied a positive esprit de corps, order, and utility. Interpersonally, the occupational therapist behaved in ways that would invite the client to participate in occupations, demonstrate standards of performance in sportsmanship and craftsmanship, and emulate the enjoyment and satisfaction that came from doing things.

Thus, during the early occupational era, the therapeutic relationship was one in which the therapist served as:

- Expert, or guide, in the performance of therapeutic activities, such as arts, crafts, and sports
- Role model for occupational engagement
- Emulator of the joy of occupation
- Instiller of confidence
- Creator of a positive physical and social milieu

To a large extent, the therapist's use of self was to set the stage for a client to wish to engage in therapeutic occupations and to have a positive experience when doing so. The therapeutic relationship required the therapist to serve as a kind of master of ceremonies who orchestrated the environment and the unfolding process of occupational engagement. The therapist also needed to get to know the client through interactions and interviews, thereby learning how to appeal to the person's innate interests and personality.

Era of Inner Mechanisms

Beginning during the 1940s, the second, mechanistic paradigm replaced the earlier humanistic one. This new perspective focused occupational therapists on remediating the internal biomechanical, neuromuscular, and intrapsychic mechanisms of the body and mind that influenced function (Kielhofner, 2004). During this time, there was an important change in emphasis on the role of the therapeutic relationship (Peloquin, 1989a).

First, this paradigm included the emphasis on eliminating pathology, borrowed from the medical model. It also included medicine's ideas about expertise and authority; these had a strong influence on occupational therapy's view of the use of self. In this framework, therapists were expected to assume an impersonal and professional attitude toward clients while at the same time commanding respect, demonstrating exceptional competence, and conveying a hope for cure (Wade, 1947). Tact, self-control, listening skills, impersonal objectivity, good judgment, and the ability to identify with a patient were emphasized as "personality qualifications" of a good therapist (Wade, 1947).

During this era, occupational therapy was also heavily influenced by psychoanalytic (i.e., Freudian and Neo-Freudian) concepts. Emotional, psychiatric, and interpersonal difficulties were considered aspects of internal pathology that needed to be treated using approaches that focused heavily on the relationship that existed between the therapist and the client. It was at this time that the term "therapeutic relationship" first emerged.

According to this new view, it was important for the occupational therapist to attend to how a client behaved toward activities within the therapeutic relationship in order to understand the client's inner motives, interpersonal feelings, and relationships with others. For example, the type of product a client chose to make in therapy and the way the client went about the activity were viewed as shedding light into the client's inner motives and feelings toward the therapist or others. Such factors as the client's choice of color, degree of dependence on the therapist, and preference for different procedures or tasks were all windows into the client's psyche.

A range of ideas was put forward about the nature of the therapy during this period, but there were two dominant themes. The first argued that the client would achieve catharsis through acting out unconscious desires and motives while performing activities and simultaneously gaining insight into these underlying issues through discussion and relating with the therapist (Azima & Azima, 1959; Fidler & Fidler, 1954, 1963). The second perspective, heavily influenced by the work of Frank (Box 1.2) used activities to establish a therapeutic relationship that would permit the person to develop healthy means of resolving intrapsychic conflict and fulfilling needs. The following quote illustrates this approach.

> The effective therapeutic approach in occupational therapy today and in the future is one in which the therapist utilized the tools of his trade as an avenue of introduction. From then on his personality takes over. (Conte, 1960, p. 3)

Given this new emphasis, the occupation or activity lost its unitary importance (Kielhofner, 2004). Instead, the central focus was on the cathartic and corrective relationship between therapist and client.

Box 1.2 Jerome Frank

In 1958 during the mechanistic era, Jerome D. Frank, a psychiatrist, introduced the term "therapeutic use of self" to the field of occupational therapy. Frank (1958) introduced psychiatry's definition of self as a term that encompasses every aspect of personality development and interpersonal behavior. Frank held that the development of a client's healthy self can be derailed by inconsistent or derogatory parental attitudes, constitutional variables (innate temperament), and physical impairments. He further argued that these interruptions in normal development of self resulted in what was referred to as a "pathological self-structure." In relationships, a pathological self-structure can manifest in one of two ways: It can result in a restricted or overly rigid use of a small set of interpersonal strategies, or it can result in a diffuse self that has not built adequate self–other boundaries and responds to the demands of all others and all situations without discrimination. In either case, Frank argued that the mechanism of repairing a client's fragmented self structure involved the self of the therapist. That is, the therapist must use his or her self as a mechanism for repairing a client's damaged self. Thus, a therapist's self structure needed to be strong enough to endure threats wrought by the demands and projections of a client's pathological self. In addition, Frank held that it was important for the occupational therapist to show competence; resist the need to reassure; act clearly, consistently, predictably, spontaneously, and flexibly; and remain ambiguous at times to force the client to cope with stress and manage problems independently.

Both approaches saw activity as augmenting the talk that took place in psychotherapy. Importantly, they carried a very different connotation about the interpersonal role of the therapist from the previous era. Whereas the therapist's role was previously to appropriately orient the client to occupations that were used as therapy, this new framework argued that the relationship between the therapist and the client was the key dynamic of therapy. These ideas, which were first developed in psychiatric settings, became the dominant way of thinking about the therapeutic relationship throughout the entire field.

Thus, during the inner mechanisms era, the therapeutic relationship was viewed as:

- A central mechanism for change
- A means by which to understand a client's unconscious motives, desires, and behavior toward others
- An avenue through which an individual could achieve catharsis through acting out unconscious desires and motives and gain insight into issues that were at the core of pathological feelings and behaviors

When relating to clients, the therapist was expected to demonstrate:

- Competence
- Professionalism
- Impersonal objectivity
- Hope
- Tact
- Self-control
- Good judgment
- Identification with the patient

Although some of these interpersonal behaviors may appear contradictory (e.g., identification with the patient versus maintaining interpersonal objectivity), they were not viewed as such at the time. According to the views of this era, the ideal therapeutic relationship involved striking an appropriate balance between having compassion for a patient and acting in an optimally therapeutic manner.

> Whereas the therapist's role previously was to appropriately orient the client to occupations that were used as therapy, this new framework argued that the relationship between the therapist and the client was the key dynamic of therapy.

It was acknowledged that this balance varied from patient to patient.

As evident in the ideas of these and other seminal contributors of the time, the closer relationship with medicine and support for the medical model was reflected in all aspects of occupational therapy practice. In the specialty area of psychosocial occupational therapy, the practice of occupational therapy was becoming strikingly similar to the practice of psychotherapy. This, in conjunction with the recognition that occupation had lost its place as the key dynamic of therapy, led some of the key contemporary leaders to reevaluate the field's identity and direction (Kielhofner, 2004; Schwartz, 2003; Shannon, 1977; Yerxa, 1967).

Return to Occupation

Beginning during the 1960s, Reilly (1962) was the first to notice that the field of occupational therapy was drifting away from a focus on occupation and away from its original values, which were based on concepts of moral treatment. Moreover, the psychoanalytical/neo-Freudian focus on the therapeutic relationship was seen as having "sidelined" the central role of occupation (Kielhofner and Burke, 1977). The view that the therapeutic relationship was the key dynamic of therapy was rejected in favor of occupational engagement as the true dynamic. Once again, the therapist was viewed as a proponent of occupational engagement who must use a variety of strategies to make occupations appealing and to support the therapy process.

Contemporary Discussions of the Client–Therapist Relationship

Alongside this contemporary emphasis on occupation, new discussions concerning the client–therapist relationship have emerged (Cara & MacRae, 2005; Cunningham-Piergrossi & Gibertoni, 1995). For example, the occupational therapy literature has argued that a collaborative relationship that is egalitarian and empowering of clients leads to improved treatment outcomes (Anderson & Hinojosa, 1984; Ayres-Rosa & Hasselkus, 1996; Clark, Corcoran, & Gitlin, 1995; Hinojosa, Anderson, & Strauch, 1988; Hinojosa, Sproat, Mankhetwit, & Anderson, 2002; Townsend, 2003).

In addition, caring, empathy, connection, personal growth, and effective verbal and nonverbal communication skills have been characterized as important qualities for successful occupational therapy practice (Cole & McLean, 2003; Devereaux, 1984; Eklund & Hallberg, 2001; King, 1980, 1994; Lloyd & Maas, 1991, 1992; Peloquin, 2005). There has been a particularly strong emphasis on the appreciative and empathic process by which the therapists come to truly understand clients' life stories and to feel deep respect for and trust in the clients' perspectives on their experiences (Hagedorn, 1995; Mosey, 1970; Peloquin, 1995, 2005; Punwar & Peloquin, 2000). Some have argued that therapist self-knowledge, self-awareness of behavior, and the ability to self-evaluate or reflect on one's practice are prerequisites for interpersonal sensitivity and the capacity for greater understanding of a client's narrative (Hagedorn, 1995; Mattingly & Fleming, 1994; Schell, Crepeau, & Cohn, 2003; Schon, 1983) (Box 1.3).

Box 1.3 Ann Mosey

In 1981, Mosey coined the term "conscious use of self." According to Mosey (1981), therapists should respond to clients in a thoughtful and planned way rather than in a spontaneous or impulsive way. Mosey (1986) explained that therapists should "manipulate" their responses to clients to accommodate the interpersonal demands of therapy. The rationale behind this approach is that each client has different interpersonal needs, and clinical situations and context may vary widely from client to client. Because of this variability, a therapist cannot respond in the same way to each client. According to Mosey, planned responses to clients can serve to reduce a client's anxiety, provide support, or obtain or share needed information. Depending on the needs of the client, the conscious use of self may include dialogue, gestures, facial expressions, touch, or the use of special talents (Mosey, 1981).

In addition to care and planning in relationships, respect for diversity and cultural sensitivity in practice were also introduced during the contemporary era. Although this area is in need of continued development, cultural competence and awareness of the potential for personal biases are considered fundamental to building effective relationships (Bonder, Martin, & Miracle, 2001; Lloyd & Maas, 1991, 1992; Wells & Black, 2000).

As can be readily seen, a variety of contemporary descriptions of the conditions necessary for an effective therapeutic relationship have been put forward. From these numerous ideas, three major themes can be gleaned in contemporary discussions of the client–therapist relationship.

- Collaborative and client-centered approaches
- Emphasis on caring and empathy
- Use of narrative and clinical reasoning

The remainder of this section summarizes the key concepts in each of these thematic areas.

Collaborative and Client-Centered Approaches

In contrast to the mechanistic era when the field emphasized professionalism, objectivity, and a more analytical approach to the relationship, a strong value of the contemporary era has been that of collaboration, mutuality, and client-centered practice.

Collaborative Approaches

Mosey (1970) was one of the first to write about the value of collaboration when planning treatment goals and evaluating therapy outcomes. Mosey (1986) emphasized a number of qualities necessary for the formation of collaborative relationships, including flexibility, humility, self-awareness, empathy, humor, honesty, and compassion. One of the central therapeutic strategies of early descriptions of collaboration involved educating clients about all aspects of the treatment process and providing them with information about the purpose and relevance of any procedure or treatment approach (Peloquin, 1988). According to this perspective, providing these rationale statements at each session was thought to facilitate increased client involvement in therapy (Peloquin, 1988).

Collaborative perspectives assume that power imbalances are inherent in all client–therapist relationships, and that therapists can seek to readjust these imbalances by facilitating client control over decision-making and by encouraging the client to become actively involved in problem-solving about his or her own situation (Hagedorn, 1995; Townsend, 2003). In support of this approach, a number of occupational therapy writers have incorporated the ideas of Schon (1983), who contrasted two types of contracts that characterized the therapeutic relationship: the hierarchical professionalism typical of the inner mechanisms era and what he labeled a "reflective contract" in which the client assumes control, becomes more educated, and joins with the professional in solving problems related to his or her situation. Rather than presuming total and complete expertise, Schon (1983) encouraged therapists to think critically about their experiences and behaviors both in the midst of performing therapy and once the practice session ended.

The collaborative approach has also been discussed with regard to relationships with parents of pediatric clients in occupational therapy (Anderson and Hinojosa, 1984; Hanna & Rodger, 2002). The rationale behind this approach is that some parents of children with disabilities may feel undermined or undervalued by therapists who focus too much on direct therapy with the child and assume an expert stance in the therapeutic relationship. Parental feelings of vulnerability may stem from difficulties accepting the fact a child is disabled, lack of

knowledge about how best to approach the child's disability, and fewer opportunities to receive positive reinforcement for good parenting skills. Because of this potential for rifts and power differentials in the therapeutic relationship, a number of researchers recommend that therapists employ collaborative strategies to enable service recipients to build a sense of their own self-efficacy as parents or caregivers (Anderson & Hinojosa, 1984; Clark et al., 1995; Hanna & Rodger, 2002; Hinojosa et al., 2002; Rosenbaum, King, Law, King, & Evans, 1998). This spirit has been reflected in the literature on family-centered care (Hanna & Rodger, 2002; Rosenbaum et al., 1998). These strategies (Anderson & Hinojosa, 1984; Hanna & Rodger, 2002; Rosenbaum et al., 1998) emphasize self-efficacy as one of the most valued anticipated outcomes (Baum, 1998).

Similar collaborative approaches have been applied to a wide range of occupational therapy clients of all ages. For example, Clark et al., (1995) researched the interpersonal behaviors of two occupational therapists interacting with caregiver-clients. Therapist behaviors were summarized in terms of four categories: caring (being supportive, friendly, and building rapport); partnering (gathering reflective feedback and seeking and acknowledging input from clients); informing (gathering, explaining, and clarifying information); and directing (providing advice and instruction) (Fig. 1.2).

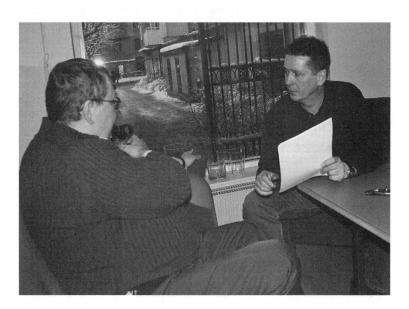

FIGURE 1.2 Roland Meisel values collaboration as an important aspect of work rehabilitation

In sum, the literature suggests that collaborative relationships are characterized by:

• Open and comfortable communication and discussion
• Highly supportive approaches that convey respect and trust in the client's perspectives, strengths, and ways of coping
• Consideration of client diversity and unique perspectives
• Establishment of shared goals and priorities
• A clear goal to address the client's difficulties together in partnership

Self-Awareness and Collaboration

In addition to emphasizing client self-efficacy, a number of writers have argued that therapist self-awareness is essential for effective collaboration (e.g., Anderson & Hinojosa, 1984; Hagedorn, 1995). Specifically, therapists are urged to recognize, control, and correct potentially nontherapeutic reactions to clients that might emerge from unresolved conflicts or their own experiences of being parented in negative ways (Anderson & Hinojosa, 1984).

Other occupational therapy researchers have expanded the definition of collaboration to include the formation of personal-professional connections with clients (Ayres-Rosa & Hasselkus, 1996; Prochnau, Liu, & Boman, 2003). These connections are described as incorporating one's own life experiences into one's understanding of the client. These connections also involve reciprocal giving and sharing between client and therapist (Prochnau et al., 2003). Acknowledging and drawing on one's personal reactions to the helping process in a constructive way and caring for patients at a fundamental human level have been described as means of deepening the process of collaboration with clients (Ayres-Rosa & Hasselkus, 1996).

Client-Centered Approach

Client-centered practice is a formal orientation to practice that emphasizes collaboration and considers clients as active agents in the therapy process (Law, 1998; Law, Baptiste, & Mills, 1995). This practice supports and values clients' knowledge and experience, strengths, capacity for choice, and overall autonomy. Clients are treated with respect and considered partners in the therapy process. Although a range of more nuanced descriptions of client-centered practice exist in the literature (e.g., Restall, Ripat, & Stern, 2003; Sumsion, 2000, 2003), the most widely recognized proponents of client-centered practice describe 13 guiding principles that enable a client's engagement in occupation within the therapeutic relationship (Law, Polatajko, Baptiste, & Townsend, 1997). The following key themes can be described as cutting across these 13 guiding principles and are held as priorities for the client–therapist relationship:

• An orientation to and value for the client's perspective, which includes the client's values, sense of meaning, natural ways of coping, and choice of occupation
• A strengths-based perspective in which clients are encouraged to problem-solve and make decisions, identify needs and set goals, envision possibilities, challenge themselves, and use their strengths and natural community supports to succeed
• Communication that involves client education, collaboration, and open and honest discussion.

The principles of client-centered practice (more recently referred to as enabling occupation) have been described as representing an ethical stance by occupational therapists because they are based on democratic ideas of empowerment and justice (Townsend, 1993, 2003). According to its founders, the ultimate aim of client-centered practice is enablement (Law et al., 1997). Enablement comprises a number of therapist behaviors that result in people having the resources and opportunities to engage in occupations that shape their lives. These behaviors include facilitating, guiding, coaching, educating, prompting, listening, reflecting, encouraging, or otherwise collaborating with clients (Law et al., 1997) (Fig. 1.3).

In summary, the ultimate functions of collaborative and client-centered approaches to the therapeutic relationship are to increase feelings of self-efficacy and ultimately to enable clients to perform occupations that hold personal significance. Collaborative and client-centered approaches continue to influence practice with a wide range of client populations in vastly diverse treatment settings throughout the world. The next section describes a second major trend concerning the client–therapist relationship in the field of occupational therapy.

Emphasis on Caring and Empathy

Whereas the collaborative and client-centered approaches emphasized those aspects of the therapeutic relationship that have to do largely with power dynamics, the emphasis on caring and empathy focus more on the affective dimensions of the therapeutic relationship. They are discussed below.

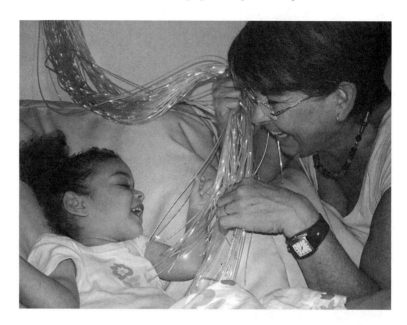

FIGURE 1.3 Being client-centered is important to Michele Shapiro's relationships with her clients

Caring

At the 60th Annual Conference of the American Occupational Therapy Association, leaders in the field called for an increase in attention to the role of caring in occupational therapy practice (Baum, 1980; Gilfoyle, 1980; King, 1980; Yerxa, 1980). This charge was in response to a belief that social change—which included decreasing value for interdependence and collectivism, a decreased sense of responsibility for the general welfare of others, and pressures and strains to focus on narrow aspects of pathology in the larger U.S. health care system—had led occupational therapy education and practice away from its core humanistic values (Baum, 1980; King, 1980; Yerxa, 1980). In essence, caring referred to:

- Knowing and responding to each client intimately as a unique individual
- Viewing clients holistically—as human beings with goals and lives outside of their specific impairments
- Being flexible in adapting to environmental and situational demands
- Harnessing the will of each client
- Connecting at an emotional level
- Restoring personal control through activity (Baum, 1980; Devereaux, 1984; Gilfoyle, 1980; King, 1980)

Caring also incorporated the following specific attitudes (Gilfoyle, 1980).

- Patience
- Honesty
- Trust
- Humility
- Hope
- Courage

Caring was described as foundational to an artful approach to therapy as contrasted with a scientific approach (Gilfoyle, 1980). From a use of self-perspective, the art of practice emphasized a mutual bond between client and therapist that enabled the client to achieve a certain depth of emotion and thereby develop affectively, engage in meaningful goal-directed activity, and undergo personal growth (Gilfoyle, 1980; King, 1980). The caring relationship was described as a partnership that respected clients' innate ability to achieve self-actualization, which was defined as the ability to achieve the highest level of motivation to fulfill their personal potentials for occupational performance (Gilfoyle, 1987). Notions of mind–body dualism in which a client's specific area of impairment was split off from recognition of the client as an entire, unique individual were considered antithetical to caring (Devereaux, 1984).

Devereaux (1984) was one of the first to acknowledge that developing a caring relationship in actual practice is not an easy task. For example, the ability to have a caring relationship with oneself as a therapist was described as one of the prerequisites for developing a caring relationship with clients (Devereaux, 1984). In addition, Devereaux acknowledged that caring, though necessary, is not sufficient to develop an effective therapeutic relationship with a client. In turn, seven additional features required for the establishment of a positive therapeutic relationship were defined (Devereaux, 1984).

- *Competence*—a therapist's duty and responsibility to practice competently and to be knowledgeable about ongoing developments in practice and about the research evidence to support these developments
- *Belief in the dignity and worth of the individual*—respecting each individual's need for mastery and control
- *Belief that each individual has the potential for change and growth*—acknowledging that each client has an innate capacity for improvement and that the therapist serves only as a facilitator or guide
- *Communication*—the ability to listen to the meaning and feelings behind a client's words, to make sensitive observations, and to send clear messages
- *Values*—knowing what can benefit a client, having expectations for behavior, and having standards for living
- *Touch*—using touch to communicate and convey sensitivity
- *Sense of humor*—using humor judiciously to bypass resistance or diffuse a tense situation

Similar notions of caring were later applied to occupational therapy practice with clients with psychiatric disorders. Psychosocial practice emphasized three central principles of caring that stood in contrast to viewing clients as anonymous and applying the same treatments indifferently across all patients (Stein & Cutler, 1998). They included:

- Individualizing treatment by carefully evaluating clients and determining what approach or technique would be most effective for each individual
- Maintaining optimism, respect, and continued care for even the most chronically and seriously ill clients—even if other health care workers have decided that treatment is not worthwhile
- Understanding and recognizing what the illness means to the client and/or caregivers

Empathy

During the late 1980s, Suzanne Peloquin began a series of arguments about the centrality of empathy in the therapeutic encounter (Peloquin, 1989b, 1990, 1993, 1995, 2002, 2003, 2005). According to Peloquin (2003), empathy was characterized by the following actions.

- Communication of fellowship
- Turning of the soul toward the client
- Recognition of how one is similar to the client and how the client is unique
- Entry into the client's experience
- Connection with the feelings of the client
- Power to recover from that connection and maintain strength to continue working with others

Like caring, empathy was also considered central to the art of occupational therapy practice and a means to convey respect for a client's personal dignity (Peloquin, 2003). Peloquin (2003) characterized the therapeutic relationship as a manifestation of artistry because it reflected a capacity to establish rapport, to empathize, and to guide clients to actualize their potential as participants within a wider social network (Fig. 1.4).

To develop empathy, Peloquin (1989b, 1990, 1993, 1995) emphasized the roles of art, literature, imagination, and self-reflection. She further argued that the fundamental characteristics required to develop one's therapeutic use of self are well conveyed through reading literature and viewing and doing art (Peloquin, 1989). She believed that providing therapists with both fictional and nonfictional poems and stories that illustrate empathy and the depersonalizing consequences of neglectful attitudes and failed communication could be a powerful motivator for the development of caring (Peloquin, 1990, 1993, 1995).

Like collaborative and client-centered approaches, caring and empathy continue to represent strong values for the field of occupational therapy, and they are studied and cited by numerous scholars. The next section describes the third and final major historical category of work related to the client–therapist relationship.

Clinical Reasoning and the Use of Narrative

As noted earlier, the caring and empathy approaches emphasized affect in contrast to the collaborative and client-centered approaches that emphasize power relationships. Clinical reasoning and narrative emphasize

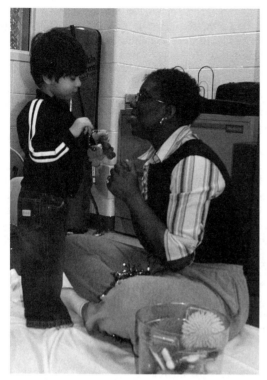

FIGURE 1.4 Caring and empathy are fundamental aspects of Belinda Anderson's interactions

thought, reflection, and understanding in the therapeutic relationship.

Clinical Reasoning

Clinical reasoning (Mattingly & Fleming, 1994; Rogers, 1983; Schell, 2003; Schell & Cervero, 1993) is a complex thought process that therapists use before, during, and after encounters with clients. It incorporates thinking about the client–therapist interaction as a component of one's overall approach to making sense of assessment findings and developing a treatment plan (Mattingly & Fleming, 1994). With concrete therapeutic action as its ultimate aim, it is the main process used to integrate assessment information and formulate an intervention plan (Mattingly & Fleming, 1994). The implicit emphasis of clinical reasoning is understanding the client and the here-and-now dynamic interplay between the client and the therapist (Cara & MacRae, 1998).

Four modes of clinical reasoning have been introduced: procedural reasoning, interactive reasoning, condi-

tional reasoning, and, later, narrative reasoning (Clark, 1993; Fleming, 1991; Mattingly, 1991, 1994; Mattingly & Fleming, 1994). The aspect of clinical reasoning that concerned the face-to-face interaction with clients was labeled interactive reasoning. The central emphasis of interactive reasoning was on collaborating or "doing with" the client and on understanding the client's experience of disability from the client's perspective. Interactive reasoning was held to be central to practice but at the same time was described as a rather mysterious "underground practice" that was often unarticulated by therapists (Fleming, 1991). More recently, however, specific information about therapists' interpersonal behaviors has been provided (Schwartzberg, 2002). In addition, information has been gathered from qualitative research studies that have focused on the interactive reasoning process. For example, based on an ethnographic study of clinical reasoning carried out by Nedra Gillette, Cheryl Mattingly, and Maureen Fleming from 1986 to 1990, six strategies have been identified as leading to effective collaboration between client and therapist.

- Providing clients with choices
- Individualizing treatment
- Structuring therapy activities such that they maximize the potential for success
- Going outside of the formal therapeutic role and doing special favors or acts of kindness for clients
- Sharing one's personal stories with clients
- Joint problem-solving

According to this perspective, careful monitoring and interpretation of one's own interpersonal behaviors and those of the client should be guided by a process of interactive reasoning. The ultimate aims of this process are to engage the client in treatment; to know the client as a unique individual; to communicate acceptance, trust, and hope to the client; and to construct a shared language of actions and meanings (Clark, 1993; Crepeau, 1991; Lyons & Crepeau, 2001; Mattingly & Fleming, 1994).

Use of Narrative

The study of clinical reasoning was accompanied by a focus on what was described as "narrative reasoning" (Mattingly, 1994). Narratives comprise information from clients that is presented and interpreted in the form of a story or metaphor. Narrative reasoning involves thinking in story form in order to discover the meaning of the disability experience from the client's perspective (Kielhofner, 1997; Mattingly, 1994). Learning to understand and nurture the client's narrative as it unfolds in light of a client's impairment was considered essential to positive therapeutic outcomes (Kielhofner, 1997).

Narrative approaches consist of various methods of data collection to understand the patient's perspective, including case histories, hermeneutic case reconstruction, life charts, life stories, narrative slopes, therapeutic employment, and other biographical methods (Jonsson, Josephsson, & Kielhofner, 2001). Using these methods, the therapist and client can create an understanding of the client's past, present, and future story together.

Narrative reasoning was considered particularly important for assisting clients to think about how disruptions in their life stories might be ameliorated or reconstituted by imagining a new or revised story (Kielhofner, 1997). In this way, a new and more hopeful vision of the future could be formed. Thus, a central aspect of narrative reasoning is story-making, which involves the creation of stories during the therapy process (Clark, 1993; Fleming, 1991; Mattingly, 1994; Schwartz, 2003). In therapy, clients are encouraged to choose and engage in activities and other occupations that have the potential to reshape their life stories. Using narrative reasoning, client's future stories are co-constructed with the therapist and constantly revised in the midst of therapy (Mattingly, 1994). In addition, therapists create clinical experiences in which a significant occurrence or event occurs during therapy such that the therapy itself becomes a meaningful short story or episode in the larger life story of the client (Helfrich and Kielhofner, 1994; Mattingly, 1994).

Summary: The Rationale for This Book

We have seen that occupational therapy's view of the therapeutic relationship has changed and developed over its history. Early perspectives of the field's first paradigm emphasized the centrality of occupation in therapy and the therapist's role in motivating the client's occupational engagement and experience. The second paradigm redefined the therapeutic relationship as a psychodynamic process that augmented or even replaced occupation as the central dynamic of therapy. This idea was rejected in favor of the contemporary, renewed focus on occupation.

During this era of heightened occupational focus, the three major themes related to the therapeutic relationship described in the prior section have been introduced. They included:

• Collaborative and client-centered approaches
• An emphasis on caring and empathy
• Clinical reasoning and use of narrative

These are important themes that offer broad and useful principles related to the therapeutic use of self.

Despite the fact that these approaches coexist with the field's returned emphasis on occupational engagement, they do not directly address the question of how the therapeutic use of self can be utilized specifically to promote occupational engagement and promote positive therapy outcomes. Their relation to an occupationally focused practice is assumed but not made explicit.

In addition, some implicitly assume that when therapists achieve a reflective, appreciative, and emotionally connected state with clients a positive therapeutic process simply emerges. This assumption is a large one that appears to be contradicted in the experience of most practicing therapists. Despite the existence of a fairly extensive contemporary literature on collaboration, client-centered practice, caring, empathy, clinical reasoning, and narrative, most practicing therapists we surveyed believe that occupational therapy does not have sufficient knowledge to support the therapeutic use of self (Taylor et al., 2007). Their perspectives suggest that something is still missing.

To date, there has been no effort to integrate all of the contemporary interpersonal approaches of occupational therapy into a coherent explanation of the therapeutic relationship. Moreover, beyond broad principles, there are few details about how the therapeutic relationship should be approached and managed in light of the central focus on the client's engagement in occupation. Consequently, there is still a lack of clarity regarding the exact definition, use, and relevance of therapeutic use of self in occupational therapy.

These observations were the impetus for this book. It was written in an attempt to clarify and to provide more detailed guidance of how to enact the therapeutic use of self in occupational therapy. It presents a conceptual practice model, the Intentional Self, that explains therapeutic use of self and its relation with occupational engagement, and it furnishes a set of concrete tools and interpersonal skills.

References

American Occupational Therapy Association (2002). Occupational therapy practice framework: domain and process. *American Journal of Occupational Therapy, 56*, 609–639.

Anderson, J., & Hinojosa, J. (1984). Parents and therapists in a professional partnership. *American Journal of Occupational Therapy, 38*, 452–461.

Ayres-Rosa, S., & Hasselkus, B. R. (1996). Connecting with patients: The personal experience of professional helping. *The Occupational Therapy Journal of Research, 16*, 245–260.

Azima, H., & Azima, F. (1959). Outline of a dynamic theory of occupational therapy. *American Journal of Occupational Therapy*, 13, 215–221.

Baum, C. (1998). Client-centered practice in a changing health care system. In M. Law (Ed.), *Client-centered occupational therapy* (pp. 29–45). Thorofare, NJ: Slack.

Baum, C. M. (1980). Occupational therapists put care in the health system. *American Journal of Occupaitonal Therapy, 34*, 505–516.

Bergin, A. E. & Garfield, S. L. (1994). *Handbook of psychotherapy and behavior change* (4th ed.). Oxford: John Wiley.

Bing, R. K. (1981). Eleanor Clark Slagle lectureship 1981—Occupational therapy revisited: A paraphrastic journey. *American Journal of Occupational Therapy, 35*, 499–518.

Bockoven, J. S. (1971). Occupational therapy—a historical perspective: Legacy of moral treatment—1800's to 1910. *American Journal of Occupational Therapy, 25*, 223–225.

Bonder, B., Martin, L., & Miracle, A. W. (2001). *Culture in clinical care*. Thorofare, NJ: Slack.

Cara, E., & MacRae, A. (1998). *Psychosocial occupational therapy in clinical practice*. Albany, NY: Delmar.

Cara, E., & MacRae, A. (2005). *Psychosocial occupational therapy in clinical practice* (2nd ed.). Albany, NY: Delmar.

Clark, F. (1993). Occupation embedded in a real life: Interweaving occupational science and occupational therapy—1993 Eleanor Clarke Slagle lecture. *American Journal of Occupational Therapy, 47*, 1067–1078.

Clark, C. A., Corcoran, M., & Gitlin, L. N. (1995). An exploratory study of how occupational therapists develop therapeutic relationships with family caregivers. *American Journal of Occupational Therapy, 49*, 587–594.

Cole, B., & McLean, V. (2003). Therapeutic relationships re-defined. *Occupational Therapy in Mental Health, 19*(2), 33–56.

Conte, W. (1960). The occupational therapist as a therapist. *American Journal of Occupational Therapy, 14*, 1–3.

Crepeau, E. B. (1991). Achieving intersubjective understanding: Examples from an occupational therapy treatment session. *American Journal of Occupational Therapy, 45*, 1016–1025.

Cunningham-Piergrossi, J., & Gibertoni, C. (1995). The importance of inner transformation in the activity process. *Occupational Therapy International, 2*, 36–47.

Denton, P. L. (1987). *Psychiatric occupational therapy: A workbook of practical skills*. Boston: Little, Brown.

Devereaux, E. B. (1984). Occupational therapy's challenge: The caring relationship. *American Journal of Occupational Therapy, 38*, 791–798.

Dunton, W. R. (1915). *Occupational therapy: A manual for nurses*. Philadelphia: WB Saunders.

Dunton, W. R. (1919). *Reconstruction therapy*. Philadelphia: WB Saunders.

Eklund, M., & Hallberg, I. (2001). Psychiatric occupational therapists' verbal interaction with their clients. *Occupational Therapy International, 8*(1), 1–16.

Fidler, G. S., & Fidler, J. W. (1954). *Introduction to psychiatric occupational therapy* (pp. 8–55). New York: Macmillan.

Fidler, G. S., & Fidler, J. W. (1963). *Occupational therapy: A communication process in psychiatry* (pp. 4–163). New York: Macmillan.

Fleming, M. H. (1991). The therapist with the three-track mind. *American Journal of Occupational Therapy, 45*, 1007–1014.

Frank, J. D. (1958). Therapeutic use of self. *American Journal of Occupational Therapy, 8*, 215–225.

Gilfoyle, E. M. (1980). Caring: A philosophy for practice. *American Journal of Occupational Therapy, 34*, 517–521.

Gilfoyle, E. M. (1987). Creative partnerships: The profession's plan. *American Journal of Occupaitonal Therapy, 41*, 779–781.

Goldstein, K., Kielhofner, G., & Paul-Ward A. (2004). Occupational narratives and the therapeutic process. *Australian Occupational Therapy Journal, 51*, 119–124.

Haas, L. (1944). *Practical occupational therapy*. Milwaukee: Bruce Publishing.

Hagedorn, R. (1995). *Occupational therapy: Perspectives and processes* (pp. 259–267). New York: Chuchill Livingstone.

Hanna, K., & Rodger, S. (2002). Towards family-centered practice in paediatric occupational therapy: A review of the literature on parent-therapist collaboration. *Australian Occupational Therapy Journal, 49*, 14–24.

Helfrich, C., & Kielhofner, G. (1994). Volitional narratives and the meaning of therapy. *The American Journal of Occupational Therapy, 48*, 319–326.

Helfrich, C., & Kielhofner, G. (1994). Volitional narratives and the meaning of therapy. *The American Journal of Occupational Therapy, 48*, 319–326.

Hinojosa, J., Sproat, C. T., Mankhetwit, S., & Anderson, J. (2002). Shifts in parent-therapist partnerships: Twelve years of change. *American Journal of Occupational Therapy, 56*, 556–563.

Jonsson, H., Josephsson, S., & Kielhofner, G. (2001). Narratives and experience in an occupational transition: A longitudinal study of the retirement process. *American Journal of Occupational Therapy, 55*, 424–432.

Kielhofner, G. (1997). *Conceptual foundations of occupational therapy* (2nd ed.). Philadelphia: FA Davis.

Kielhofner, G. (2004). *Conceptual foundations of occupational therapy* (3rd ed.). Philadelphia: FA Davis.

King, J. (1994). Our patients, ourselves: Will the therapeutic relationship survive health care reform? *Journal of Hand Therapy, 7*, 226–231.

King, L. J. (1980). Creative caring. *American Journal of Occupational Therapy, 34*, 522–528.

Law, M. (1998). *Client-centered occupational therapy*. Thorofare, NJ: Slack.

Law, M., Baptiste, S., & Mills, J. (1995). Client-centered practice: what does it mean and does it make a difference? *Canadian Journal of Occupational Therapy, 62*, 250–257.

Law, M., Polatajko, H., Baptiste, S., & Townsend, E. (1997). Core concepts of occupational therapy. In E. Townsend, S. Stanton, M. Law, H. Polatajko, S. Baptiste, T. Thompson-Franson, et al. (Eds.) *Enabling occupation: An occupational therapy perspective* (pp. 29–56). Ottawa, Ontario: Canadian Association of Occupational Therapists.

Lloyd, C., & Maas, F. (1991). The therapeutic relationship. *British Journal of Occupational Therapy, 54*, 11–13.

Lloyd, C., & Mass, F. (1992). Interpersonal skills and occupational therapy. *British Journal of Occupational Therapy, 55*(10), 379–382.

Lyons, K. D., & Crepeau, E. B. (2001). The clinical reasoning of an occupational therapy assistant. *American Journal of Occupational Therapy, 55*, 577–581.

Mattingly, C. (1991). The narrative nature of clinical reasoning. *American Journal of Occupational Therapy, 45*, 998–1005.

Mattingly, C. (1994). The narrative nature of clinical reasoning. In C. Mattingly & M. H. Fleming (Eds.). *Clinical reasoning: Forms of inquiry in a therapeutic practice* (pp. 239–269). Philadelphia: FA Davis.

Mattingly, C., & Fleming, M. H. (1994). *Clinical reasoning: Forms of inquiry in a therapeutic practice* (pp. 178–196). Philadelphia: FA Davis.

Meyer, A. (1922). The philosophy of occupational therapy. *Archives of Occupational Therapy, 1*, 1–10.

Mosey, A. C. (1970). *Three frames of reference for mental health*. Thorofare, NJ: Slack.

Mosey, A. C. (1981). *Occupational theapy: Configuration of a profession*. New York: Raven Press.

Mosey, A. C. (1986). *Psychosocial components of occupational therapy* (p. 400). Philadelphia: Lippincott, Williams & Wilkins.

Orlinsky, D. E. (1994). Research-based knowledge as the emergent foundation for clinical practice in psychotherapy. In P. F. Talley, H. H. Strupp, & S. F. Butler (Eds.) *Psychotherapy research and practice: Bridging the gap*. New York: Basic Books.

Peloquin, S. M. (1988). Linking purpose to procedure during interactions with patients. *American Journal of Occupational Therapy, 42*, 775–781.

Peloquin, S. M. (1989a). Moral treatment: Contexts considered. *American Journal of Occupational Therapy, 43*, 537–544.

Peloquin, S. M. (1989b). Sustaining the art of practice in occupational therapy. *American Journal of Occupaitonal Therapy, 43*, 219–226.

Peloquin, S. M. (1990). The patient-therapist relationship in occupational therapy: Understanding visions and images. *American Journal of Occupational Therapy, 44*, 13–21.

Peloquin, S. M. (1993). The depersonalization of patients: A profile gleaned from narratives. *American Journal of Occupational Therapy, 47*, 830–837.

Peloquin, S. M. (1995). The fullness of empathy: Reflections and illustrations. *American Journal of Occupational Therapy, 49*, 24–31.

Peloquin, S. M. (2002). Reclaiming the vision of reaching for heart as well as hands. *American Journal of Occupaitonal Therapy, 56*, 517–526.

Peloquin, S. M. (2003). The therapeutic relationship: Manifestations and challenges in occupational therapy. In E. B. Crepeau, E. S. Cohn, & B. A. Boyt Schell (Eds.). *Willard & Spackman's occupational therapy* (10th ed.) (pp. 157–170). Philadelphia: Lippincott, Williams & Wilkins.

Peloquin, S. M. (2005). The 2005 Eleanor Clarke Slagle Lecture: Embracing our ethos, reclaiming our heart. *American Journal of Occupational Therapy, 59*, 611–625.

Peloquin, S. M., & Davisdon, D. A. (1993). Interpersonal skills for practice: An elective course. *American Journal of Occupational Therapy, 47*, 260–264.

Prochnau, C., Liu, L., & Boman, J. (2003). Personal-professional connections in palliative care occupational therapy. *American Journal of Occupational Therapy, 57*, 196–204.

Punwar, J., & Peloquin, M. (2000). *Occupational therapy: principles and practice* (pp. 42–98). Philadelphia: Lippincott

Reilly, M. (1962). Occupational therapy can be one of the great ideas of the twentieth century [Eleanor Clark Slagle Lecture]. *American Journal of Occupational Therapy*, 23, 299–307.

Restall, G., Ripat, J., & Stern, M. (2003). A framework of strategies for client-centered practice. *Canadian Journal of Occupational Therapy, 70*, 103–112.

Rogers, J. C. (1983). Clinical reasoning: The ethics, science, and art: 1983 Eleanor Clarke Slagle lecture. *American Journal of Occupational Therapy, 37*, 601–616.

Rosenbaum, P., King, S., Law, M., King, G., & Evans, J. (1998). Family-centered service: A conceptual framework and research review. In M. Law (Ed.). *Family-centered assessment and intervention in pediatric rehabilitation* (pp. 1–20). Binghamton, NY: Haworth.

Schell, B. A. (2003). Clinical reasoning: The basis of practice. In E. B. Crepeau, E. S. Cohn, & B. A. Boyt Schell (Eds.) *Willard & Spackman's occupational therapy* (10th ed.) (pp. 131–152). Philadelphia: Lippincott, Williams & Wilkins.

Schell, B. A., & Cervero, R. M. (1993). Clinical reasoning in occupational therapy: An integrative review. *American Journal of Occupational Therapy, 47*, 605–610.

Schell, B. A., Crepeau, E. B., & Cohn, E. S. (2003). Professional development. In E. B. Crepeau, E. S. Cohn, & B. A. Boyt Schell (Eds.) *Willard & Spackman's occupational therapy* (10th ed.) (pp. 141–144). Philadelphia: Lippincott, Williams & Wilkins.

Schon, D. A. (1983). *The reflective practitioner: How professionals think in action*. New York: Basic Books.

Schwartz, K. B. (2003). The history of occupational therapy. In E. B. Crepeau, E. S. Cohn, & B. A. Boyt Schell (Eds.). *Willard & Spackman's occupational therapy*, (10th ed.) (pp. 5–13). Philadelphia: Lippincott, Williams & Wilkins.

Schwartzberg, S. L. (2002). *Interactive reasoning in the process of occupational therapy*. Upper Saddle River, NJ: Pearson Education.

Schwartzberg, S. L. (1993). Therapeutic use of self. In H. Hopkins & H. Smith (Eds.). *Willard & Spackman's occupational therapy* (8th ed.). Philadelphia: Lippincott, Williams & Wilkins.

Shannon, P. D. (1977). The derailment of occupational therapy. *American Journal of Occupational Therapy*, 31, 229–234.

Slagle, E. C. (1922). Training aides for mental patients. *Archives of Occupational Therapy 1,* 11–17.

Stein, F., & Cutler, S. K. (1998). *Psychosocial occupational therapy: A holistic approach* (pp. 11–12). San Diego: Singular

Sumsion, T. (2000). A revised occupational therapy definition of client-centered practice. *British Journal of Occupational Therapy, 63,* 304–309.

Sumsion, T. (2003). Focus on research: Defining client-centered occupational therapy practice. *British Journal of Occupational Therapy, 66*, 218.

Taylor, R. R., Lee, S. W., Kielhofner, G., & Ketkar, M. (2007). *Therapeutic use of self: a nationwide survey of practitioners*. Manuscript submitted for publication.

Townsend, E. (2003). Reflections on power and justice in enabling occupation. *Revue Canadienne D'Ergothera-pie, 70,* 74–87.

Tracy, S. (1912). *Studies in invalid occupation.* Boston: Whitcomb & Barrows.

Wade, B. D. (1947). Occupational therapy for patients with mental disease. In H. S. Willard & C. S. Spackman (Eds.). *Principles of occupational therapy* (pp. 81–117). Philadelphia: JB Lippincott.

Wells, S. A., & Black, R. M. (2000). *Cultural competency for health professionals.* Bethesda, MD: American Occupational Therapy Association.

Yerxa, E. J. (1967). Authentic occupational therapy [Eleanor Clarke Slagle Lecture]. *American Journal of Occupational Therapy,* 21, 1–9.

Yerxa, E. J. (1980). Occupational therapy's role in creating a future climate of caring. *American Journal of Occupational Therapy, 34,* 529–679.

WHAT DEFINES
A GOOD THERAPIST?

Clearly many variables contribute to becoming an effective occupational therapist. Most therapists would agree that they include such things as a sound theory base and good technical skills. Moreover, as seen in Chapter 1, it also requires being able to manage the interpersonal aspects of therapy. When considering this crucial dimension of being a good therapist, some questions come to mind: What qualities define interpersonal success in therapy? What distinguishes a therapist with highly effective interpersonal skills? Is there a particular interpersonal style that defines good therapeutic use of self?

To address these questions, this chapter introduces 12 occupational therapists from around the world. All of them were nominated by their occupational therapy colleagues as exemplifying outstanding use of self in therapy. During the past 2 years, I visited each of them to understand better why their colleagues considered them exceptional. I observed them practicing with an interpersonally complex client and conducted an in-depth qualitative interview about their approach to the use of self in therapy.

These therapists are quite diverse in terms of practice areas, client populations, and preferred theoretical orientations to practice. Intriguingly, they differ drastically in personality styles and in their attitudes about what constitutes effective interpersonal practice with a given client population. None of the therapists featured in this chapter was self-nominated. Perhaps as a result there was substantial variation among them in terms of their personal convictions about their own interpersonal efficacy in therapy. A few of them were so prone to self-examination that they often expressed doubt about why they were nominated, whether a given interpersonal decision was the best one

to take, or whether I agreed with a given interpersonal action they took in therapy. After watching them practice, the source of their self-doubt was a mystery to me. I found it ironic that such talented individuals would doubt their own capacities. Although there is likely a threshold beyond which self-questioning becomes counterproductive rather than helpful to therapists, I found the self-questioning nature of these therapists matched historical accounts and my own convictions that the most effective therapists are the ones with the greatest ability to evaluate continually their communications and other interpersonal behaviors in therapy.

Although the therapists featured in this chapter are quite diverse in personality styles, they have one thing in common. Each was capable of providing powerful examples of therapeutic encounters from their own practice that illustrated exceptional judgment and care in highly challenging interpersonal situations. These examples, coupled with personal narratives illustrating their unique interpersonal approaches to therapy, provide a complex and variegated response to the major question framing this chapter. They illustrate that therapists can be equally effective in managing interpersonal challenges of therapy regardless of differences in age, sex, orientation to practice, and personality style. In the sections below, I have relied mainly on their own narratives of an interpersonal challenge they faced and their descriptions of their therapeutic strengths and styles. It should be noted that I have not highlighted under each therapist all the traits that characterize their therapeutic approach. Rather, I included those that stood out as most prominent in my observation of each person and/or in their self-description.

Kim's Interpersonal Challenge: The Emotionally Charged Therapy Task of Bladder Management with Maggie

I was working with Maggie,[1] a young North African woman with paraplegia from a gunshot wound. She was referred to occupational therapy for rehabilitation related to activities of daily living. Due to the political situation in her country, she was forced to immigrate to the United States 5 years before the injury. She had been working as a secretary and was living alone.

Maggie was a talented, proud, and attractive woman who, at the very beginning of her adult life, was completely devastated by her injury. She experienced being in a wheelchair as very devaluing, and she seemed con-

---

[1]All client names and geographic information have been changed.

Box 2.1

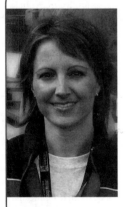

Therapist:	Kim Eberhardt, MS, OTR/L
Practice Location:	Chicago, Illinois, USA
OT Roles:	Practitioner and Fieldwork Supervisor, Rehabilitation Institute of Chicago
	Adjunct Professor of Occupational Therapy, University of Illinois at Chicago
Years Experience:	11 years
Populations Served:	Adolescents and adults with spinal cord injury

sumed by feelings of shame and humiliation. Throughout the course of therapy, she made very little eye contact with me and spoke softly in a very low tone of voice. I saw her as an outpatient, and she missed a lot of therapy. Though bladder management was one of the priorities for the interdisciplinary team, we all avoided working on it with her for a long time. I had a feeling that it would be very difficult for her to learn this in my (or anyone's) presence. Instead, we worked on a number of other activities in therapy, including homemaking, money management, and mobility and travel training. She learned that she could be self-sufficient with daily activities, and we built trust like that.

Interpersonal Solution

Despite my attempts to postpone it with this client, eventually the time came when we were forced to work on toileting. The physician's recommendation was to progress from an indwelling catheter and teach Maggie to perform intermittent catheterization so that she could use the toilet regularly. I deliberately saved this until the last phase of therapy after Maggie had a number of successful experiences performing other activities. I wanted to wait until I felt she knew that I would respect her privacy and dignity.

I began with a graded approach by first getting her interested in traveling into the community. At the same time, I introduced the idea of the necessity of and benefits to learning this approach to toileting. We decided not to make it the focus of any single session but, instead, to spend just a little time on it over a period of several sessions and then rewarding her for progress made by working on other activities that she preferred. I have learned that if you hit it so hard with people it becomes a chore and I didn't want it to be like that for her.

For a time we began by just practicing getting onto and off a chair. We treated it as a kind of dry-run simulation until she felt very competent at this. We also went shopping for clothing, which was an activity that she ended up enjoying a lot. Once she was interested in purchasing something, we practiced going into a dressing room and changing clothes together. This gave me some idea of her level of comfort with being unclothed, and it allowed us to build trust. We also set a goal to visit a restaurant, making this approach to toileting training very relevant to our activities. I had to draw upon activity analysis and grading, and I had to structure it to ensure success at each level. I used a lot of empathy and reassurance. Even though I knew she could do it, I told Maggie, "I think you can do it, I have a lot of faith in you." I made her feel valued, and I provided her incentives; I told her that if she could do this she could go back to work. We planned that ultimately we would go to a restaurant where she would use a public toilet for the first time. Eventually, Maggie agreed to try it, but she clarified that she would attempt it only with me; she did not want other members of the treatment team to be involved.

Outcome

She was able to do it. It took extra time, planning, and practice, a lot of reassurance, and having successful progressive experiences. Finally, we celebrated by going to a public restaurant where Maggie used the bathroom on her own.

About Kim

Before this book was formulated I knew Kim because she is adjunct instructor in the occupational therapy program at the University of Illinois. Following a solicitation I sent out for Chicago-area nominations, I was not surprised when multiple people suggested Kim to be featured in this book. When we met for the interview, our working relationship came immediately easily and felt entirely natural. Kim has a unique quality of making one feel entirely accepted and comfortable in her presence. She approached the interview with genuine interest and curiosity, and she was utterly task focused and oriented toward the questions and ideas. She has a placid elegance about her and conveys an implicit faith in the talents and capacities of others.

I asked Kim for her own perceptions of her strengths as a practitioner. Some of her replies and the themes they reflect are below.

Trustworthy

I'm a good, active listener and I'm patient … loyal and committed. I always follow through on what I say I will do. Patients know they can count on me as the person who will get things done quickly. This links into issues of trust. Right away if I say to a patient that "I'll be back," I will…. If I promised we would go on an outing, we will…. If patients see right away that they can count on you, they never forget it. It builds consistency…. I am very consistent, very structured, and very immediately responsive to my clients. You have one chance with people; and if you blow the first chance, you lose their trust and investment forever. I have seen that some professionals are not so good at this, and I have seen the consequences in terms of trust.

Motivating

I know how to balance pushing and supporting people. I know when to challenge clients, cheerlead, or push them a little bit to accomplish their goals, and I know when to stop the process and provide support, empathy, incentives, hope, or encouragement.

Empowering

I use this same view of balance to slowly teach patients to be more aware of themselves and their achievements over time. I carefully pace what I highlight or reinforce, and then I withhold my input and direct patients' attention to themselves. By doing this, patients learn how to observe and evaluate their own performance and develop an internal locus of control. I allow them to take credit for their own achievements. For example, when they first learn to eat, they may take an hour and result in a lot of food on their clothing. Over time, they are taking 30 minutes to eat and not getting as much on themselves. This would go unnoticed and would not be a big accomplishment for them unless they saw it. I think it's important to teach people how to notice their own accomplishments because they will have to use this strategy to empower themselves when they leave the hospital. An internal locus of control is what will sustain their efforts over time.

Empathetic

When I get different reactions to therapy, as when patients tell me "I'm too tired today," "I'm depressed," "I'm in pain," "I'm afraid," "I'm not into this—my mind is not here," I try to think of an instance where I felt the same thing or a family member said something like this to me. Most of the time if I look deeper I see that they are depressed or very anxious. I also try to think of patients from the past who said these things and remember what I did in those situations. I ask myself questions like, "Do I need to stop and be responsive and build the trust?" I draw most heavily on my empathic side with challenging clients. I remember relatives with cancer and arthritis who told me they had days like these.

Energetic

I put a lot energy into my practice, and I convey this energy to my patients when appropriate.

As a therapist, Kim embodies the image of a steady yet gentle guide. Solid, loyal, dependable, dedicated, sincere, efficient, and industrious are other adjectives that come to mind. No doubt her clients appreciate the comfortable, warm feeling one gets from simply being around her. Kim also has a highly refined sense of the dialectical aspects of client–therapist interactions. She knows precisely when to challenge clients and when to provide support. She knows when to provide incentives and highlight strengths and when to pull back and allow clients to become inspired and notice their own achievements in therapy. Her relationships leave people hopeful, stronger, and enriched (Box 2.1).

René's Interpersonal Challenge: Managing a Difficult Emotional Pattern with Madam Gauthier

I worked with a 47-year-old woman of European origin. She had been divorced for 12 years and was living with her 18-year-old son, a full-time student. Madam Gauthier was diagnosed with active borderline personality disorder and had a history of bipolar disorder with psychotic features (now stabilized) and a diagnosis of multiple sclerosis. In the past she performed janitorial work for a hospital, but she was then receiving disability income. I worked with Madam Gauthier as an outpatient for more than 2¹/₂ years with some brief intermissions. I still see her periodically for follow-up appointments.

During our work together, Madam Gauthier exhibited a specific pattern of interpersonal behavior. She was

---

Box 2.2

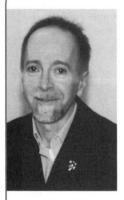

Therapist: René Bélanger, OTR, MBA
Practice Location: Quebec City, Quebec
   Province, Canada
OT Roles: Practitioner, Hôtel-Dieu de
   Lévis Hospital
   Clinical Professor of Rehabili-
   tation, Laval University
   Fieldwork Supervisor
Years Experience: 24 years
Populations Served: Adolescents, adults, and eld-
   erly with severe psychiatric
   disorders

---

referred for occupational therapy because of difficulties with passive-aggressive behavior, elevated and overly dramatic affect, and absence of goal-directed behavior. She often showed up at the hospital spontaneously in-between sessions and presented with a dramatic emotional crisis. She had lost her self-confidence, and her reactions were to behave in interpersonally intrusive and regressive ways such that she became difficult to relate to and overly dependent on friends and family. This ultimately led others to withdraw from her, leaving her very isolated, depressed, almost paranoid, and virtually immobile in terms of her daily living routines.

Each time we began the therapy session, Madam Gauthier spoke very rapidly about a wide range of subjects but mostly focused on her frustrations in daily living. At that time, I always had the feeling she didn't listen to me (my verbal interventions), and she left me very little room for input to guide her to become more stable and centered in her interactions with others. Each session started with this period of free ventilation and excessive talking without listening, rejecting all of my attempts to introduce notions of problem-solving. After a while during this first part of therapy, she would become very sad and would begin to cry. A few seconds later she seemed surprisingly open and became available to work on some specific problematic aspect of her life. She would then begin to apply my suggestions and initiate the actions necessary that would enable her to decrease her daily living dissatisfaction. Throughout the course of therapy, this pattern did not change significantly.

Interpersonal Response

Although Madam Gauthier learned to exert more control over this pattern, she still seemed to find it very important to keep and repeat this pattern at the beginning of each therapy session. Frequently, I made many attempts to avoid, skip, or shorten this first part of the therapy. I perceived her enactment of this pattern as wasted time because it did not leave me enough room during the sessions to work directly on the heart of my objective: to provide support and to assist Madam Gauthier in exploring ways to decrease her excessive emotionality, establish a routine for daily living, and improve upon her ways of relating with others. At first, I was always unsuccessful and unproductive when I confronted her or pushed her to make this first part of free ventilation shorter. The result of my pressure was that it was always impossible to work on what I perceived as the true objectives of therapy.

It took me a while to understand this pattern and to consider Madam Gauthier's engagement in this process as a facilitator for our work rather than an impediment to therapy. Once I recognized this, I negotiated specific boundaries within therapy in which Madam Gauthier was provided a specific amount of time at the beginning of therapy to vent about her problems with the condition of respecting my therapy-oriented part of the session.

Outcome

Interestingly, occupational therapy was the only long-term therapeutic approach that Madam Gauthier was able to tolerate and sustain active participation and investment in at our hospital. At the end of therapy, she was able to preserve some stability in her daily living environment and she had stopped showing up at the hospital in-between therapy sessions presenting with a big drama and storm whenever she was frustrated with her life. For the first time in a long time, she has not had an inpatient hospitalization. She has been able to maintain relative emotional stability and quality of life, despite the complexity of her psychiatric and physical conditions. She has made genuine progress in mobilizing a daily living routine, reintegrating in the community, and improving her relationships with others despite her other health problems.

About René

I first met René when he was visiting and lecturing in Chicago. Subsequently, I spent some time observing his work and getting to know him more in Quebec City. One of the most striking qualities about René is that he is amazingly honest and frank about life. Immediately, I was struck by the juxtaposition of relaxed kindness in his face as it was blended with an air of dignified formality, determination, and shrewdness of intellect. René holds himself with a very straight posture, and is parsimonious with words. He moves very slowly, giving the impression that his every action is precise and deliberate. There is a distinct calmness and stability about him. Although he tends to maintain a certain degree of guardedness in relation to others, he never comes across as cold or rejecting.

I began our interview by asking him to describe the personal strengths he draws upon when doing therapy. Some of his responses and the themes they reflect are below.

Calm

I'm calm with a certain level of distance. This means I do not express my feelings too much at the beginning of the relationship. Instead, I am neutral but remain invested and slightly oriented toward the idea of working on the client's dissatisfaction or need for change. I think this invites people to be centered and also to trust that I will not push or burden them with my own needs or agenda.

Assertive

When the time is right, I am good at providing clear directions and setting clear expectations.... It's easy for me to put feelings into words and to directly name situations.

My thought process is very structured and I think it's easy for clients to understand what I am saying to them. At the beginning, I use short, direct, and simple sentences to make sure clients won't be distracted or disturbed by their cognitive and communication impairments.

René is a very precise and controlled, yet very human, therapist. Stable, dignified, calm, and comforting, he is the type of person with whom one enjoys spending time. He is always present and available but never imposing. Observing him, one is struck with how masterfully he interacts with a client. His demeanor speaks volumes about the interweaving of clarity, honesty, and interpersonal self-discipline in therapeutic interactions (Box 2.2).

Michele's Interpersonal Challenge: Motivating Assaf and the Bubble Machine

Assaf, a child with severe developmental delay, was about five when I began treating him. He was markedly passive and showed no interest in anything. I would bring him to the regular occupational therapy room and try hard to arouse his interest in something in the room. I worked very hard and creatively to inspire his interest in anything I could think of. During our first and second sessions in the Snoezelen[2] room, he did nothing. He was characteristically passive and quiet. He just stared at the wall.

During his third session, Assaf started tearing at his clothes and emitting loud sounds of distress. I thought he might be anxious, and I became somewhat alarmed. Gradually it occurred to me that Assaf's behavior was not random. He was, in fact, trying to attract my attention. He kept pulling me.

---

[2]*Snoezelen* (which comes from the Dutch words that mean to "sniff" and "doze") was developed by an art therapist in Holland. It refers to a multisensory room that typically incorporates: a) lighting effects such as projectors and spotlights that disburse light patterns in the room, bubble lamps, and star panels; b) soft items on the floor such as mats, pillows, or beanbags; c) aromatic items such as aromatherapy fans and oils; and d) sound effects such as music and nature or animal sounds. It also incorporates sensory activities such as blowing bubbles, along with tactile experiences such as touching and feeling cotton balls, bubble wrap, or feathers, along with switches that allow control of the environment and objects that provide visual effects, vibrate, make noise, or have a tactile feel.

Box 2.3

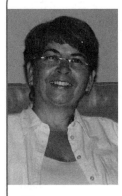

Therapist: Michele Shapiro, OTR, Doctoral
                         Student
Practice Location: Raanana, Israel
OT Roles: Practitioner and Fieldwork
                         Supervisor, Beit Issie Shapiro
                         Community Organization
                         Director of Snoezelen and Envi-
                         ronmental Design
                         Lecturer, Trump International
                         Institute of Higher Learning
Years Experience: 33 years
Populations Served: Infants, toddlers, and children
                         with a wide range of develop-
                         mental, physical, and neuro-
                         psychiatric impairments

Interpersonal Response

At first I resisted but then I let myself be pulled. I found that he was guiding me in the direction of a tall vibrating bubble unit. When we drew near to it, I was surprised to see Assaf extend his arm to touch it. It was incredible; I'd never before seen Assaf reach out to anything! Instead of coaxing him to do things or trying to attract his interest, I began to track his behavior. My total strategy shifted from one of trying to control the therapeutic interaction to trying to understand and go wherever Assaf led me. I am convinced that this change in my style of handling the interaction is what led to the breakthrough in our treatment. It was only when I changed my behavior that Assaf, somehow, felt free enough or safe enough to begin tentatively to explore.

Outcome

Assaf has severe impairments, which have remained. Nonetheless, the experience in the Snoezelen gave light to Assaf's likes and dislikes. We changed our educational strategy for him by adding more sensory-based stimuli to his daily routine. His parents and class caregivers noticed a considerable change in his motivation and investigation. He went from being totally passive to an investigator! From lying in one spot for hours, to crawling around and opening every single door on the way, removing pots and pans from his mom's kitchen cupboards.

About Michele

I first encountered Michele while giving a series of challenging lectures at Hebrew University in Jerusalem. When I think of her, the first image that comes to mind is that of a strong, wise face sending me her confidence and energy from among numerous unfamiliar faces in the auditorium. Without knowing me, Michele implicitly took on the role of serving as a kind of emotional anchor for me during those lectures. It is not surprising that Michele was the person in the audience who noticed that I could use the support of her obviously approving nods and gestures. She has a natural inclination to notice and orient herself toward the most subtle emotional needs of others—a remarkable level of interpersonal sensitivity. She conveys her support through a quiet and tacit presence. Michele notices the smallest detail about you and makes an unobtrusive and attentive comment about it, letting you know she is paying attention and that she cares. Michele is a deeply spiritual person who gives of herself to others unquestioningly. Clients, strangers, friends, family, and colleagues all readily enjoy Michele's emotional generosity. Her faith in humanity is remarkable.

When I asked her to describe some of her own interpersonal strengths as a therapist, she had many thoughts, but over and over again she emphasized one theme.

Positive

I love people and believe in them. I believe in making things work. I have an insatiable need for knowledge, especially about human behavior, and I enjoy following my clients and trying to understand the details of their communication. In nursery school I loved a line from the Wizard of Oz: "It depends upon, it begins and ends upon, it depends on how you look at things." I believe that there is always a positive and a negative way to see a situation, and I prefer to see the positive one. This applies to people too. Some people say I am a "Pollyanna." Well, I have decided to take that as a great compliment and wish more people saw the good in others. I often hear myself saying to a child in treatment "I knew you could do that!" and I really did believe in that child. I also have patience during treatment and can wait for things to happen.

Michele is no Pollyanna. She has acquired the wisdom to realize that relationships are priceless. She acts on that belief on a moment-to-moment basis. Michele's self-description is rich with a number of implications. She has a steadiness of faith in the good intentions, strengths, and capacities of her clients, her keen ability to observe what her clients need in order to learn and make progress, and a predisposition to emphasize the positive aspects of a challenging situation where many others would be more inclined to focus on the problematic aspects (Box 2.3).

Anne's Interpersonal Challenge: Boundary Testing—A Hug From Mr. Klien

Mr. Klien is a remarried elderly man in his late fifties. He was referred to occupational therapy for a conversion disorder involving intermittent paralysis and spasms in his right arm. He also has a history of psychosis and numerous traumatic separations and losses beginning early in life. Mr. Klien is an intelligent man who has served in a variety of professional capacities, including owning and managing his own restaurant. He is now retired and living in a home for the elderly. Mr. Klien has particular difficulty with self–other boundaries and tends to lack an appropriate level of social distance from others. After a few sessions together, Mr. Klien startled me by embracing me at the end of the therapy. When he repeated this behavior at the next session, I knew that it was my responsibility to show him that he was making me uncomfortable and that this type of intimacy was not appropriate for the situation. Nonetheless, I had a feeling that if I had said this to him directly and right away, he would have felt rejected and that I was insulting his intelligence. He has seen many therapists, and on some level he knows the rules of conduct but chooses to test the boundaries.

Interpersonal Response

Because the need to embrace me seemed so important to him, I decided against my first impulse, which was to discuss his emotional needs as they contrasted with my need for limits. I sensed that this could have jeopardized the formation of trust in this early stage of therapy. It seemed that by hugging me he was mainly trying to make a human connection and to express gratitude. So, I decided to use nonverbal communication as a means of intervention. That meant that the next time Mr. Klien moved to embrace me, I simply began to assert my hand into the space between us and shake his hand with a warm expression on my face.

Outcome

Mr. Klien followed this new ritual and after a while he no longer tried to embrace me. By maintaining consistency with the handshake, Mr. Klien eventually recognized that a handshake is enough to say good-bye. Now at the end of therapy, he shakes my hand whenever he feels the need. I still feel that this particular client is not yet ready to talk about the meaning of his need for connection with me explicitly. His extensive history of poor coping with loss makes him vulnerable to misinterpreting explicit statements about rules and boundaries as rejection. However, we are now able to talk about boundary norms and rules of conduct as they relate to other people, so in that way we are slowly making progress.

About Anne

Anne and I first met over lunch in Bad Elster, a quiet and immaculate spa town in what was formerly East Germany. Because Anne speaks primarily German and I do not, we relied mostly on a translator for conversation. Additionally, my nonverbal interactions and observations of

---

Box 2.4

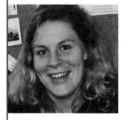

Therapist:	Anne Reuter, State-Approved Occupational Therapist
Practice Location:	Plauen, Germany
OT Roles:	Practitioner, In Motio Outpatient Rehabilitation Center
Years Experience:	8 months
Populations Served:	Children, adults, adolescents, and elderly with a wide range of physical, cognitive, and psychiatric impairments

Anne gave me a feeling for her personality. Anne appears slightly older than her 24 years, and her tall physique coupled with her gentle mannerisms gives her a warm but powerful presence. Anne appears very content and peaceful. She demonstrates a level of awareness about life that is way beyond her years. She obviously uses this awareness to exhibit restraint, patience, and appreciation for others during her therapy.

Observing Anne with one of her clients on a snowy winter day in Plauen, I realized why faculty at the school had nominated a young therapist with less than a year of experience to be featured in this book. Anne has an uncanny ability to anticipate how her clients might interpret or react to a statement or action before it takes place. In this way, her clinical reasoning is significantly more anticipatory than it is reactive.

At the same time, Anne combines a youthful lightheartedness with an authoritative sense of structure, firmness, and an empowerment-oriented approach to her clients. On many occasions, she and her client would chuckle together at an ironic or humorous aspect of the therapy, as if they were sharing a private joke. The next moment they would be back to the business of working through the tasks of therapy.

She is detail-oriented when it comes to reading and understanding her clients and at the same time highly conscious about how even the most nuanced differences in her own daily experiences might affect her use of self in therapy. When I asked Anne to give me her take on her interpersonal approach to her clients, she emphasized the following themes.

Attentive

I believe that establishing trust between the client and therapist is the primary and most important aspect of therapy. I base all of my treatment approaches on this singular prerequisite.... Giving clients choice in terms of what they want to accomplish and respecting that choice is also very important.... I believe that there are good days and bad days in the life of each person and that experiences a person has from day to day influence how one does therapy each time. On the other hand, I believe that it is very important to keep one's personal life out of therapy. At each session, I always try to concentrate fully on the problems of each client and not let any other thoughts or circumstances intrude.

Friendly

I'm sociable and enjoy interacting with a wide variety of people.

Flexible

I'm flexible in that I can adapt myself to almost any type of person and his or her mood of the day.

Despite the short time I had to know Anne and despite our language difference, I was grateful to have had the opportunity to observe her work. Watching her raw interpersonal talent unfold in a highly complex clinical situation is inspiring. Anne exhibits an impressively high level of clinical reasoning, grace, and ease of communication with her clients (Box 2.4).

Roland's Interpersonal Challenge: Helping Mr. Olson Reframe His Views on Working

Mr. Olson is a Swedish man in his early forties who has never been married, has no children, and lives with his aging mother in an apartment in a town just south of

---

Box 2.5

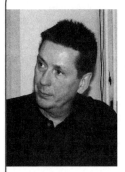

Therapist:	Roland Meisel, MS, OTR/L
Practice Location:	A-Rehab, Inc. Stockholm, Sweden
OT Roles:	President of A-Rehab, Inc.
	Evaluation and practice in work rehabilitation
	Designer of customized assistive technologies for the workplace
Years Experience:	25 years
Populations Served:	Adults with a wide range of impairments that have led to work disability

Stockholm. He has lived with his mother for most of his life. His diagnoses include type I diabetes, morbid obesity, major depression, and chronic neuropathic pain, particularly in his feet. Mr. Olson has been receiving disability income for the past 5 years. Previously, he worked as a cook (in his early adulthood) and as a machine operator (in his middle adulthood). He discontinued work as per the recommendation of his employer and his physician, both of whom felt that his work was too stressful for him and that his ongoing fatigue and periodic symptoms of confusion, dizziness, and disorientation were putting him at risk for injury on the job. At that time it was recommended that Mr. Olson pursue a diabetes management program and psychotherapy, but he never followed through with that recommendation. I was hired by Mr. Olson's long-term disability insurance company to determine whether Mr. Olson was capable of returning to any type of work.

The insurance company provided me only two sessions to evaluate Mr. Olson's work capacity and, if indicated, to find an appropriate job placement for him. I often have to work within these very tight time frames to get a multidimensional idea of what a client might be interested in and capable of doing. Because of this temporal horizon, I have learned to work swiftly and to be very direct and respectfully confrontational with clients, when necessary.

During the initial session, Mr. Olson consistently denied interest or capacity for any type of work activity. He focused on describing his impairments and complained about his chronic pain. He maintained that his main occupations were to maintain the apartment where he and his mother were living and to serve as a caretaker for his mother, who was aging. He reported that he does enjoy reading, doing crossword puzzles, and playing other games of logic involving mathematics. He maintained that he could perform these kinds of activities for hours at a time. Given his responses, there seemed to be an inconsistency between his ability to do caretaking and other activities he reported and his avowed lack of interest or ability for work.

Interpersonal Response

By using a series of questions that were aimed to gently nudge Mr. Olson to honestly think out loud about his situation, I was able to guide him to think through things in ways that I'm not sure he had fully done before. I was straightforward but not accusatory in pointing out inconsistencies between things he had said. I gave him opportunities to reframe his conclusions or statements as we explored his situation together.

Outcome

As our discussion unfolded, Mr. Olson admitted that he might be able to function at a desk job that involved basic office work, such as filing, sorting, assembling mailings, and perhaps bookkeeping. After the careful process of examining Mr. Olson's logic and rationale for why he would be unable to perform such a job, it became clear to both him and me that his main motivation for remaining on disability was so he could stay home and care for his mother. By the end of the interview, Mr. Olson was able to admit that he could probably perform a basic office job, if required, and if alternative arrangements could be arranged for the care of his mother.

He was also able to acknowledge that, on an emotional level, it would be very difficult for him to be away from his mother for most of the day, nearly every day, for a long period of time. In the spirit of collaboration, we both decided that the recommendation to the insurance company would be that Mr. Olson would attempt to work in the proposed work situation on a preliminary trial basis for a defined period of time if the appropriate arrangements could be made. If the situation did not work for any reason, Mr. Olson would be eligible to continue receiving disability income.

About Roland

I first met Roland at a social gathering during the World Federation of Occupational Therapy conference in Stockholm. Through the evening, he entertained several of us with a series of amusing stories and jokes. At one point during the interaction, I observed him to pick up on an argument between two persons in our group. During the argument, Roland served as a kind of facilitator and mediator. Boldly, he intervened. With tremendous empathy, he ensured that each person's perspective was heard and responded to until the conflict was resolved. When I later learned that, as the president of A-Rehab Incorporated, part of his job is to evaluate individuals' capacity to return to work for insurance companies, it was difficult for me to conceive of him dealing with the often contentious issue of whether people merit benefits for being unable to work. Roland is a very easygoing humorous, flexible, empathic, and emotionally generous person.

I later got to know Roland professionally and had the chance to observe him in a professional capacity. Then, a more nuanced picture emerged. Beneath Roland's easygoing style is a sophisticated, worldly, persuasive, and savvy interpersonal style. He is a reasonable yet strong leader. One can readily see how he could be president of a very successful rehabilitation company. When I asked Roland to describe his interpersonal style at work, he replied with the following themes.

Logical

I use a lot of cognitive behavioral strategies, reasoning, and logical questioning to raise people's consciousness about the ways in which they might be underestimating themselves or dismissing their capacity to engage in meaningful work.

Firm

I focus on volition and try to shift the power back into the hands of the client, even if they resist taking responsibility for themselves at first. I am firm. I use the evidence from their performance and behavior to show them they are capable of doing something.

Collaborative

If I detect resistance or discover certain barriers and obstacles to return to work, we discuss those challenges openly together and try to get to the root of them.... We work things out together.

Humorous

Sometimes when situations get tense I try to break the tension a little by using humor. Generally, I will say something self-effacing to let the client know that I am human, too.

Persausive

Most of the time I assert myself as the one with expertise in this area. I believe strongly in structure and in the use of formal authority to deliver the reality of the situation to my clients. Up front the clients know that I am hired by their insurance company and that the interest of the insurance company is to get them to return to work. If I think they are in any way capable of performing some type of work, I attempt to persuade them to think about the health and quality of life benefits of work. This is because, fundamentally, I believe that work is therapeutic for people if they are capable.

Roland's interpersonal efficiency and skill are very much a product of the context in which he works. The fast-paced and demanding nature of simultaneously serving as a consultant for insurance companies and as an equipment designer requires that he have a strong work ethic and be a multi-tasker. At his company, he proudly showed some of his latest custom-designed assistive technologies that allow workers with motor impairments to return to work. At any given time, Roland has several simultaneous contracts and projects underway. However, beneath these more pragmatic qualities is a very honest and compassionate man who clearly strives to guide his clients toward the best paths possible and who genuinely cares about empowering individuals to function at their best within the community in which they live (Box 2.5).

Belinda's Interpersonal Challenge: Overcoming Jacob's and his Grandmother's Resistance

When I first started working with Jacob, he was an 18-month-old boy with a visual impairment that would eventually progress to total blindness by age 10 or 11.

Box 2.6

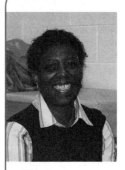

Therapist:	Belinda Anderson, MEd, MS, OTR/L
Practice Location:	Select Medical, Skokie, Illinois, which subcontracts to: Chicago Lighthouse for the Blind and Visually Impaired, Chicago, Illinois and the Chicago Board of Education
OT Roles:	Practitioner and school consultant, Chicago Lighthouse and Chicago Board of Educaiton Fieldwork Supervisor
Years Experience:	14 years
Populations Served:	Multiply-disabled children and adolescents with visual impairments Early intervention with infants and toddlers 0–3 years of age

He was referred for occupational therapy because he was so sensory defensive that he did not want anything or anyone to touch him except his grandmother.

During the initial stages of treatment, Jacob refused to engage in therapy in any way. He would just sit in his grandmother's lap. When I got within any close physical distance, he would scream and cry. If I tried to touch him while he was on his grandmother's lap and work toward a relationship in a graded way, he would still cry loudly and would not stop until I withdrew my hand. To complicate matters, his grandmother would not say anything reassuring or encouraging to him that might facilitate his engagement with another person.

Grandmother was reluctantly cooperative about taking him off of her lap for treatment. Once off of her lap, Jacob would cry the entire time without stopping until he was returned to his grandmother's lap. It would not matter what I tried to do with him in therapy—soothe him, sing to him, try to make him laugh, point out body parts to orient him in space, take his shoes on and off—he would cry indiscriminately. All of my fail-safe approaches that worked with even the most fearful or reluctant children were not working with Jacob.

Interpersonal Response

I realized that the first, most difficult but most critical step in getting Jacob to relate to me differently would be to change his view of me. I had to redefine what my role was in his life. Until this point, he had been viewing me as a threatening person who was taking him away from his grandmother. I had to remove grandmother from the picture and teach him to relate to me as a new and independent person rather than as a "kidnapper." The first goal was to try to convince grandmother that she had to leave Jacob in the treatment room alone with me. That is really hard for parents and grandparents. I was straightforward with grandmother about why I thought this approach would work. I told her that she was playing a role in preventing Jacob from relating to others by overprotecting him. I had to educate her about the importance of giving Jacob reassurance and encouragement to relate with others. At the clinic I have a two-way window so grandmother could observe the entire process. I prepared grandmother that Jacob's crying was likely to get worse before it became better and that he would probably cry even harder at first.

Outcome

It was difficult to get grandmother to collaborate with me at first. She would become anxious when Jacob cried in her absence. However, eventually she saw that the process worked. It took months before he stopped crying. I worked with Jacob on being able to tell me if he was "ready" for

therapy. Eventually, he became more assertive. Interacting with him became the coolest thing. He would come into the therapy room, and he would tell me whether he was ready. Some days he would just walk into the room and get on the swing or climb over something, but most days he would say, "I'm not ready" in a defiant tone. My response would be "Well you better get ready!" in a very loud voice. Each time we had this exchange, he would crack up laughing. He must be 5 years old now. His mother, who I also worked with, called me last year. The mother moved away with Jacob because grandmother continued to try to be too dominating and protective of Jacob, and it was not in his best interest.

About Belinda

Belinda is a strong and confident person who evokes feelings of warmth, security, and appreciation. Her strength is obvious in her proud stance and engaged way of speaking, both of which command respect. At the same time, Belinda is also fun and friendly, always ready to share a laugh. These are useful qualities for any therapist, but they are particularly important in pediatrics. When I asked Belinda to describe the strengths of her approach in her own words, she offered the following.

Open

I'm open. People seem to tell me everything. Sometimes I wonder if I have the word "therapist" written on my forehead.… I try to find something personal about people, and in return I am more of an open, revealing person. I give of myself and let people know about me to the extent that it's appropriate.… I also accept feedback from people very well. People can tell me anything, and I'll deal with it. At the same time, I am not afraid to give people feedback. A speech therapist told me one time that she appreciated that I am upfront. She said: "You can tell someone how you feel, they tell you how they feel, and you're finished with it."

Respectful

I don't tend to see hierarchies in human relationships— only a need for mutual respect. No matter what role I am in I get my hands dirty and do the work that needs to get done.

Playful

I am playful too, and I can do that in therapy with kids. I like to sing in my therapy sessions. I might even dance with kids during the therapy sessions. Singing and dancing not only comfort, they encourage people to participate. With kids, you sing their instructions, and then they'll do something they wouldn't otherwise do. It makes it more fun for them.

Easygoing

I think I get along with all different types of people and personalities. In milieu situations, I tend to be the therapist who the most difficult clients will listen to and respond to.

Belinda is a therapist who is at once interpersonally sensitive and fearless, able to come across as both vulnerable and strong. In therapy she draws upon her characteristics to be variously confident and dignified as well as open, entertaining, and fun. Balance, timing, and judicious use of the right ingredients are words that come to mind when explaining her interpersonal approach in therapy (Box 2.6).

Stephanie's Interpersonal Challenge: Lois's Surgery

Lois, one of my adolescent clients, had a sexually transmitted disease so severe that she needed surgery to remove a mass near her genitals. She was in pain and discomfort for most of her hospitalization. Her peers on the psychiatric unit distanced themselves as she required an adapted

seat, and she had a distinct odor. The day she got back to the unit from her surgery, she was lying in bed and clearly uncomfortable and unhappy. It was the end of my work day, and generally I do not spend time with patients as they have evening programming. However, Lois was not going to groups, and I knew she was likely to be feeling low.

Interpersonal Response

I stopped by and talked to her that evening about how she was feeling. She wasn't very talkative; but when I would try to end the conversation, she would do or say something to get me to stay. Finally, she asked if I could stay and read from her book while she closed her eyes and rested.

Outcome

I started reading to her, and within minutes she was asleep. As I left the hospital I felt a deep sadness about her situation and cried for her and all that she had experienced as such a young person. I still reflect back on this powerful experience as representative of how important allowing yourself to feel for the client is to being an effective therapist.

About Stephanie

It takes a unique person to work full-time on a locked psychiatric unit with adolescents who have severe psychopathology. Each day, Stephanie works with clients who have had histories of significant trauma and who normally live in foster care or in group homes under State custody. Many of them have had repeated hospitalizations over a period of years. Because these teens often have difficulty forming stable attachments to others, it takes a significant amount of generosity of heart and spirit to pursue an approach to therapy that hinges almost entirely on effective therapeutic use of self.

Because Stephanie works in the same department as I do, I have known her for several years. She always seems a bit understated yet clearly centered. In professional relationships, Stephanie comes across as a gentle yet assertive, no-nonsense kind of person. She is known by her peers as always being reliable. In conversation, she conveys what she is thinking, and one always knows where one stands with her.

When I asked her what she thought the fundamental ingredient was to effective therapy with this population, Stephanie responded that empathy was the key to successful relationships. She described her approach as providing various forms of empathy and support within a structured framework consisting of clear boundaries, psychoeducational strategies, and graded approaches to facilitating

---

Box 2.7

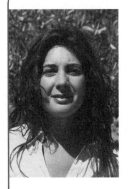

Therapist:	Stephanie McCammon, MS, OTR/L
Practice Location:	University of Illinois Medical Center, Chicago, Illinois, USA
OT Roles:	Practitioner, Adolescent Psychiatric Inpatient Unit Fieldwork Supervisor
Years Experience:	6 years
Populations Served:	Adolescents with severe psychiatric disorders

occupational engagement. In her own words, she summarized her approach as follows:

Empathetic

I feel that I have a strong sense of empathy and the ability
to make people comfortable when talking with me. I make
a concerted effort to find what is interesting or unique
about a person and find that they feel more relaxed and
accepted when asked about things that matter to them. I
also feel that I actively listen to others and know when to
just listen or be more specific in my responses. These
interpersonal skills definitely come into play in my relationships with both coworkers and clients. Our kids being
teenagers generally do not feel listened to, and this particular population is marginalized even further. I find that
providing an opportunity to talk about their thoughts/feel-
ings/ideas without judgment is useful for establishing
therapeutic rapport with my clients.

Attentive

I find myself searching for an internal motivator within the
client, something I can draw on to help me connect on a
more practical level. I have found that taking the time to
seek out even a minor or superficial interest can help to
establish some temporary rapport with hard-to-reach
clients. I also find that my ability to allow the client to
direct the activity (within boundaries) also has a positive
impact on my therapeutic rapport.

Stephanie is that special kind of therapist who
patiently stands by her clients as they experience the necessary rewards and failures that always go along with
forming relationships. Stephanie's work requires steadfast
consistency, thoughtfulness, and dedication to her young
clients. It is not often accompanied by explicit rewards,
significant amounts of progress, or expressions of gratitude. Therefore, Stephanie manages to notice and capitalize on the smaller signs of improvement in her clients. It is
clear that her clients believe she understands them, and
they know they can always rely on her as an ally and a
guide each time they visit the unit (Box 2.7).

Vardit's Interpersonal Challenge: Reading Zoe's Nonverbal Clue

I began to treat Zoe when she was $1\frac{1}{2}$ years old. She had
severe developmental delay in all areas including speech.

Box 2.8

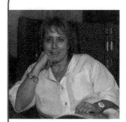

Therapist:	Vardit Kindler, OTR/L, MEd
Practice Location:	Dvora Agmon Preschool, Israel
	Elwyn, Jerusalem, Israel
	Mish'aul—The Israeli Center
	for Augmentative Communi-
	cation and Assistive Devices,
	Jerusalem, Israel
	Private Practice, Jerusalem,
	Israel
OT Roles:	Practitioner
	Assistive Device Consultant
	Bobath/NDT Instructor
	International Lecturer
Years Experience:	31 years
Populations Served:	Infants and children with a wide
	range of physical, cognitive,
	and sensory/communication
	impairments

At that point she was receiving physiotherapy, and the
parents wanted to add occupational therapy in order to
work on development of her play skills. Zoe was severely
dystonic with a lot of grimacing and involuntary movements. The constant grimacing had the effect of making
her appear unaware of things around her.

Interpersonal Response

As I carefully watched Zoe, her eyes indicated that she
was fully aware. Despite the grimacing, she was able
to focus and control her eyes in a manner that I saw
as communicative. My "reading" of her communication
with her eyes prompted me to introduce a single message
voice output communication aid (VOCA) to give her the
possibility of controlling the therapeutic process (i.e.,
requesting to continue a specific activity, in this case
swinging on the swing). I would swing with her and then
stop, and she would have to operate the VOCA, which
she did by hitting it with her foot, in order to ask me to
continue.

Outcome

Even on the first trial, Zoe burst out laughing, showing how much she enjoyed being able to control me. This was an extremely emotional moment for her mother who was present and who was in tears at witnessing her daughter's newfound ability. The building of Zoe's communication skills within play then became the focus of my therapy intervention with her, and this was carried over into the home as well. Zoe's ability to communicate changed her family's view, expectations, and acceptance of her as a child with abilities together with her disability.

About Vardit

Vardit is a seer. She recognizes and understands communication in a highly detailed and multidimensional way—so much so that she can often relate to her pediatric clients in unprecedented ways. She is logical, reserved, and highly competent in her areas of expertise. By nature a team player and a better listener than talker, Vardit is at the same time a highly effective leader in both her professional interactions and her work with her clients. She has well developed principles and opinions about what her clients need interpersonally and an exceptional understanding of children. When asked about her therapeutic skills, she emphasized the following.

Watchfulness

Being watchful involves giving enough *time* for a child to show a response. I believe that, even with lower functioning clients, the ability to respond is always there, it's just my job to identify it.

In the observation during the interaction, I wait for a response that shows attentiveness to the stimulus I provide. The stimulus can be auditory, visual, or vestibular—a song, a poem, a toy, motor activity of the child, motor activity of the therapist, sensory stimulation, among others. I look for the response by scanning for a shift or change in the child's state: The child might begin focusing visually, his eyes may show an awakening or tension. He may exhibit a different breathing rate, a change in muscle tone or tone of voice, being still, and so on.

It is very important for me to give the child the feeling of control. Quite often I see that the child can't handle being the "center" of attention. That is when I have to be extra attentive to the signs I pick up from him: body language, facial expression, a glance, a sound or tone of voice.

Playfulness

My general style of relating is very informal. I accept everyone as an equal. I look at people's strengths without being overly critical. I like interacting with people and find them interesting. I enjoy making new friends and being a part of what's going on.

My belief is that play in itself is interaction. I believe that therapy should be fun and that each child has his own strengths—and in therapy I aim to build on these strengths. It's an ingrained part of my personality, and it is what I bring into therapy. I myself enjoy playing and constantly "feel" its therapeutic benefits.

What is apparent from Vardit's work is that she has developed special intuition in her interactions with children. This higher intuition involves seeing and hearing a child's most subtle nuances—an unvarnished openness to what Vardit described as "what is seen and isn't seen, to what is heard and isn't heard." Vardit also has a unique ability to be entirely synchronized with others, especially children. She explained, "I go with the child to where he's at…. That's when he feels safe… No pressure. I show him that I don't expect him to be somewhere else where he's not." Vardit explained that "this requires accurate tuning into the child's "dance"—the motion, rhythm, gestures, posture, voice, tone, and all other forms of expression." According to Vardit, in order to be synchronized with a child, one must put oneself aside, make no preliminary assumptions whatsoever, and enter completely into the child's world. She described this as "the courage to see what there is, without giving a value." She explained: "I am inconspicuous, and my movement is minimal with a soft and quiet voice as if I'm the child's voice that is talking with the child. It is as if, for a moment, I'm the child." Vardit feels that her inconspicuous presence allows the child to access himself, and from there he feels secure to act. "If a child is at a certain cognitive level, he will probably feel curious. If not, he will feel safe—safe so he can "flower" the way he is. It all depends on accepting the child for who he is. The child learns his own boundaries (not rules that are external or confounding). Maybe this is because I know my own boundaries."

Vardit creates an environment with so much trust that the child can grow from there. This is possible only if the child is in the center in terms of being allowed to be curious, to play, or just to be. Then, in order to see, Vardit explained "it's not just patience, time, and nonanticipation, it's the accuracy of interpretation and finally the attempt to give it meaning." This is a comfortable interaction characterized by integrity, an honest dialogue that invites the child to be who he is (Box 2.8).

Kate's Interpersonal Challenge: A Disclosure from Kayla

The following scenario comes from my direct observation.

Kayla is a 12-year-old student with whom Kate has been working since the age of five. She was referred for occupational therapy for work on functional mobility, motor control, activities of daily living, physical endurance, and needs related to assistive technologies. Kayla is a spirited, energetic, and opinionated young woman who lives with her mother (a Mainer), father (Cherokee), and two younger siblings in a small rural community. Kate described Kayla as a "spiritual giant" because of her unusual level of interpersonal wisdom and maturity. Kate also disclosed that Kayla is "her own OT" because Kayla is comfortable setting her own goals and agenda for therapy. It is clear that Kate adores Kayla, enjoys working with her, and is very intense and focused when it comes to Kayla's well-being.

Box 2.9

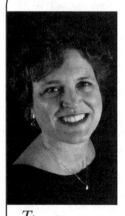

Therapist:	Kathryn (Kate) M. Loukas, MS, OTR/L, FAOTA
Practice Location:	Raymond School District, Raymond, Maine, USA
OT Roles:	Practitioner
	School consultant
	Adjunct Professor, University of New England
Years Experience:	21 years
Populations Served:	Children and adolescents with physical, cognitive, and psychiatric impairments

---

Following a vigorous swim therapy session, Kate and Kayla began spontaneously to share memories they had about their 5-year therapy relationship. Kate had a memory of saving Kayla from becoming injured by one of the unbroken horses on a horse farm. Kayla had a memory of accidentally getting pudding or yogurt on Kate's shirt when they were doing a lot of feeding work together. The sharing was heartfelt and very touching to watch. Kayla did not remember being rescued from the horse, and Kate did not remember having her shirt soiled. Following this exchange, Kayla casually said to Kate, "love ya."

Interpersonal Response

Kate: "Kayla, I've noticed you've said that to me a few times over the years… I was wondering—do you say that to everyone?"

The Outcome

Kayla: "Do I say what to everyone?"

Kate: "Love ya … you just said 'love ya' to me"

Kayla: "NO!!!! Only to three people other than my parents, my two friends, and you."

Kate: (becoming noticeably tearful) "That's so sweet, Kayla, I'm really touched that you say that to me sometimes. It means a lot to me."

Kayla: "Well I mean it."

About Kate

I first met Kate when she picked me up at my hotel in Portland, Maine to drive me to a community pool where she was going to do therapy with a longtime client. As we drove, Kate became my tour guide pointing out local sites. It struck me that she was deeply rooted there and shared the quiet dignity of the locale. Kate has a way of listening that makes you feel valued and taken very seriously. You get the feeling that you can rely on her as a trusted confidant and friend, and that she would have no problem defending your interests if she ever had to go to bat for you.

When I asked Kate to describe some of her other strengths in her own words, she disclosed the following.

Caring

I allow myself to become emotionally involved with clients, but I also know when to set boundaries around that.

Giving

Some giving is not very difficult. It just involves putting extra time and effort in for a person during the times you know they need it and it will make a difference.… Most therapists would probably not dedicate time in a summer to look for a mentor for a client or put in the kind of gas and mileage on their personal vehicles to take a client to the swimming pool she prefers.... Settings, personal resources, and workload are also factors that come into play in my ability to do that.

Direct

I believe most issues should be discussed openly and that leaving things unaddressed is burdensome to clients.

Before the observation, Kate told me she works best with people with significant physical or central nervous system dysfunction because she feels "they are stronger than [she is]." The admiration Kate has for children and their parents has an empowering effect and comes across in her interactions. When I asked her, Kayla told me that she appreciates Kate's presence in her life as a strong adult who, when necessary, can protect her, take control, and advocate on behalf of her best interests. She also appreciates Kate's softer side, which comes through in her caring, emotionality, and ability to stop and listen when she detects that Kayla has something to say. Although Kate brings many technical and interpersonal strengths to her work, the other significant strength I observed is that she is unafraid to openly discuss interpersonal issues when they become relevant to the therapy, even if discussing them might be awkward or might place her in a position of vulnerability (Box 2.9).

Krissa's Interpersonal Challenge: Annalina's Shame

Annalina is a 48-year-old Swedish woman with Down's syndrome, impaired vision, impaired speech (it is slurred), and occasional urinary incontinence. She comes to the activity center voluntarily to participate in occupations that have meaning for her and to be with others. She enjoys participating in a wide range of activities, including swimming, hiking, gardening, and many others. She also enjoys the social aspects of coming to the center. However, Annalina tends to be nervous about what other people think of her.

One day on a hiking trip Annalina lost bladder control midway through the hike. She burst into tears of shame. I had to take her down the hill back to the activity center because we did not bring a change of clothes for her. She had to walk all the way down wet and uncomfortable. On the way down, it was difficult to soothe her or help her contain her emotions. Afterward, she became apologetic, sad, and anxious for having cried. She said

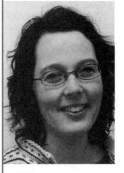

Box 2.10

Therapist:	Kristin (Krissa) Alfredsson Ågren, MScOT, RegOT
Practice Location:	Dagcenter Valla, Linköping, Sweden (community-based daytime activity center)
OT Roles:	Practitioner
Years Experience:	9 years
Populations Served:	Adults with moderate and severe learning (developmental) disabilities

things like: "You get mad? Do you?" or "Are you angry?" This eagerness to please and subsequent shame when she feels she has let others down is evident in many other situations around the center.

Interpersonal Response

During this event, I was careful to say soothing words to Annalina and to reassure her that she had not done anything wrong. I did not try to stop her from crying or from expressing herself. I remained a supportive witness to her experience and made sure she was clean, dry, and comfortable as soon as we got back to the center.

Outcome

Over time, I have learned that if Annalina becomes ashamed, she will suddenly burst into tears. I believe it has something to do with her self-esteem and with her past life. She has spent many years interacting with staff in various institutions. I suspect that she has been shamed in the past for some of the behaviors related to her impairment (e.g., incontinence, dropping something) or that she has been ignored and rejected a great deal. Now, whenever Annalina cries I make it a point to tell her that it is OK to cry and to reassure her that I am not angry with her. She is slowly beginning to make choices of her own, rather than trying to please staff and make the choices she thinks we want her to make. I think she is beginning to learn that my appreciation of her as a person is not related to her choices and behaviors and that she has the right to make choices of her own and also to change her mind.

About Krissa

I spent several hours observing Krissa working with her clients at the activity center in Linköping. Krissa is a quiet woman but persistent in pursuing her convictions. In the center, she constantly strives to improve the treatment milieu for her clients and their access to resources. She described this as follows: "Sometimes the organization around you is rigid and difficult to change,... I have found that I really need to work with organizations in a slow, patient, but persistent way on behalf of our clients." Krissa clearly is not willing to accept "no" for an answer if she believes a change is needed to improve the lives of her clients. When I asked her to describe some of her strengths, she offered the following.

Patient

I have patience, in many aspects. Working with clients with learning disabilities is a lifelong work. You can never lose hope in them and their ability to gain new experiences.

Collaborative

I work together with my clients. I try to discuss with other staff about the importance of choice and of working with clients' volition.

Clearly, Krissa is always respectful and patient with her clients; but more than this, she considers her clients coworkers within a working setting, which makes her therapeutic style extremely empowering. She continually reinforces their sense of dignity and self-respect by encouraging them to function as autonomously as possible (Box 2.10).

Carmen's Interpersonal Challenge: Knowing When to Self-Disclose

Mario is a man in his late forties with a diagnosis of schizophrenia. He lives alone in a low-income neighborhood in Santiago, Chile. He independently sought out occupational therapy treatment with me at our community-

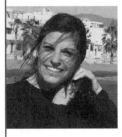

Box 2.11

Therapist:	Carmen-Gloria de Las Heras, MS, OTR/L
Practice Location:	Reencuentros, Santiago, Chile
OT Roles:	Director of Reencuentros, a community-based outpatient and residential facility for individuals with severe mental illness
	Private Practitioner
Years Experience:	25 years
Populations Served:	Adolescents and Adults with Severe Mental Illness

based occupational therapy program, Reencuentros, after his psychiatrist told him about us. Since then I have been seeing him intermittently for nearly 10 years. When he first came for treatment, Mario had a very difficult time trusting others. Although he had many capacities and strengths, he could not talk about his concerns openly. I tried to encourage him to follow a structure in which he would tell me what was wrong first and then focus on setting goals and achieving them through activity. However, his difficulties with trust continued to prevent him from opening up.

Interpersonal Response

Because Mario's issues with trust were not getting any better over time, I decided to tell him that I had depression and that I was in treatment just like him. When I told him, he began to ask me questions, which I answered with honesty. I normalized the situation to the greatest extent possible. I was calm, and told my story as part of my life without any exaggeration. I described the situations that happened to me that were similar to his feelings and the ways I managed them.

Outcome

As I answered his questions, I could see that he began to relax immediately. I felt it was necessary for him to believe in someone who understood his pain. After that time, he became more confident, and he knew he could tell me about his moments of anxiety or about the content of his obsessive thinking. Now, it is easier for him to begin the sessions and to follow the structure that I had originally desired. He tells me what is wrong first, he receives and trusts my validation, and then we focus on his goals and achievements.

About Carmen

When I first met Carmen, she rushed up to give me a warm hug and a big kiss. In addition to being very open with her affection, Carmen is an utterly honest, transparent, and emotional individual. This comes across very clearly in her work with clients.

When I asked her to describe her interpersonal style in therapy, Carmen emphasized the following characteristics.

Spontaneous

In the institutions in which I worked in the past, people had a tendency to "put the coat on" [referring to the white coat that helps establish authority and a professional distance from patients]. Instead, my theme is "take the coat off." You've got to be real with people. If I think a patient or the parent of a patient needs it, I show intense emotion with that person. I do not try to restrain myself. I show whatever reaction I have to that person at that time. I flow easily inside and outside therapy. I keep my way of being, I am spontaneous and generous. I am firm when I have to be. I adjust my style according to the needs of others, but in the end I keep my personality. I am myself with clients as I am with everyone else.

Humble

I have the humility to accept feedback and not personalize others' judgment of me.

Carmen's style is uniquely courageous in that she believes in having unbridled and highly honest interactions with those with whom she works. It is clear from observing her work that she has a high regard for her clients' dignity, and she is keen on recognizing anyone's needs for love and affection. These ingredients allow individuals, who would otherwise be emotionally trapped and unmotivated to interact, to trust Carmen and open themselves to the process of participating in occupational therapy (Box 2.11).

Jane's Interpersonal Challenge: Resolving Power Struggles with Cecile

Cecile is a woman in her forties who is divorced and lives alone. In the past, Cecile worked in a department store but was fired from her job, which she describes as one of many significant losses in her life. Cecile was referred for occupational therapy during a stay at an inpatient psychiatric unit. Her diagnosis has been difficult to determine,

---

Box 2.12

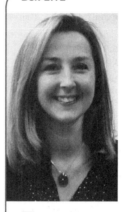

Therapist:	Jane Melton, MSc (Advanced OT), DIPCOT (UK)
Practice Location:	Gloucestershire Partnership National Health Service Trust Gloucestershire England, UK
OT Roles:	Consultant Occupational Therapy Practitioner
	Honorary Lecturer in occupational therapy at the University of the West of England, Bristol
	Head Research Practitioner for the GPT partnership with the UK Centre for Outcomes Research and Education
	Training consultant for Harrison's Associates
Years Experience:	20 years
Populations Served:	Adults with learning disabilities (developmental disorders) and adults with severe mental illness

but Cecile has a long history of depression and anxiety with features of both borderline and narcissistic personality disorder.

Before she was referred to occupational therapy, Cecile had been using the psychiatric inpatient unit repeatedly during the previous 3 years. Cecile's behavior was also characterized by a tendency to lose favor with her health care workers. She often made strong and repeated demands for support and assistance but then became dismissive of any attempts to meet these demands. At times she has been known to become rejecting or subtly hostile toward care workers. Her nonverbal messages matched her verbal communication, which conveyed that she was defensive, hopeless, or angry. She often twisted facts about her care and distorted or ignored attempts at support from family, friends, and caregivers. Her communication was redundant with statements such as, "I cannot carry on like this" or "You are not helping me" or "This is not making me better." In therapy, Cecile lacked curiosity and explored new environments only hesitantly. Though she was a highly capable person, she did not take pride in any current achievement or seek out challenges. She was reluctant to show preferences, engage with others, complete activity, sustain focus, or show that any activity was significant to her. This was particularly true when she was aware that staff were observing her but were not prompting, instructing, or encouraging her. Because of her attitude and behaviors, many health care workers have become weary of providing support, and some have refused to work with her.

Interpersonal Response

Quickly I realized that issues of power were dominating our interactions. Cecile would say something that indicated a desire to change (e.g., "I want to be myself again"), and shortly thereafter she would tell me my approach was not working. Because this dynamic occurred repeatedly despite my many efforts to change my approach or incorporate her feedback, I interpreted this pattern's true meaning as, "I can say your intervention is not making me better and therefore I am powerful over you, even though I tell you that I want to change." This played out in other ways. For example, we once shared a joke when visiting a local café, and Cecile smiled. Because she rarely smiled, I pointed out that I enjoyed seeing her smile. She immediately returned to a mask-like expression. On another occasion I was gently questioning Cecile about her interests and achievements, and she quickly became tearful and insisted we stop the conversation.

One of the central tasks of our work together involved understanding this power dynamic as an indication of Cecile's need for control. I then had to work with this dynamic to maximize Cecile's feelings of control so she could develop other aspects of volition. On some occasions, this meant occasionally giving in to the dynamic and sometimes becoming vulnerable in her eyes. For example, I might use some self-disclosure about how her behavior affects me. I did this with the hope of stimulating her self-reflection about our conversation and raising her awareness of how her use of power in this way affects other people.

On other occasions, I have worked with the power dynamic by standing my ground and providing a rationale for why my approach might assist her. I often validate Cecile's desire for me to see that she is deeply troubled, but I also remind her that if and when she is ready to build strength I will be there to assist her. On some occasions, we have also agreed to take short, planned breaks from our work together. The reason for these breaks is to give her space from the therapy process, to allow her time to reflect upon the responsibility that she holds within the therapy relationship, and to enable me to reform with ideas and energy to maintain the relationship. Aside from working with the power dynamic in these ways, an overarching aspect of my approach has been to not take any of Cecile's behaviors or comments personally.

Outcome

Cecile was discharged after an 8-month stay in the hospital. A structured and sophisticated support network was designed and implemented including regular occupational therapy appointments. Activities were set up and undertaken with the aim of engaging Cecile in making choices, taking control over her activities, regaining interest in past activities, and formulating a pattern within her occupations. Cecile's motivation for doing did not develop any further than what she needed to maintain independent functioning. Importantly, however, it was maintained at the same level; and now, many months since her last hospitalization, Cecile has not yet felt the need to return to the hospital.

About Jane

I met Jane Melton in her native Glouchester in the West of England. Her tone of voice, posture, dress, and use of language all reflect a sense of propriety, politeness, and dignity often characteristic of British culture. She has an endearing ability to laugh at herself and find humor in the irony of challenging situations. Yet Jane never comes across as superficial, distancing, or intimidating. To the contrary, she has a way of making one feel accepted and respected. I asked Jane to describe her interpersonal strong points as she perceived them. Among others, she identified the following.

Reliable

I have a natural optimistic belief in people and compassion and empathy for my clients. Personally, I have qualities of good humor, loyalty and reliability. In my work, I demonstrate high levels of self-management and personal integrity.

Gentle

I am honest, tactful, resilient, but gentle in my approach. By gently challenging both clients and my colleagues and by encouraging reflective thinking, I think in a nonthreatening way I am able to invite people to be reflective and analytical when considering complex cases and dilemmas.

Jane is a circumspect therapist who has mastered the delicate art of walking on eggshells without breaking them. Her judgment about what people need, particularly when they are feeling vulnerable or threatened, is precise and a quality that any therapist would admire. The story above illustrates that Jane's level of sophistication in managing more difficult interpersonal issues within therapeutic relationships is highly developed. She emanates kindness, grace, and gentleness (Box 2.12).

Summary

The variety of interpersonal challenges described in this chapter illustrate how varied are the circumstances that require a careful therapeutic use of self. Moreover, the responses to these challenges illustrate the wide range of behaviors that make up therapeutic use of self. Some are instantaneous, whereas others unfold over a long period. They may involve a variety of empathic, guiding, humorous, confronting, informing, revealing, collaborating, empowering, limiting, questioning and other behaviors. In each case, the therapists understood what was needed and had the self-awareness and self-control to enact it.

In this chapter, I also highlighted some of the traits that therapists reported as characterizing their approach to therapy.[3] They are intended simply as self-descriptions to illustrate the range of ways that therapists think about their own therapeutic use of self. I have labeled these traits in this chapter and in the exercises in the Activities section, which you are encouraged to complete once you have read the chapter.

Although some of the therapists' traits overlap, each of the therapists discussed in this chapter has a distinctive personality. Some are quite different than others. This illustrates an important fact that different therapists bring quite different innate abilities, strengths, and weaknesses to the therapy process. How, then, can therapists with such different personalities and abilities all manage to be excellent interpersonal therapists? There are many answers, but I believe the essential one is that all of these therapists are clearly aware of their own personality and style of doing therapy. They have carefully chosen practice situations in which they can be highly effective. Many of these therapists may likely not thrive in all the situations or with the populations that others handle with ease. They have carefully chosen their own right niche. Moreover, each therapist has developed ways of using his or her innate strengths in the most advantageous way in the therapy situation. In the end, what characterizes all these therapists is that their use of self is intentional. Consequently, if there is one overarching answer to the question that began this chapter it is the following: One factor that makes a good therapist is the ***intentional use of self***.

---

[3]The labels I have given therapist's traits are intended only to be descriptive or summative. They are not proposed as a taxonomy for two reasons. First, they are not entirely mutually exclusive categories. Second, no attempt has been made here to arrive at an exhaustive list of therapeutic traits.

ACTIVITIES FOR LEARNING AND REFLECTION

In this chapter we learned about the unique combinations of interpersonal characteristics, or traits, that each of the therapists drew upon in practice. Not every one of these traits comes naturally or can work for everyone. You can achieve interpersonal excellence only within the context of your personality. As we will see later in the book, you can learn a range of strategies and styles of doing therapy—but only within the constraints of your natural abilities and those that you clearly work hard to foster and develop.

This section contains two exercises designed to encourage thinking about your current interpersonal traits and to allow for creativity in developing goals for broadening your capacity to relate to a wider range of people.

EXERCISE 2.1

Identifying Your Interpersonal Traits

Chapter 2 identifies a number of traits that characterize interpersonally effective occupational therapists. As the chapter indicates, no single person possesses all of these traits. Moreover, they are not all required for interpersonal effectiveness in therapy. What is important is to develop an awareness of your own unique profile.

This exercise is designed to help you think about and identify:

• Your own interpersonal strengths (what comes naturally to you and that you tend to do often)
• Your interpersonal abilities (things you can do but that take a bit more awareness or effort)
• Your interpersonal challenges (things that are more difficult for you, that do not come naturally)

As we will see later in the book, you can learn a range of strategies and styles of doing therapy—but only within the constraints of your natural interpersonal tendencies, abilities, and challenges. This exercise should help you bring into greater awareness what your interpersonal tendencies, abilities, and challenges are.

In the form below the interpersonal traits that were identified in the chapter are listed along with brief suggested definitions. You should examine each one and decide whether it is an interpersonal strength, an ability, or a challenge for you. To honestly reflect on these traits, you should try to think of at least one recent situation that illustrates whether this trait is one of your strengths, abilities, or challenges. You might also find it helpful to put in your own words how you think your characterization is true (for example, what is it about yourself that makes this a strength, ability, or challenge).

My Interpersonal Traits					
Trait	**Definition**	**Strength**	**Ability**	**Challenge**	**Personal Example: Is this a situation where the trait came naturally? Did it require some effort on my part? Did it require tremendous effort? How frequently and consistently am I reminded of this trait? Do others notice this about me?**
Trustworthy	Can be counted on, consistent and reliable in interactions, keep commitments				
Motivating	Challenge, support, encourage others, instill hope, cheer and applaud				
Empowering	Support others to be more aware of their personal strengths, give clients power and control				
Empathetic	Recognize and strive to understand others' emotions and perceptions without judgment				
Energetic	Put forth and convey energy/enthusiasm				
Calm	Quiet presence, neutral, interpersonally centered, and composed				
Assertive	Give directions clearly, explain my perspective, take a stand on issues, provide others with feedback				
Positive	Optimistic view of other people, tendency to see strengths and positives over weaknesses				
Attentive	Notice things about others' behaviors, thoughts, and feelings				
Friendly	Outgoing, sociable, seek out contact, easy to relate to				
Flexible	Adaptable to different kinds of people, emotions, and interpersonal situations				

Trait	Definition	Strength	Ability	Challenge	Personal Example: Is this a situation where the trait came naturally? Did it require some effort on my part? Did it require tremendous effort? How frequently and consistently am I reminded of this trait? Do others notice this about me?
Logical	Help others make sense of things, reasonable, skilled at clearly identifying problems and solutions				
Firm	Able to state expectations, set limits, and have personal boundaries				
Collaborative	Readily work with others, share power/ responsibility, provide choice, educate clients				
Humorous	Find humor, funny, amusing, entertaining, or witty				
Persuasive	Convincing, persistent, influential, believable, credible				
Open	Approachable, hear, accept and share ideas, experiences, worldviews, and emotions				
Respectful	Polite, courteous, appropriately deferential, aware of others' rights, admire others' capacities				
Playful	Fun loving, light-hearted, child-like, unrestrained, mischievous				
Easygoing	Good-natured, get along with different personalities, unbothered by small dilemmas				
Caring	Sensitive, share in people's life stories, can be vulnerable with clients, can take emotional risks				
Giving	Do things for others, share or provide resources, exceed average expectations for relationships or service provision				

(table continued on page 42)

My Interpersonal Traits (continued)					
Trait	**Definition**	**Strength**	**Ability**	**Challenge**	**Personal Example: Is this a situation where the trait came naturally? Did it require some effort on my part? Did it require tremendous effort? How frequently and consistently am I reminded of this trait? Do others notice this about me?**
Direct	Openly discuss what's on my mind with others				
Patient	Wait for things to happen in therapy, unbothered by slower pacing of therapy, tolerate others' behaviors and emotions				
Spontaneous	Actively share and react to clients in the moment				
Humble	Able to admit mistakes, receive feedback gracefully, aware of limitations				
Loyal	Maintain relation- ships, defend primary others' best interests, keep confidences, con- sistent in relating				
Gentle	Mild, tactful, nonthreatening, tender, kind				
Watchful	Being inconspicuous and entering into others' worlds in order to notice nuances of expression and behavior				

After completing the Interpersonal Traits form, you might find it useful to record your self-ratings on the form below, My Interpersonal Profile, so you can easily see your own profile.

My Interpersonal Profile														
Trustworthy	**Motivating**	**Empowering**	**Empathetic**	**Energetic**	**Calm**	**Assertive**	**Positive**	**Attentive**	**Friendly**	**Flexible**	**Logical**	**Firm**	**Collaborative**	**Humorous**
S	S	S	S	S	S	S	S	S	S	S	S	S	S	S
A	A	A	A	A	A	A	A	A	A	A	A	A	A	A
C	C	C	C	C	C	C	C	C	C	C	C	C	C	C
My Desired Interpersonal Profile														

My Interpersonal Profile														
Persuasive	**Open**	**Respectful**	**Playful**	**Easygoing**	**Caring**	**Giving**	**Direct**	**Patient**	**Spontaneous**	**Humble**	**Loyal**	**Gentle**	**Watchful**
S	S	S	S	S	S	S	S	S	S	S	S	S	S
A	A	A	A	A	A	A	A	A	A	A	A	A	A
C	C	C	C	C	C	C	C	C	C	C	C	C	C
My Desired Interpersonal Profile														

S, strength; A, ability; C, challenge

These interpersonal traits will reflect some tendencies that may have been innate in your personality from childhood. Others may be ways of interacting you learned along the way through various experiences. As you review your profile, consider whether any of your self-ratings are different from what you would like them to be. If they are, you can write in the last row what you would like that trait to become for you (e.g., an ability or a strength). For example, if something is a challenge and you prefer that it would be an ability or a strength, mark the final row corresponding to that trait with an "A" or an "S." Like all other traits, those you plan to develop more must be practiced to become a personal trait. One way to help ensure that you practice them is to identify some short-term goals. For example, let us say you rated the item, "Open" as a challenge, and you would like it to become an ability. You might begin by considering some situations in which you would like to be more open in your interactions. Think about what you could say or do more of in those situations and then write down your plan in Exercise 2.2.

EXERCISE 2.2

Goals for Trait Development

My long-term goal: to be more:

_____

The situations in which I would most prefer to enact this trait:

_____

My short-term goal (tangible steps) is to:

_____

Remember to consider what exactly you will do, when, how frequently, with whom, and with what result.

CHAPTER 3

A MODEL OF THE INTENTIONAL RELATIONSHIP

Therapeutic use of self involves a highly personal, individualized, subjective decision-making process. For some therapists, the process is driven by emotional reactions to clients and a perceived reliance on an innate or nurtured intuitive capacity. Others perceive the process as largely rational and grounded in the disciplined application of a set of interpersonal guidelines. Irrespective of such viewpoints, therapeutic use of self is, in large part, a product of the extent to which one possesses a knowledge base and interpersonal skills that can be applied thoughtfully to common interpersonal events in practice. Accordingly, therapeutic use of self is an occupational therapy skill that must be developed, reinforced, monitored, and refined.

This chapter presents a model that conceptualizes the processes involved in therapeutic use of self. The rationale, conceptual background, and underlying principles of this model are presented. The model explains how components of the client–therapist relationship interact and can be enhanced in the face of everyday challenges to that relationship. Finally, a set of principles that guide the implementation of this model in practice are outlined.

> The central question that a conceptualization of the therapeutic relationship in occupational therapy must answer is this: How can one's therapeutic use of self be utilized specifically to promote occupational engagement and promote positive therapy outcomes?

Explaining the Therapeutic Relationship: Need for a Conceptual Practice Model

As noted in Chapter 1, there has been discussion of the therapeutic relationship throughout occupational therapy's history. Although numerous recommendations have been made regarding the requisite training, characteristics, feelings, and behaviors necessary for effective interpersonal practice in occupational therapy, they have not been integrated into a coherent explanation of the therapeutic relationship. Moreover, there are few details about how the therapeutic relationship should be approached and managed in light of the field's central focus on the client's engagement in occupation. Educators, supervisors, students, and staff may benefit from a vocabulary with which to discuss and describe the interpersonal phenomena that have an ongoing impact on everyday practice.

The central question that a conceptualization of the therapeutic relationship in occupational therapy must answer is: how can one's therapeutic use of self be utilized specifically to promote occupational engagement and promote positive therapy outcomes?

The intentional relationship model is intended as a conceptual practice model (Kielhofner, 2004). It was developed to explain the therapeutic use of self in occupational therapy and how that relationship can facilitate or hinder a client's occupational engagement. The model is designed to guide interpersonal reasoning for addressing dilemmas and challenges to the therapeutic relationship that arise in everyday practice. Finally, the model illustrates how best to develop relationships that embrace the fundamental values and ethics of occupational therapy practice.

Conceptual Background for the Model: How Therapeutic Use of Self in Occupational Therapy Differs from Psychotherapy

Many of the concepts for the intentional relationship model have their origins in theory underlying psychotherapy. However, the model recognizes a fundamental difference between occupational therapy and traditional psychotherapy. Figure 3.1 portrays the traditional psychotherapy process. As it shows, interpersonal relating between client and therapist is the central focus. Moreover, interpersonal communication is typically the only activity that occurs during psychotherapy.

In occupational therapy, particularly when conducted outside of mental health, the client–therapist relationship should not pretend to emulate the intensity, duration, and complexity of a traditional psychotherapy relationship. By contrast, the central focus of occupational therapy is occupational engagement. The unique role that the therapeutic relationship plays in occupational therapy is diagrammed in Figure 3.2. As shown, the occupational therapist employs a number of therapeutic strategies usually rooted in existing models of practice to facilitate the client's engagement in occupation. Depending on the occupational needs, capacities, and diagnosis of the client, any number of occupational therapy practice models might be employed alone or in combination to promote occupational engagement. However, this main task of promoting occupational engagement through employing the specific methods and strategies of occupational therapy does not exist in isolation of a larger process of relating that occurs between client and therapist.

The *intentional relationship model* explains the relationship between client and therapist that is part of the overall process of occupational therapy. Accordingly, the model is intended to complement existing occupational therapy conceptual practice models rather than to replace any single model. It explains the detailed and overarching aspects of the client–therapist relationship, an aspect of occupational therapy not addressed thoroughly or extensively by other conceptual practice models. Figure 3.3 shows how the intentional relationship is designed to supplement the use of other occupational therapy conceptual practice models. As

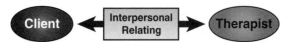

FIGURE 3.1 Client–therapist relationship in traditional psychotherapy

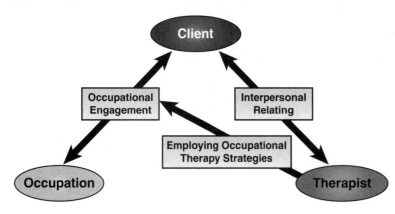

FIGURE 3.2 Unique relationship between client, therapist, and occupation in occupational therapy

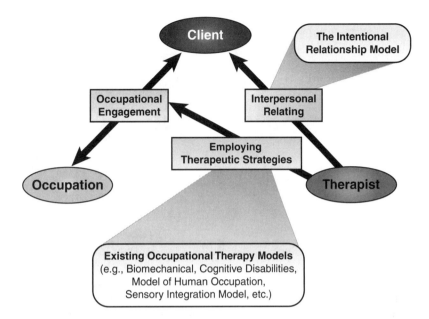

FIGURE 3.3 Intentional relationship model as a complement to existing occupational therapy models

shown, the intentional relationship model should complement the usual concepts and strategies of occupational therapy that are directly aimed at facilitating occupational engagement.

The model's utility for occupational therapy lies in addressing the otherwise unarticulated aspects of the interpersonal relationship that occur during the therapy process and that influence both occupational engagement and therapy outcomes. The next section defines the elements of this model and provides an explanation of how the elements interact to optimize the circumstances for a successful client–therapist relationship in occupational therapy.

To reiterate, the intentional relationship model is not a free-standing model of practice for occupational therapy. If a therapist utilized only this model, the essential work of occupational therapy would not occur. Instead, the model was designed to fill a gap in our practical knowledge about how to manage the interpersonal aspects of therapy, particularly the more challenging ones. This

model should complement the field's existing methods and models by making the process of establishing a successful relationship with clients easier, clearer, and more straightforward.

Elements of the Intentional Relationship Model

The intentional relationship model (IRM) views the therapeutic relationship as being comprised of four central elements.

1. The client
2. The interpersonal events that occur during therapy
3. The therapist
4. The occupation

A summary diagram of the model is presented in Figure 3.4. The model explains the requirements for a functional client–therapist relationship, and it incorporates guidelines for responding to common interpersonal events

> The intentional relationship model is intended to complement existing occupational therapy conceptual practice models rather than to replace any single model.

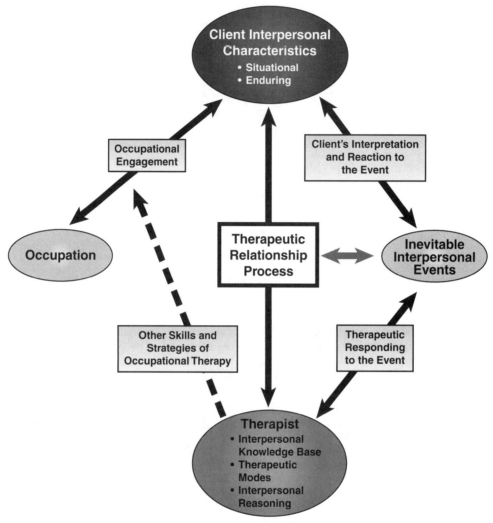

FIGURE 3.4 Model of the intentional relationship in occupational therapy

that frequently occur during therapy. The relevant aspects of each element of the model and their relations with one another are described in the following section.

The Client

According to the IRM, the client is the focal point. It is the therapist's responsibility to work to develop a positive relationship with the client and to respond appropriately when interpersonal events occur. To develop this relationship and respond appropriately to the client, a therapist must work to understand the client from an interpersonal

perspective. This involves getting to know the client's interpersonal characteristics. According to IRM, a client's interpersonal characteristics can be understood according to two dimensions.

• Situational characteristics
• Enduring characteristics

Situational characteristics are interpersonal characteristics that are generally inconsistent with how a client typically and consistently behaves when interacting with others. Instead, they reflect a client's acute emotional reaction to a specific situation. Typically, a client's situational characteristics attract our attention when that client is encountering a situation that is somehow painful, frustrating, or stressful. For most of us, stressful situations result in some negative emotional state that makes it temporarily difficult for us to engage in occupations as planned. Thus, a client's situational characteristics are likely to surface when they interfere with the client's ability to engage in the activities of therapy as planned.

A client's situational characteristics are most likely to reveal themselves in therapy when the client is facing a situation where some immediate aspect of the impairment and/or the environment is experienced as stressful. Impairments, particularly when they are new or when there is a medical crisis or exacerbation in severity that disrupts one's usual relationship with the environment, often cause people to experience stress. Therapists are encouraged to assume, on some level, that a client's impairment situation and/or the client's interaction with an unaccommodating or difficult environment causes the client to be more vulnerable to experiencing a variety of emotional reactions, many of which may be perceived as negative or at least atypical for that individual. For example, feelings of loss are common among newly disabled individuals, and they may manifest in terms of sadness, irritability, anxiety, insecurity, or anger. A therapist's interpersonal behavior, if perceived as insensitive, judgmental, or uncaring, may also serve as a source of stress and cause the client to interact in a manner that is generally inconsistent with his or her personality. It is important for new therapists to recognize that these and other acute emotional reactions are normative. In fact, they are "givens" in many health care situations. They bear no reflection on the client's character or personality. However, they do have the potential to play out within the therapy relationship, and the way in which a therapist chooses to respond to them is often vital to the future of that relationship (Fig. 3.5).

By contrast, ***enduring characteristics*** are more stable and consistent aspects of the client's interpersonal behavior. They are not necessarily related to the situation of acquiring an impairment or to the environment's reaction or lack of accommodation to that impairment. Instead, they comprise an interpersonal profile that is idiosyncratic to the client. Enduring interpersonal characteristics include such things as a client's preferred style of communicating, capacity for trust, need for control, general orien-

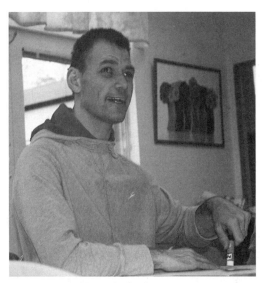

FIGURE 3.5 The client is the focal point

tation to relating, and usual way of responding to change, challenge, or frustration.

Because they coexist in each client, situational and enduring characteristics are mutually informative. Behavior that reflects one's acute emotional reaction to a stressful event may temporarily attenuate, alter, or intensify one's interpersonal behavior in what are usually more stable categories. For example, a client who normally responds to a challenging situation adaptively may become irritated when the therapist recommends a more challenging activity if, earlier in that day, the client underwent a painful biopsy and then discovered she did not have enough money to cover the insurance co-pay fees upon leaving the physician's office. The rationale for distinguishing the two categories of interpersonal characteristics is to help inform therapists' understanding of the client in stressful and nonstressful situations so therapeutic responses can be appropriately tailored and modulated. Both situational and enduring client characteristics and how to assess them are described in more detail in Chapter 5.

Interpersonal Events of Therapy

An ***interpersonal event*** is a naturally occurring communication, reaction, process, task, or general circumstance that occurs during therapy and that has the potential to detract from or strengthen the therapeutic relationship. During therapy, these events may be precipitated by the following circumstances.

- Client resistance (e.g., a client refuses or feels unable to participate in some activity)
- Therapist behavior (e.g., the therapist asks a question that the client perceives as intrusive or emotionally difficult to face)
- Client display of strong emotions in therapy (e.g., an elderly client begins crying during transfer training or a child client runs up to the therapist and hugs her in the midst of sensory motor activity)
- A difficult circumstance of therapy (e.g., a client is embarrassed because of losing bladder control or becomes frustrated or fearful in the midst of an activity)
- A rift or conflict between client and therapist (e.g., the client is offended by a comment made by the therapist)
- Differences concerning the aim of therapy (e.g., a client insists on a goal that the therapist believes is not attainable, or the therapist recommends a goal that the client rejects)
- Client requests that test the boundaries or limits of the therapeutic relationship (e.g., the client invites the therapist to attend her wedding)

These situations, of course, are only a few of the myriad possible interpersonal events that occur during the course of occupational therapy (Fig. 3.6).

When interpersonal events of therapy occur, their interpretation by the client is a product of the client's unique set of interpersonal characteristics. Sometimes the event has a significant effect on the client, whereas at other times a client is unaffected or minimally affected. When such events occur, what is important is that the therapist be aware that the event has occurred and take responsibility for responding appropriately.

Interpersonal events are:

- Inevitable during the course of therapy
- Ripe with both threat and opportunity

Interpersonal events are part of the constant give and take that occurs during a therapy process. They are distinguished from other events or processes in that they are charged with the potential for an emotional response either when they occur or later upon reflection. Consequently, if they are ignored or responded to less than optimally, these events can threaten both the therapeutic relationship and the client's occupational engagement. When optimally responded to, the events can provide opportunities for positive client learning or change and for solidifying the therapeutic relationship. Chapter 2 presented a series of therapists' stories about particularly challenging moments of therapy. Each was an example of a significant interpersonal event. Chapter 6 describes and gives examples of interpersonal events that have been found from our research to occur with a high level of frequency in occupational therapy. Because they are unavoidable in any therapeutic interaction, one of the primary tasks of a therapist practicing according to the intentional relationship model is to respond to these inevitable events

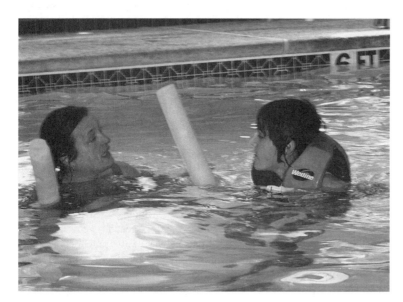

FIGURE 3.6 Kathryn Loukas and a client pause to discuss a difficult circumstance during therapy

in a way that leads to repair and strengthening of the therapeutic relationship.

The Therapist

Within the IRM, the therapist is responsible for making every reasonable effort to make the relationship work. Specifically, the therapist is responsible for bringing three main interpersonal capacities into the relationship.

• An interpersonal skill base
• Therapeutic modes (or interpersonal styles)
• Capacity for interpersonal reasoning

This section provides a brief description of each of these interpersonal capacities. The first capacity involves development and application of a wide-ranging interpersonal knowledge base.

The therapist's *interpersonal skill base* is comprised of a continuum of skills that are judiciously applied by the therapist to build a functional working relationship with the client. The perspective of the model is that, depending on the unique experiences, knowledge, and innate capacities of the therapist, some of these skills come naturally whereas others require significant effort and practice to develop.

These interpersonal skills are summarized in terms of nine categories.

• Therapeutic communication
• Interviewing skills and strategic questioning
• Establishing relationships with clients
• Families, social systems, and groups
• Working effectively with supervisors, employers, and other professionals
• Understanding and managing difficult interpersonal behavior
• Empathic breaks and conflicts
• Professional behavior, values, and ethics
• Therapist self-care and professional development

The first category, therapeutic communication, involves activities such as verbal and nonverbal communication skills, therapeutic listening, assertiveness, providing clients with direction and feedback, and seeking and responding to client feedback. Interviewing skills comprise another skill set that involves being watchful and intentional about the way in which one approaches the process of asking a client questions. Strategic questioning is a specific approach to questioning borne out of cognitive psychology (e.g., Beck, 1995). It involves asking questions

in a way that guides the respondent to think more broadly or differently. Establishing relationships with clients includes rapport building, matching your therapeutic style to the interpersonal demands of the client, managing a client's strong emotion, judicious use of touch, and cultural competence.

Because many clients have caregivers, family members, or other individuals with whom they have regular contact, understanding and working with families, social systems, and groups is an essential aspect of occupational therapy practice. It includes using the guiding principles of IRM in combination with prominent systems theories to gain the collaboration of partners, parents, other family, and friends to serve the goals of therapy. It also involves understanding the structure, process, and interpersonal dynamics of group therapy.

Another fundamental skill involves knowing how to work collaboratively with supervisors, employers, and other professionals. It involves knowing how to communicate with other professionals about clients both in the presence and in the absence of those clients. Additionally, it requires understanding the power dynamics and value systems that underlie supervisor/student and employer/employee relationships. Understanding and managing clients' difficult behavior is another category of necessary interpersonal skills required in many practice situations. It involves knowing how to respond effectively to behaviors that involve manipulation, excessive dependence, symptom focusing, resistance, emotional disengagement, denial, difficulty with rapport and trust, and hostility. Responding effectively helps limit the extent to which this behavior disrupts the goals and processes of therapy.

Knowing how to resolve conflicts and empathic breaks (or rifts in understanding between client and therapist) is another fundamental skill set that can salvage a failing relationship or repair minor threats to an otherwise functional relationship. Professional behavior and ethics encompass knowledge of how your own values are consistent or inconsistent with the occupational therapy core values, ethical behavior and decision making, behavioral self-awareness around clients, being reliable and dependable, upholding confidentiality, and setting and managing professional boundaries. Therapist self-care incorporates knowing and managing your own emotional reactions to clients and being accountable to those reactions, a general capacity for self-reflection, an ability to manage your personal life and seek support when necessary, and the capacity to maintain perspective regarding client outcomes. More information about all of these skills, which comprise

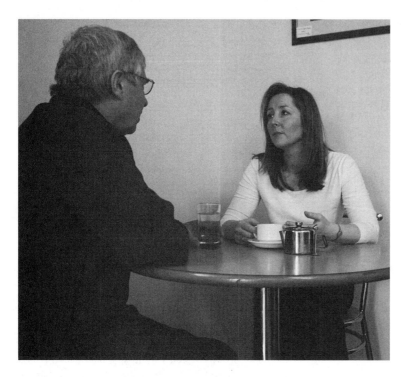

FIGURE 3.7 Therapists such as Jane Melton assume responsibility for developing a wide range of interpersonal skills to be used in therapy

a therapist's interpersonal skill base, is provided in Chapters 8 through 16 (Fig. 3.7).

The second interpersonal capacity that a therapist brings to the client–therapist relationship is her or his primary therapeutic mode or modes. A *therapeutic mode* is a specific way of relating to a client. The IRM identifies six therapeutic modes: advocating, collaborating, empathizing, encouraging, instructing, and problem-solving. A brief synopsis of each mode and examples of how Jane Melton used each mode in practice, are presented in Table 3.1.

They are defined and elaborated in more detail in Chapter 4.

Therapists naturally use therapeutic modes that are consistent with their fundamental personality characteristics. For example, a therapist who tends to be more of a listener than a talker and believes in the importance of understanding another person's perspective before making a suggestion would likely utilize empathizing as a primary therapeutic mode in therapy. Therapists vary widely in terms of the range and flexibility with which they use modes in relating to clients. Some therapists relate to clients in one or two primary ways, whereas others draw upon multiple therapeutic modes depending on the interpersonal characteristics of the client and the situation at

hand. One of the goals in using the IRM is to become increasingly comfortable utilizing any of the six modes flexibly and interchangeably depending on the client's needs. A therapeutic mode or set of modes define therapist's general *interpersonal style* when interacting with a client. Therapists able to utilize all six of the modes flexibly and comfortably and to match those modes to the client and the situation are described as having a *multimodal* interpersonal style.

According to the IRM, a therapist's choice and application of a particular therapeutic mode or set of modes should depend largely on the enduring interpersonal characteristics of the client. In addition, certain events or interpersonal events in therapy may call for a mode shift. A *mode shift* is a conscious change in one's way of relating to a client. Mode shifts are frequently required in response to interpersonal events in therapy. For example, if a client perceives a therapist's attempts at problem-solving to be insensitive or off the mark, a therapist would be wise to switch from the problem-solving mode to an empathizing mode so he or she can better understand the client's reaction and the root of the dilemma. An interpersonal reasoning process, described in the following paragraph, can be utilized to guide the therapist in deciding when a mode

Table 3.1 **Brief Definitions of Therapeutic Modes and Practice Examples from Jane Melton**

Mode	Definition	Example
Advocating	Ensuring that the client's rights are enforced and resources are secured. May require the therapist to serve as a mediator, facilitator, negotiator, enforcer, or other type of advocate with external persons and agencies.	Lobbying to secure adequate resources for the provision of ongoing support and environmental adaptation. This enabled a man with learning disabilities to participate safely in self-care and domestic activities in his own home environment.
Collaborating	Expecting the client to be an active and equal participant in therapy. Ensuring choice, freedom, and autonomy to the greatest extent possible.	Setting recovery-oriented occupational goals with a man who had been through an inpatient detoxification program for alcohol misuse. The service user reported that the structured routine for healthy activity choices coupled with feedback to the therapist helped to build his sense of personal responsibility for achieving the goals.
Empathizing	Ongoing striving to understand the client's thoughts, feelings, and behaviors while suspending any judgment. Ensuring that the client verifies and experiences the therapist's understanding as truthful and validating.	Taking care to appreciate fully the occupational requests and sensitivities of a woman experiencing psychotic symptoms. This approach enabled her to reclaim her values of being a vegan and being very environmentally conscious throughout her therapeutic recovery experience.
Encouraging	Seizing the opportunity to instill hope in a client. Celebrating a client's thinking or behavior through positive reinforcement. Conveying an attitude of joyfulness, playfulness, and confidence.	Spontaneously responding to a woman attending an occupational therapy group session who, inspired by some background music, started to dance. Therapeutic connection was enhanced by this small gesture to join with her joy of the activity.
Instructing	Carefully structuring therapy activities and being explicit with clients about the plan, sequence, and events of therapy. Providing clear instruction and feedback about performance. Setting limits on a client's requests or behavior.	Enabling a withdrawn woman with little belief in her own abilities to undertake self-care activities. This was achieved by talking the woman through the task, all the while reinforcing verbally the support available with the task if required.
Problem-solving	Facilitating pragmatic thinking and solving dilemmas by outlining choices, posing strategic questions, and providing opportunities for comparative or analytical thinking.	Allowing a young man with Asberger's syndrome to undertake the activities of value to him that also supported his well-being. This involved analyzing options and negotiating with his family, who were concerned about his extraordinary choices of some occupations and his neglect of others.

shift might be required and determining which alternative mode to select. Because the interpersonal aspects of occupational therapy practice are complex and require a therapist to have a highly adaptive therapeutic personality, the IRM recommends that therapists learn to draw upon all six of the therapeutic modes in a flexible manner according to the interpersonal needs of each client and the unique demands of each clinical situation (Fig. 3.8).

The third therapist interpersonal competence involves the capacity to engage in an *interpersonal reasoning* process when an interpersonal dilemma presents itself in therapy. Interpersonal reasoning is a stepwise process by which a therapist decides what to say, do, or express in reaction to the occurrence of an interpersonal dilemma in

therapy. It includes developing a mental vigilance toward the interpersonal aspects of therapy in anticipation that a dilemma might occur and a means of reviewing and evaluating options for responding. A full description of the steps of interpersonal reasoning and examples of its application in practice are provided in Chapter 7.

Desired Occupation

As noted earlier, occupational therapy is unique in that the crux of the therapy process is the client's occupational engagement. The *desired occupation* is the task or activity the therapist and client have selected for therapy. Desired occupations may include a wide range of tasks and activities, such as dressing oneself, driving, shopping, gross

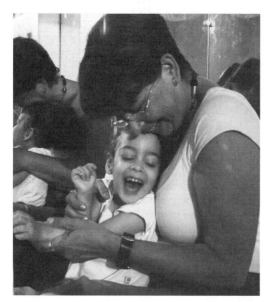

FIGURE 3.8 Multimodal therapists such as Michele Shapiro are able to answer a variety of interpersonal demands in therapy

motor play, participating in a goal-setting group, completing a craft activity, or engaging in a simulated or modified work task. The selection of the occupation and support for occupational engagement is primarily informed by other occupational therapy conceptual practice models such as the biomechanical model, the sensory integration model, or the model of human occupation (Kielhofner, 2004).

The primary function of the IRM is to enable the therapist to manage the interpersonal dynamic between the client and the therapist that also occurs as part of the therapy process. This interpersonal dynamic influences the occupational engagement and also serves as an arena in which the emotional reactions that stem from or influence occupational engagement can be positively managed. Thus, according to the IRM, the therapeutic relationship has two functions.

- A support to occupational engagement
- A place where the emotions and coping process associated with the client's impairment and its implications for occupational participation can be addressed

Relationships Within the Model

According to the IRM, the client and therapist relationship can be viewed at two levels or scales.

- The usual therapeutic relationship process that consists of the ongoing rapport and patterns of interaction between client and therapist. This relationship is enduring, and it occurs outside of any unusual circumstances or stressors (macro level).
- The therapeutic relationship process that is influenced by interpersonal events of therapy, or the stressors or highlights that have the potential to challenge or enrich the relationship depending on how they are responded to and resolved (micro level).

The ***therapeutic relationship*** is a socially defined and personally interpreted interactive process between the therapist and a client. It is socially defined in that the therapist and the client are engaged in an interaction within publicly understood roles. The therapist is recognized as bringing a certain kind of expertise, ethical guidelines, and values into a relationship. The client is recognized as a person receiving service to address a particular need. The relationship is understood to exist for the sole purpose of achieving improvement in the client's situation. These parameters are given and provide an important definition of the relationship. Therapist and client are in a particular relationship that can be differentiated from other kinds of relationships such as friendships. At the same time, this relationship has a personal side. The client and therapist are human beings who encounter each other with the same potential range of thoughts and emotions that occur when any two people interact (Fig. 3.9).

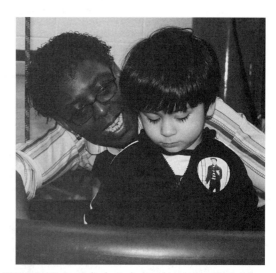

FIGURE 3.9 For Belinda Anderson the relationship is fully human

Consequently, the therapist's responsibility is to ensure that:

• The appropriate definitions and boundaries of the therapeutic relationship are sustained
• Positive interpersonal relating, such as trust, mutual respect, and honesty, characterize the relationship

Sustaining the therapeutic relationship is an ongoing task that does not focus solely on interpersonal events. The therapeutic relationship process that occurs outside of the interpersonal events is the macro dimension of the interpersonal process of therapy.

Responding to the immediate events that occur during therapy is the micro dimension. Responding to these interpersonal events of therapy requires that the therapist detect the occurrence of an event, read the client's reaction to the event, and decide on an appropriate way to address the event with the client.

> It is the therapist's responsibility to manage and continually strive to fortify the therapeutic relationship and to seek optimal resolutions to interpersonal events in therapy.

Both the micro and macro scales of therapeutic interaction play a critical role in the overall process of occupational therapy. Moreover, they are interrelated. That is, the nature of the therapeutic relationship has an influence on how the client interprets and how the therapist responds to interpersonal events; and, in turn, interpersonal events and their resolution either enhance or detract from the therapeutic relationship.

In some cases, the two scales of interaction are difficult to differentiate. For example, some therapy relationships last only one or two sessions. In these cases, a therapist must work to respond to a client and to interpersonal events with much more vigilance and self-control because a more stable underlying therapeutic relationship does not yet exist. Moreover, the interpersonal events and their resolution during the therapy sessions are the major determinants of the therapeutic relationship.

In most cases, however, therapy continues over a period of weeks or months, allowing the development of some kind of predictable pattern or usual way of interacting within the therapeutic relationship. That therapeutic relationship is infused and shaped by interpersonal events that occur in the moment-by-moment therapy process. It is

also influenced by the characteristics and behaviors the client and therapist bring to the relationship as well as by the circumstances surrounding the relationship. These circumstances include such factors as the nature and unfolding of the client's impairment and the context (e.g., school, rehabilitation setting, home, work) in which the therapy takes place.

It is the therapist's responsibility to manage and continually strive to fortify the therapeutic relationship and to seek optimal resolutions to interpersonal events in therapy. The stability and success of a therapeutic relationship cannot be assumed. Rather, it begins early in treatment with attempts by the therapist to build rapport, followed by other efforts to develop a relationship that meets the client's immediate interpersonal needs and is appropriate in terms of the circumstances of therapy and the demands of the treatment setting. Recognizing and sustaining a successful therapeutic relationship might include such things as:

• Sharing certain interpersonal rituals that facilitate bonding (e.g., paying a visit to a garden or other favorite locale within the client's setting each time before the ending of therapy)
• Witnessing the client enjoying or benefiting from therapy
• Sharing mutual feelings of respect, admiration, or appreciation
• Feeling interested and engaged in the therapy process
• Being open and comfortable digressing during therapy for discussion, venting, or advice-seeking about events in his or her personal life (without interfering with progress toward goals)
• Being able to discuss and overcome the interpersonal events that might otherwise challenge the relationship
• Having a long-standing private joke with a client
• Sharing a certain intensity of eye contact that communicates mutual trust
• Noticing a certain way a client laughs that conveys her appreciation of the therapist

These are only a few examples among myriad factors that might contribute to a successful therapeutic relation-

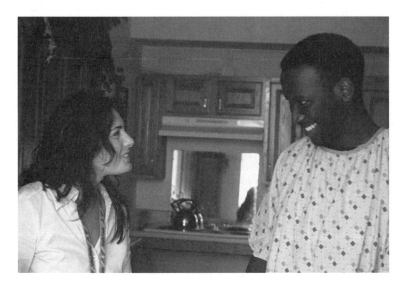

FIGURE 3.10 Signs of a successful relationship between Stephanie McCammon and a client

ship. It is the responsibility of the therapist to be vigilant to explore, identify, and sustain the factors that contribute to a relationship that supports positive therapy outcomes (Fig. 3.10).

This is not to say that the client does not make positive contributions to the therapeutic relationship. In most instances, clients bring important or essential characteristics and behaviors into the relationship. However, the fundamental difference is that it is the therapist who must assume the ultimate responsibility for ensuring that the relationship is positive. By assuming this responsibility, the therapist creates a space in the relationship wherein a client can be vulnerable, distressed, frustrated, or angry without fearing that the relationship will be ruptured. Moreover, this does not mean that the therapist assumes an expert or authoritative stance in the relationship. Rather, it means that the therapist must assume responsibility for the caring within the relationship.

The enduring aspects of the therapeutic relationship are systematically built and fortified as a result of naturally occurring variables in the relationship (similar personality styles or interpersonal chemistry or other optimal circumstances and timing) and as a result of the therapist's consistent efforts to build the relationship in the face of the inevitable interpersonal events and challenges that occur. If the therapist's efforts to build a relationship are successful and the client is not particularly sensitive, untrusting, or otherwise vulnerable, the therapeutic relationship becomes

stronger over time and is more likely to withstand interpersonal events that would otherwise challenge or strain the relationship.

For any number of reasons, however, the therapeutic relationship may not develop adequately to endure threats caused by the interpersonal events that routinely emerge during therapy. Signs that there is difficulty in the therapeutic relationship may include, but are not limited to:

- Change in affect, attitude, or interpersonal behavior
- Becoming disengaged from therapy
- Appearing/feeling impatient, irritable, or angry
- Therapy is experienced as "boring"
- Utility of the therapy becomes questionable
- Questioning or criticism feels excessive
- Taking therapy "home"
- Dreading or becoming apprehensive about the next appointment
- Having a desire to refer or terminate prematurely
- Conflict with the client
- Client's attendance pattern changes or declines

There are a number of potential reasons that difficulty may emerge within the therapeutic relationship. For example, a client may bring a particular interpersonal history into the treatment relationship that makes it difficult for the therapist to establish rapport in ways that usually work. Conversely, the client may be mistrustful of the therapist because of the circumstances under which he is being seen. For example, a client may have been mandated by an insurance company to receive an evaluation for work potential, and the client perceives that the therapist has tremendous power to influence his life (i.e., whether he continues to receive disability support). Alternatively, a therapist may have a negative reaction to a client because the client reminds the therapist of someone with whom the therapist has had a difficult relationship in the past. General sources of difficulty within the relationship may include, but are not limited to:

- Client brings a difficult interpersonal history into the relationship or has an Axis II diagnosis.
- Circumstances under which client is being seen are threatening or pressured (i.e., an evaluation is being conducted for the purpose of verifying disability to an insurance company).
- There is a poor match between client and therapist's interpersonal styles.
- There is an inability to overcome challenges caused by differences in culture, values, or world view.
- Client or therapist remind each other of someone with whom they have had a negative experience.
- Client or therapist disappoints or fails to meet expectations.
- Client or therapist inadvertently says or does something that is perceived as injurious, and the situation is not processed and resolved.

These and other obstacles to a more stable enduring relationship with a client are only intensified by inevitable interpersonal events. Examples of events that are likely to further stress an already-vulnerable therapy relationship include such things as a therapist's unanticipated absence for a period of time, a common misunderstanding that occurs between client and therapist, a comment or question that is perceived by the client as insensitive or inappropriate, or an unexpected personal crisis that causes the client to regress or temporarily relinquish treatment goals. Although they are normal and inevitable examples of difficult aspects of therapy, the way in which the therapist responds to them is a powerful mediator of the final outcome.

Irrespective of the extent to which the therapeutic relationship process is stable and strong, the process of therapeutic responding to interpersonal events is essential to good therapy. If a therapist does not respond adequately to interpersonal events or challenges to the relationship, the process of occupational engagement may suffer, and the therapeutic relationship process quickly erodes.

For the duration of the therapy process, the therapist must engage in a process of interpersonal reasoning. ***Interpersonal reasoning*** is the process by which a therapist consciously and reflectively monitors both the therapeutic relationship and the interpersonal events of therapy in order to decide on and enact appropriate interpersonal strategies. Chapter 7 discusses the interpersonal reasoning process in detail.

Intentional Relationship Model: Underlying Principles

The IRM defines the most critical components of the client–therapist relationship as it occurs in occupational therapy. In addition to its central elements and mechanisms, 12 fundamental principles underlie the conceptualization of this model (Table 3.2). They are explained in the following sections. Each principle specifies unique assumptions about how the client–therapist relationship is approached. Collectively, the principles should be kept actively in mind anytime the model is applied during an interaction with a client.

Table 3.2 **Underlying Principles of the Intentional Relationship Model**
1. Critical self-awareness is key to the intentional use of self.
2. Interpersonal self-discipline is fundamental to effective use of self.
3. It is necessary to keep head before heart.
4. Mindful empathy is required to know your client.
5. Therapists are responsible for expanding their interpersonal knowledge base.
6. Provided that they are purely and flexibly applied, a wide range of therapeutic modes can work and be utilized interchangeably in occupational therapy.
7. The client defines a successful relationship.
8. Activity focusing must be balanced with interpersonal focusing.
9. Application of the model must be informed by core values and ethics.
10. Application of the model requires cultural competence.

Principle 1: Critical Self-Awareness is Key to the Intentional Use of Self

Developing *critical self-awareness* involves having a working knowledge of your interpersonal tendencies while interacting with clients of different personality styles and under different conditions and circumstances. These interpersonal tendencies may manifest in one's emotional reactions to others and in one's verbalizations and nonverbal behavior. Critical self-awareness also requires understanding how your interpersonal reactions and behaviors change, become attenuated, or become amplified in awkward, tense, or stressful situations. Understanding yourself in these highly detailed and variegated ways is not easy to achieve. Nevertheless, this understanding is critical to developing interpersonal skills that are perceived as therapeutic by clients.

The difficulty involved in achieving critical self awareness is illustrated by research findings that therapists are usually not accurate in their self-estimation of the extent to which they convey an attitude of care and empathy toward their clients (Burns & Auerbach, 1996; Orlinsky, 1994). In studies of psychotherapy, empathy was linked to positive outcomes only if it was perceived by the client; therapist self-ratings of empathy were not associated with positive outcomes (Burns & Auerbach, 1996). Because therapists are not always accurate self-estimators of their own interpersonal capacities, merely considering oneself to be a caring and empathic therapist does not offer adequate assurance that an effective interpersonal process has occurred in therapy. Many of us have probably had the opportunity to know someone whose caring behavior toward us was fully spontaneous, sincere, and heartfelt but nevertheless largely missed what we most needed at the time.

Truly effective use of self hinges on *ongoing critical awareness* of your interpersonal behavior and emotional reactions to clients. This includes a mindfulness concerning:

- What you are communicating verbally (content, choice of words, types of questions asked)
- What you are communicating nonverbally (stance or sitting posture, positioning of arms and legs, angle of torso and head in relation to the client, gestures, extent and pace of body movements)
- What you are communicating emotionally (tone, tenor, and volume of voice; facial expression; extent to which emotion is shown or shared)

- What you are withholding, limiting, or otherwise not communicating and the implications of these kinds of noncommunication for the therapeutic interaction

Principle 2: Interpersonal Self-Discipline is Fundamental to Effective Use of Self

Achieving critical self-awareness is necessary for effective therapeutic relationships, but it is not sufficient. Therapists must also have the courage to seek and respond to interpersonal feedback from clients in a manner that reflects a dynamic, second-by-second recognition of what the client needs at any given moment. These abilities to anticipate, measure, and respond to the effects of ongoing communications with a client are most succinctly characterized as *interpersonal self-discipline*. Interpersonal self-discipline is fundamental to the use of self because it allows a therapist to develop stable, predictable relationships with clients. It allows a client to trust that the therapist has the ability to place his or her own interpersonal reactions and expectations aside to best fulfill what the client wishes to take from the relationship.

A critical aspect of interpersonal self-discipline involves acting on your awareness of your reactions to interpersonally challenging clients whose interpersonal behavior does not meet your expectations or tends to be negative. These clients may be particularly emotional, hypersensitive, defensive, demanding, critical, manipulative, difficult to manage, or otherwise vulnerable. Therapists differ among and within themselves regarding:

- What kinds of client behaviors and emotions are experienced as difficult
- The extent to which they feel comfortable managing these different types of difficult interpersonal behaviors

Some therapists find it easier to work with an emotionally sad client than an angry client, whereas the opposite may be true for another therapist. Interpersonal self-discipline involves knowing the types of clients and the situations that are most likely to test your interpersonal resolve and emotional perspective. Once you are familiar with your own vulnerabilities, you can more effectively prepare yourself emotionally and psychologically before interacting with these clients. In addition, you can more readily seek support, advice, and guidance from mentors and peers when treating difficult clients.

Collectively, the actions you take toward self-preparation and self-management in the face of interpersonally difficult clients helps ensure that the ways in which you choose to interact with these clients will be optimally therapeutic. This decreases the likelihood that you will unwittingly act out your own negative feelings toward a difficult client. For example, a therapist once shared that she felt less guilty about precipitously changing an appointment with a client in order to meet an out-of-town friend for lunch because the client tended to behave in demanding ways and had recently questioned her approach. Changing an appointment with a client for a nonurgent matter is not a disciplined way of managing one's feelings toward a client. Moreover, changing the appointment with an already-difficult client may lead to increased tension in the relationship. Another example is the extent to which one may make special efforts on behalf of a client. It is generally easier to make these extra efforts for clients whom one likes and sees as investing a great deal in the therapy. However, depriving the difficult client or the client who is not invested in therapy of one's extra effort is not justified ethically.

Table 3.3 contains additional examples of difficult interpersonal behaviors that clients commonly exhibit, typical emotional reactions a therapist might have to such behavior, and undisciplined versus disciplined ways in which therapists can behave in response.

In addition, Exercise 3.1 in the Activities section of this chapter provides a blank copy of this table so you can furnish your own examples of difficult interpersonal situa-

tions, note your own reactions, and judge for yourself what would be a disciplined versus an undisciplined response.

Another important aspect of interpersonal self-discipline is that therapists avoid viewing the relationship as a potential source of self-esteem or as a barometer by which to measure their own interpersonal competence. Regardless of whether a relationship is successful or unsuccessful, the extent to which a therapist can truly control what occurs during a clinical interaction is limited. Therapists must keep their successes and failures in perspective and work to manage their needs to feel connected with, approved of, or celebrated by clients. Investing too much of one's own interests in having a relationship with a client can result in deep feelings of disappointment when a positive connection does not occur. Importantly, more intuitive clients may detect subtle hints toward the therapist's need for connection or approval and may withdraw further because they feel pressured or emotionally suffocated. When clients do not meet a therapist's expectations, some may detect underlying feelings of disappointment or frustration in the therapist. Over time, not keeping therapeutic relationships in perspective can also lead to emotional exhaustion or burnout in therapists.

A final aspect of interpersonal self-discipline in the therapy process involves perspective and responsibility-taking. According to the IRM, it is the therapist's responsibility to manage the more challenging aspects of the relationship and continually strive to fortify the relation-

Table 3.3 Examples of Disciplined Versus Undisciplined Responses to Interpersonally Difficult Clients

Client's Behavior	Effect of Client's Behavior	Undisciplined Response	Disciplined Response
Critical of new approach	Feel judged by client	Avoid trying new approaches in the future	Discuss pros and cons before recommending new approach
Emotionally over-reactive	Feel emotionally drained	Become less engaged with the client over time	Assist client in verbalizing or describing feelings when they occur
Distant and uninvolved	Feel I am not trying hard enough to build rapport with the client	Try harder to build rapport	Identify possible explanations for client's lack of involvement
Entitled and demanding	Feel anger toward client	Set more limits with this client than with others	Discuss different perceptions about therapy expectations with client
Needy and manipulative	Feel guilty and sorry for client	Respond inconsistently – occasionally do more for this client than for others	Respond consistently within reasonable limits/boundaries

ship with the client. This aspect of interpersonal self-discipline is particularly relevant to working with more frustrating clients who are interpersonally sensitive, difficult, or otherwise vulnerable. Even if a client misperceives a therapist's good intentions, attempts to break professional boundaries, or becomes upset with the therapist for no apparent reason, it is the therapist's responsibility to respond to the client in a way that is ethical and maximally therapeutic given the client's interpersonal characteristics and the circumstances of therapy. More information about therapeutic responding is provided in Chapter 7.

Principle 3: It is Necessary to Keep Head Before Heart

Responding to clients from the heart—that is, intuitively, spontaneously, and emotionally—should be considered an indulgence and a privilege earned by therapists rather than an entitlement. Responding from the heart must be accompanied by sufficient development of critical self-awareness and interpersonal self-discipline. With sufficient experience and practice, therapists become aware of the various types of positive therapeutic communication of which they are capable. By the same token, therapists become familiar with the many potential ways in which their communication (or lack of communication) has the potential to become nontherapeutic, psychologically risky, ambiguous, or (at worst) emotionally harmful to clients. With sufficient practice, a disciplined and systematic process of therapeutic responding becomes automatic and intuitive. Over time, therapists feel as if they are responding to their clients spontaneously and intuitively, even though each of their more critical communications is accompanied by a sophisticated process of interpersonal reasoning (Fig. 3.11).

According to this principle, it is incorrect to assume that so long as your heart is in the right place you naturally react and behave appropriately in therapy. Instead, it is important to know that each of us has certain tendencies that do not always play out positively for a client simply because we care, have compassion, or can appreciate the client's life story. To be sure, these are all important attitudes for a therapist to sustain, but they are not a replacement for thoughtful self-knowledge and self-discipline.

Principle 4: Mindful Empathy is Required to Know Your Client

As reviewed in Chapter 1, the centrality and importance of empathy to the client–therapist relationship is supported by a number of occupational therapy scholars and practitioners. A therapist's capacity for empathy is a prerequisite for a functional client–therapist relationship. However, the IRM differs from prior discussions of empathy in the occupational therapy literature in that it treats empathy as a mindful process rather than a predominantly affective one. The concept of mindful empathy was developed based on Heinz Kohut's (1984) underlying theory of self psychology.

Mindful empathy is an objective mode of observation in which the therapist comes to feel and understand a client's underlying emotions, needs, and motives while at the same time maintaining an objective viewpoint. Kohut labeled the empathic process of accessing a client's internal world "vicarious introspection," and he consistently emphasized the importance of evaluating each client's experiences and behaviors from the client's unique perspective (Gardner, 1991; Kohut, 1984). The idea of mindful empathy, which was influenced by some of these

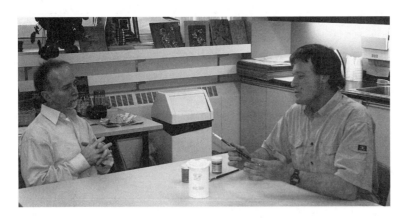

FIGURE 3.11 René Bélanger putting head first as a client discusses a significant occupational concern

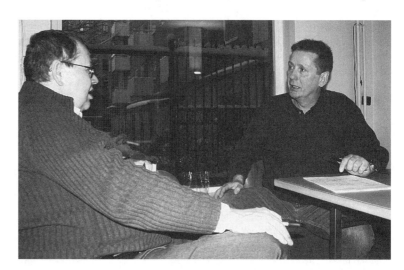

FIGURE 3.12 Roland Meisel relies on mindful empathy when striving to understand a client's views about returning to work

ideas, assumes that the client is the expert on the meanings that he or she attaches to his or her experiences in therapy (Fig. 3.12).

According to the IRM, mindful empathy is fundamental to interpersonal reasoning. It guides both the therapist's response to interpersonal events and the therapist's efforts to sustain the therapeutic relationship. For instance, mindful empathy is necessary to interpret accurately a client's reactions to a given interpersonal event. Achieving an understanding of the client's cognitive interpretation and emotional and behavioral reactions to the event must be accomplished through empathically based listening and questioning. Although the client's interpersonal characteristics are likely to play a role in his or her interpretation and reactions to the event, assumptions about a client's reaction and needs should not be made until the client's reactions have been verified through reflective listening and an explicit conversation about the event that has occurred. Assumptions should not be based entirely on prior knowledge of the client's interpersonal characteristics. Mindful empathy is an advanced skill in the therapist's interpersonal knowledge base. More information about this skill and examples of how therapists have employed mindful empathy in practice is presented in subsequent chapters of this book.

Principle 5: Grow Your Interpersonal Knowledge Base

Interpersonal communication is as complex as the limits of human understanding. From client to client, communica-

tion is as variegated and unique as are the differences between and within individuals, families, social networks, communities, neighborhoods, nations, cultures, geographies, climates, and governments. For these reasons, therapists benefit from knowing as much about human behavior as possible, particularly as it pertains to more commonly occurring events in the client–therapist relationship.

The IRM describes skills that are essential to meeting the basic interpersonal demands of practice, such as listening effectively, communicating clearly, overcoming basic conflicts and events, and being reliable and predictable in interactions. The model describes additional skills that are required to achieve a level of communication with a client that responds to his or her interpersonal needs. This continuum of skills is described in detail and accompanied by clinical examples in Chapters 8 through 16.

Principle 6: Provided that They Are Purely and Flexibly Applied, a Wide Range of Therapeutic Modes can Work and be Utilized Interchangeably in Occupational Therapy

Individuals who enter the profession of occupational therapy have a side to their personalities that is oriented toward others and desires to support, uplift, empathize with, motivate, advocate for, guide, or otherwise empower people. At the same time, each therapist has a unique combination of interpersonal characteristics that largely derive from innate temperament or personality and from life experience. These characteristics influence the therapist to have a natural therapeutic mode or modes (i.e., particular ways of relating to a client in a given situation). As already mentioned, the six interpersonal therapeutic modes are the advocating mode, collaborating mode, empathizing mode, encouraging mode, instructing mode, and problem-solving mode. The therapeutic mode or set of modes that characterize a therapist's general approach to interacting with clients is referred to as the therapist's interpersonal style.

An underlying principle of the IRM is that no particular mode or interpersonal style is superior to another. Two therapists with diametrically opposite personalities, who use different combinations of modes, can be equally effective. However, certain interpersonal styles tend to work better with different populations and circumstances. Thus, therapists who are critically self-aware choose areas of practice most suited for their interpersonal style.

More importantly, effective use of self depends on the flexible and appropriate use of modes depending on the client and the situation. A therapist who relies heavily on only one therapeutic mode is effective with a narrower range of circumstances and clients than a therapist who can employ a variety of modes in response to changing interpersonal circumstances. Thus, the IRM recommends that therapists make an ongoing effort to expand their capacity to use different modes as demanded by individual differences between clients and the unique features of specific interpersonal events that may occur during therapy.

When a therapist decides to invoke a particular mode, it is important that the mode is communicated to the client accurately in its pure form. To achieve the pure, accurate use of a mode, it is recommended that the therapist remain within that mode for as long as it takes to communicate and ensure that the client has received the intended interpersonal message (e.g., that the intention for the moment is solely to empathize, solely to instruct, solely to problem solve, or what have you). If a therapist attempts to blend modes so two interpersonal messages are being communicated simultaneously, it is likely to weaken the intended communication of both modes and to result in the client becoming confused. For example, if a therapist's true intention is to address a client's behavior by using the instructing mode but, instead, begins to question the client about the reasons behind the behavior in a way that conveys disapproval, the therapist is blending the problem-solving mode into the instructing mode. The result is that the client receives a confused message about the desirability of the behavior (e.g., does the therapist want me to stop the behavior, or might it be okay if I explain to her why I am doing this?). Similarly, if a therapist shifts modes too

rapidly it may also lead to confusion or weakening of the communication, depending on the cognitive level and emotional maturity of the particular client. Although the IRM acknowledges the need for therapists occasionally to share mixed feelings with a client and send complex messages to clients that involve many mode shifts, this approach to communication must be done with great circumspection. These and other issues pertinent to shifting modes are discussed in more detail in Chapter 7.

Principle 7: The Client Defines a Successful Relationship

Clients differ widely in terms of what they are seeking from their relationships with health care professionals. For instance, some clients prefer a relationship that is professional, hierarchical, and relatively distant in which the therapist provides specific instructions, technologies, or resources to assist in the accomplishment of occupational goals and objectives. Other clients desire a relationship that involves a more personalized connection and results in feelings of emotional support as well as tangible occupational outcomes. Still others wish for a collaborative relationship in which mutual planning and problem-solving take place.

What is considered a successful relationship in occupational therapy must be defined by the client rather than the therapist. A successful client–therapist relationship must be based on the achievement of the type of therapeutic relationship the client needs most and is capable of during the time he or she is in therapy. This means that a successful therapeutic relationship is not defined by a feeling of closeness, or connection, unless the client clearly wants it as a feature of the relationship. Although in many circumstances these variables are associated with the client's perception of a successful relationship, for some clients a successful relationship may mean one that involves a certain level of professional distance or some other kind of interaction that is consistent with the client's prior experiences with health care professionals and cultural expectations.

A corollary to this principle is that clients may change over time in their desires for the therapeutic relationship. The following are some examples. A client who at first desires a more hierarchical and therapist-structured relationship following a traumatic event resulting in impairment, may wish for a more collaborative relationship later during the course of therapy. A long-term client seen first as a child may wish to achieve more distance as he or she comes into adolescence. A client who previously insisted on a highly collaborative relationship may, following an exacerbation of an impairment or symptom or during a crisis, need an empathic and supportive relationship. Such changes in a client's desires for the therapeutic relationship may reflect such factors as responses to stress, personal growth, or natural development. They must be respected and accommodated by the therapist.

Principle 8: Activity Focusing must be Balanced with Interpersonal Focusing

One way to determine what a client needs from the therapy relationship is by evaluating his or her preference for interpersonal interaction during therapy. Not all clients benefit from the same level of emotional intensity or closeness in the therapeutic relationship. For this reason, interpersonal self-discipline is required on the part of the therapist to ensure that *activity focusing* must be well balanced with *interpersonal focusing* in occupational therapy.

Activity focusing refers to strategies of responding to interpersonal events that emphasize "doing" issues over "feeling" or "relating" issues. *Interpersonal focusing* refers to strategies that emphasize the latter over doing issues. The difference can be illustrated through the following examples. Let us say a client becomes upset, frustrated, or fearful when trying a new activity. Activity focusing would involve modifying the activity or the environment or encouraging a client to try another activity. By contrast, interpersonal focusing would involve addressing the client's emotional reaction to what the therapist is saying or doing. In this instance, it might mean interrupting the activity to discuss the client's emotional reaction to therapy, or it may involve strategic questioning that reveals the client's inner feelings about the activity or to the overall therapy approach (Fig. 3.13).

This balance between activity focusing and interpersonal focusing varies from client to client depending on the client's progress in therapy, expectations from therapy, construal of the relationship, and reactions to the therapist. To accomplish this balance, a large measure of interpersonal reasoning and self-discipline is required. Interpersonal reasoning and self-discipline allow the therapist to keep the client's unique needs in focus to interpret the appropriate balance clearly. If a therapist achieves this balance, he or she does not rely too much on using activities to avoid direct discussion of interpersonal issues or, by contrast, does not overemphasize discussion of interpersonal issues when it is not comfortable for that particular client or appropriate for the situation.

Principle 9: Application of the Model must be Informed by Core Values and Ethics

Occupational therapy core values (AOTA, 1993) and ethics (AOTA, 2005) must inform application of the IRM in practice. As each component of the model is covered in

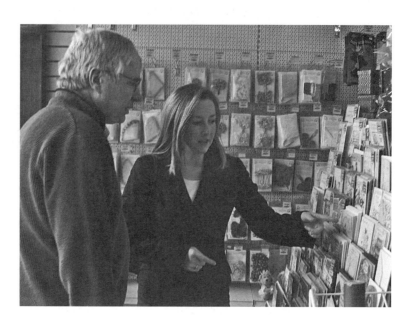

FIGURE 3.13 Jane Melton is careful to attend to both the activity and interpersonal dimensions of the therapy process

subsequent chapters of this book, examples of how occupational therapy core values and ethics inform application of model are provided. In addition, Chapter 14 overviews the occupational therapy core values and ethics, highlights the importance of the use of self in applying ethical principles, and specifies the numerous associations between ethical principles and the model. Examples of ethical dilemmas from clinical practice and possibilities for resolution are provided.

Principle 10: Cultural Competence is Central to Practice

Therapeutic use of self must be informed by human diversity. In client–therapist relationships, human diversity is defined by differences in sex, age, race, ethnicity, socioeconomic status, religious views, sexual orientation, disability status, and a wide range of other social and cultural dimensions. Developing cultural competence is fundamental to effective use of self in occupational therapy. For this reason, cultural competence is considered a central skill that must be developed and incorporated into every therapist's interpersonal knowledge base. Chapter 9 summarizes existing knowledge about cultural competence in the field of occupational therapy and provides additional recommendations for professional development in this area.

✴Summary

A rationale for the need of the intentional relationship model was provided, and the primary elements of the model were described. Ten principles underlying the model were also elaborated. Formulation of these principles was influenced by a number of sources, including information provided by the contributing therapists and direct observations of their behavior in practice, my own training and clinical experience as a psychotherapist, occupational therapy core values and ethics, and general principles derived from the occupational therapy and psychology literature and existing knowledge bases. The remainder of this book describes the intentional relationship model as one explanation of what occurs during our relationships with clients. Clinical examples of this model in action that were provided by the 12 featured therapists are incorporated throughout the book to illustrate how the concrete skills and concepts of this model can be utilized in practice.

References

American Occupational Therapy Association (AOTA) (1993). Core values and attitudes of occupational therapy practice. *American Journal of Occupational Therapy, 47*, 1085–1086.

American Occupational Therapy Association (AOTA) (2005). *AOTA: Occupational therapy code of ethics.* Bethesda, MD: AOTA. http://www.aota.org/.

Beck, J. (1995). *Cognitive therapy: Basics and beyond.* New York: Guilford Press.

Burns, D. D., & Auerbach, A. (1996). Therapeutic empathy in cognitive-behavioral therapy: Does it really make a difference? In P. M. Salkovskis (Ed.), *Frontiers of cognitive therapy* (pp. 135–164). New York: Guilford Press.

Gardner, J. R. (1991). The application of self psychology to brief psychotherapy. *Psychoanalytic Psychology, 8*, 477–500.

Kielhofner, G. (2004). *Conceptual foundations of occupational therapy* (3rd ed.). Philadelphia: FA Davis.

Kohut, H. (1984). *How does analysis cure?* Chicago: University of Chicago Press.

Orlinsky, D. E. (1994). Research-based knowledge as the emergent foundation for clinical practice in psychotherapy. In P. F. Talley, & H. H. Strupp (Eds.), *Psychotherapy research and practice: Bridging the gap.* New York: Basic Books.

ACTIVITIES FOR LEARNING AND REFLECTION

Personal Examples of Disciplined Versus Undisciplined Responses to Interpersonally Difficult People/Clients

This exercise is designed to allow for self-reflection about interpersonally difficult situations so you may become increasingly self-disciplined in your responses in actual practice situations. If you are a student who has not yet had a significant amount of practice experience, you are encouraged to furnish examples of difficult behavior of other people you have met or known and to reflect upon your reactions and responses to that behavior using this table.

Client's Behavior	Effect of Client's Behavior	Undisciplined Response	Disciplined Response

CHAPTER 4

KNOWING OURSELVES AS THERAPISTS:
Introducing the Therapeutic Modes

A *therapeutic mode* is a specific way of relating to a client. Six therapeutic modes have been identified as occurring with a high level of frequency in occupational therapy practice relationships. In this chapter, each of these six modes is described and examples are provided to illustrate the multiple ways in which the primary modes can be combined and utilized during therapeutic interactions with clients. Strengths and cautions associated with each mode are noted. Moreover, the chapter provides a rationale for the importance of the modes to the intentional relationship model (IRM).

At the end of the chapter, a self-assessment is provided for you to begin to gain a greater understanding of the modes you might tend to utilize most frequently in a practice situation. **It is recommended that you complete the Self-Assessment of Modes Questionnaire before reading any further.** This questionnaire is presented in Exercise 4.1 in the Activities section. After responding to the questions in the exercise, you should continue reading the chapter. After reading the chapter, it is recommended that you score your responses to Exercise 4.1, complete the Personal Modes Profile, and then complete Exercise 4.2. It is not recommended that you score your responses until you have finished reading the chapter.

Personality

Our personalities are comprised of a unique set of emotional experiences, a distinct pattern of interpersonal behavior, and a stable psychobiological profile (Kagan, 2000). Personality begins forming early in life and is a product of genetics, biology, and experiences interacting within one's family and in the broader social community. These variables converge and contribute to the development of a relatively stable and unique temperament (Carlson, 1998; Kohut, 1984). Almost a century of research has taught us that personality, and more specifically an individual's basic temperament, does not change significantly over the life span (Kagan, 2000).

Although our personalities may be relatively fixed, how we relate to others in our day-to-day lives may vary as a function of current mood state, social and environmental context, and the interpersonal behavior of others in the social environment. Thus, whereas our personality is relatively stable over time, our interpersonal behavior and way of being in a given social group vary with context. Psychologically healthy individuals utilize a wide range of natural interpersonal strategies to adapt to the social demands of living (Beck et al., 1990). Examples of these strategies are empathy, compassion, hopefulness, altruism, kindness, assertiveness, competitiveness, deference, dominance, passivity, resistance, avoidance, emotionality, restraint, power, aggression, suspiciousness, emotional disengagement, and isolative behavior.

Individuals with well-functioning personalities draw upon these and other strategies in an ever-changing and flexible manner in an attempt to adapt to the social demands of life (Beck et al., 1990). For example, a woman who is otherwise outgoing and gregarious at parties may significantly limit the extent to which she talks and socializes at a funeral if the social atmosphere is such that it requires silence and solemnity.

By contrast, individuals with chronic interpersonal difficulties or poorly functioning personalities tend to overutilize a small set of interpersonal strategies in inflexible, maladaptive, or compulsive ways (Beck et al., 1990).

For example, an individual whose primary objectives in relating to others involve self-preservation, resource acquisition, and a desire for power over others may consistently come across as confident, charming, competitive, and dominant.

Although a primary personality style like this is likely to work well in some competitive work or sporting situations, it does not work well in group situations where people value the sharing of power and other mutually supportive behaviors. If the individual described above is unable to demonstrate other characteristics necessary for collaborative activities, such as deference, thoughtfulness, kindness, and empathy, negative consequences are likely to result when these characteristics are needed. For example, an individual with a more fixed style may become emotionally fatigued, may struggle to move into alternative roles within the group, or may even act to interfere with someone else's attempt to move into a position of power. Others in the group may grow fearful or resentful if they are not able to witness this person's humility, vulnerability, or attempts to share and be supportive.

An individual with greater capacity to draw on a wider range of characteristics is better able to establish appropriate relationships in both social situations. Thus, although our personalities are relatively stable, they function best if they allow us to utilize interpersonal strategies in a flexible way and adapt to a wide range of individuals in a variety of social situations.

Personality and Therapeutic Modes

Therapists' personalities are reflected in:

• Their fundamental motivation to serve others
• Their preferred approach to serving
• The values they hold while serving

Therapists' personalities are also reflected in the specific ways in which they behave and interact with clients. Consequently, each therapist's personality is reflected, in part, in preferred styles of interacting with clients (i.e., therapeutic modes). Consequently, our personalities are the first and most natural determinants of the modes we use during therapy.

Chapter 3 noted that the process of therapy is optimal when therapists are able to draw on a variety of modes consciously and flexibly. This has several implications. First, therapists should develop an awareness of their natural modes (i.e., the ones that flow from their personalities). Second, they should develop the self-discipline to use these modes in response to client needs rather than in response to their own internal comfort levels. Third, therapists should be aware of the limits of the modes they use and, in some instances, develop the capacity to use modes beyond those that come naturally (Fig. 4.1).

Six Therapeutic Modes

The six therapeutic modes used most frequently in occupational therapy practice include:

• Advocating
• Collaborating
• Empathizing
• Encouraging
• Instructing
• Problem-solving

Because therapists naturally select and use modes that are most consistent with their personalities, the use of therapeutic modes is as diverse and complex as therapists' personalities.

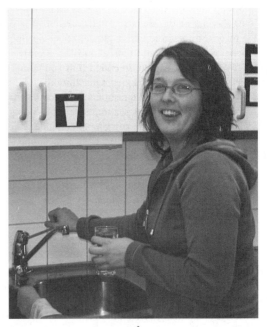

FIGURE 4.1 Kristin Alfredsson Ågren draws on a wide range of modes while working at a community-based daytime activity center in Sweden

All modes have equal potential to enable a functional therapeutic relationship. However, any mode may have a negative effect on a client's attitudes and feelings toward the therapist if used:

- Too frequently or inflexibly
- When the timing is not right for the client
- When the mode is not consistent with the client's personality as a whole
- When the mode is not changed so as to be more consistent with the client's interpersonal needs of the moment

In the worst cases, overreliance on a particular mode with a client can result in negative consequences for the therapy process and for the client (Box 4.1).

The previous chapter argued that your *therapeutic style* is defined by the primary mode or set of modes that you tend to utilize most often during interactions with clients. It is important to recognize that some therapists' styles reflect use of one primary mode or set of modes, whereas other therapists incorporate a much wider range of modes into their approach. For this reason, the therapeutic modes are presented in this section in alphabetical order to underscore that no one mode is superior to another. Key points regarding each of the modes are summarized in Table 4.1.

The points describing each mode are guidelines, not rules. They were included to stimulate creative thinking about a wide range of interpersonal behaviors that could potentially converge to form a therapeutic style. As you learn more about each mode, you may begin to form some of your own thoughts and ideas about interpersonal behaviors that you typically utilize that reflect a given mode but are not explicitly described in this section. This type of thinking is encouraged because it promotes critical self-awareness and greater insight into your own unique therapeutic style.

Advocating Mode

The *advocating mode* is becoming more prevalent as therapists become aware of and embrace the perspective that disability is a function of environmental barriers rather than client impairments. Therapists using the advocating mode work to ensure that clients have the personal, material and interpersonal resources they need for maximal participation in productivity, leisure, and all other daily life activities. It includes ensuring that clients have access to housing, transportation, education, equal opportunities for employment, assistive devices, personal assistants, and any other resources pertinent to their independence and well-being. Functioning in the mode of advocate often involves being a facilitator or defender of justice, rather than in the more traditional roles in which the occupational therapist guides, questions, listens, or administers a service (Fig. 4.2).

Therapists functioning in the advocating mode are quick to recognize and respond to the physical, social, and occupational barriers that their clients encounter. They are careful not to undermine their clients' autonomy, dignity, sense of personal power, and capacity to judge what is in their own best interest by functioning in an expert role. They are also careful about being misperceived by clients as someone interested in fixing or rehabilitating them. At the same time, therapists functioning as advocates can be ardent and forceful activists and promoters on behalf of their clients when the circumstances require it. Some engage in consciousness-raising with their clients about their legal rights, and some utilize their professional capacity to testify on behalf of a client in a legal situation or to broker access to services or resources to which a client is entitled (Box 4.2).

Box 4.1   Mode Preference is Relative to Each Client's Need: Advocating Mode

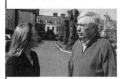

Jane Melton and a client discuss how to request reasonable accommodations after visiting a potential worksite

The idea that a therapist merely needs to select the correct mode to produce a desirable outcome has an important caveat. Each mode is subject to the interpretation of the client, who is the receiver of that mode. Thus, the same mode can produce two opposing reactions in two different clients. A client's reactions are less a function of the mode choice and more a function of the interpersonal characteristics and immediate needs of the client. One example of this involves use of the instructing mode. I once had a client who misinterpreted my well-intentioned attempt to guide him in baking a pizza as undermining, whereas a different client I had earlier that same day found a similar approach to instruction to be helpful and supportive. It is important to keep in mind that modes are *perceived, relativistic, and subjective*. As such, they are best interpreted through the mind's eye of the client. Rather than the mode itself, the client's interpretation and experience of the mode is what determines which mode is most desirable at any given time.

—**Renee Taylor**

Table 4.1 **Summary Description of the Six Therapeutic Modes**			
Mode	**Style/Strategies**	**Strengths**	**Cautions**
Advocating	· Ensure clients have needed material and interpersonal resources. · Tends toward roles of facilitator or consultant. · Ensures opportunities for participation and access. · May engage in consciousness-raising with clients about legal rights, barriers to access, and obstacles to independence. · May be willing to become involved in civil rights or legal activities on behalf of their clients. · Approach interpersonal difficulties by adjusting and accommodating the needs of the client.	· Provide clients access to vital resources. · Client may be more likely to regain self-esteem and develop a positive identity as a disabled person if treated by a therapist who does not view disability as a tragic outcome but, instead, embraces it and believes that the true problem is not the impairment but the social attitudes and environmental barriers that exist outside the individual.	· May be premature or inconsistent with client needs to raise awareness about injustices they would rather deny or discover in their own time. · Focusing therapy on changing social and environmental obstacles may limit the amount of time that can be spent on remediation and/or accommodation of client problems.
Collaborating	· Make decisions jointly with clients. · Involve clients in one's reasoning during therapy. · Expect clients to actively participate. · Solicit ongoing feedback from clients. · Encourage autonomy and independence. · Approach interpersonal difficulties by empowering the client to use his or her own judgment and by allowing the client to take the lead in the therapy process.	· Likely to convey their belief in their clients' capacities, dignity, and independence. · Likely to promote self-confidence and independence in clients. · Less at risk for encouraging dependent or regressive behavior. · Honest style increases likelihood to gain clients' trust. · May be less defensive in that they are able to embrace and utilize client feedback to improve the therapy process.	· May favor clients who are more willing to take responsibility and assume independence. · May work less effectively with clients who do not embrace joint decision-making or those who do not take responsibility for their own progress in therapy. · Clients from cultures that view the patient–provider relationship in a more hierarchical fashion may misperceive the therapist as lacking expertise. · May overestimate client strengths and capacities, rush the pace of therapy, and/or miss a client's occasional need for direction, empathy, or emotional security. · Collaboration may result in diffusion of responsibility or uncertainty regarding who is responsible for which part of the therapy process. It may also cause confusion about roles within the therapeutic relationship.
Empathizing	· Put a significant amount of time and effort into striving to understand a client's perspective as accurately as possible. · Listen carefully, watch what clients are communicating, and adjust their approach depending on the client's needs. · Use intermissions from "doing" for processing and communicating with clients. · Able to notice and respond to	· Due to their patience and ability to listen, validate, and accept negativity, these therapists are able to work with a wide range of clients. · Able to work effectively with even the most challenging, reluctant, negative, critical, or resistant clients. · By modeling empathy, they enable clients to empathize with themselves, self-reflect,	· Overutilizing empathy may lead to overprotecting clients if therapists listen and validate at the expense of questioning or challenging them to engage in occupations in which they may otherwise be ready to engage. · Owing to the slower pace of therapy and the time dedicated to listening and communication, some of the fundamental occupational and activity-related tasks of therapy may not be accomplished. This is most likely

Mode	Style/Strategies	Strengths	Cautions
	nuances in clients' affect and behavior. · Accepting and validating of clients' negative emotions and self-reported difficulties and do not rush to alter or fix. · Utilize striving for understanding as a means for resolving rifts, obstacles, and conflicts that occur during therapy. · Pacing of introducing activities, providing feedback, and making recommendations tends to be slower due to the focus on listening. · Show tremendous discretion when deciding whether to reveal their spontaneous heartfelt reactions to clients or whether to put themselves aside to allow full space for clients' reactions and reported experiences.	and gain insight into their emotional reactions and behaviors. · Most likely to gain resolution of conflicts, rifts, and misunderstandings that inevitably occur during therapy. · Clients more likely to feel responded to, cared about, and respected by these therapists. · Therapists are more likely to achieve open and honest communication with clients, improving trust and resulting in a stronger therapeutic relationship.	to happen with resistant or reluctant clients who require extensive use of empathy before engaging in the tasks of therapy. · If empathic approaches are used with clients who are not accustomed to having someone empathize with them or with those who have difficulty trusting the therapist, some clients may recoil or withdraw from what they see as too much intimacy or emotional involvement in therapy. · Use of empathy may lead to confusion in some clients regarding the role of the therapist and the objectives of occupational therapy. This may make negotiation and setting of appropriate professional boundaries between client and therapist more challenging.
Encouraging	· Instills clients with hope, courage, and the will to explore, participate, or perform a given activity. · Examine the extent to which clients value and are interested in a given activity carefully to determine what might motivate them to engage in a particular occupation. · Focus on selecting and altering activities to make them more appealing, pleasurable, or attractive to the client. · Frequent use of positive reinforcement, positive feedback, humor or entertaining antics, cheering, coaxing, compliments, applause, motivational words.	· Able to identify and celebrate even the smallest of clients' accomplishments during therapy. · Skilled at conveying their optimism and hope to clients. · Keen observers of motivational issues in their clients. · Skilled at selecting and adapting activities so they better correspond with what motivates their clients. · Because of their emphasis on motivation, therapists are effective at enlisting participation from even the most reluctant or resistant clients. · Some therapists are skilled at using humor and may convey an entertaining, cheerful, and playful attitude, which many clients appreciate when timed appropriately. For example, children, in particular, appreciate therapists who are playful and entertaining.	· Because of their optimism and belief that all clients have the capacity to improve in some way, some therapists overfunction during therapy with the hope of seeing positive outcomes. · If overused, some clients may become desensitized to efforts to motivate them. · If overused, some clients over-rely or grow dependent on the therapist's efforts to motivate them and do not develop intrinsic motivation to engage in occupation. · Some clients reject outward efforts to motivate, encourage, or cheer them. One reason for this is that they may misinterpret the therapist's efforts as manipulative. Other clients may view a well-intended therapist's humor or other attempts to cheer or encourage them as foolish or insincere.
Instructing	· Emphasize educational aspects of therapy and assume a teaching stance in client–therapist interactions. · Skilled at sharing information and structuring the therapy process and activities.	· Convey confidence to clients and have strong ideals, opinions, and assertions about what a client needs to accomplish during therapy to maximize the likelihood of a positive outcome. · Have a sense of conviction about their assessment findings, thera-	· If this mode is overused, some therapists are at risk of overfunctioning during therapy sessions, making premature, anticipatory statements about client performance, or overprotecting their clients to prevent them from experiencing failure.

(table continued on page 72)

Table 4.1 **Summary Description of the Six Therapeutic Modes** (continued)			
Mode	**Style/Strategies**	**Strengths**	**Cautions**
	· Comfortable with an active and directive style using training and coaching and providing feedback to clients. · Not afraid to state their professional opinion, set limits, provide feedback, or disagree with clients. · Skilled at gentle or finessed confrontation. · Approach interpersonal difficulties with clients by restating their own point of view, educating clients about the value of their perspective, providing more of a rationale for their perspective, and (if the client continues to disagree) agreeing to disagree.	peutic approach, and interpersonal values. As a result, they do not waiver in the face of a difficult or demanding client and are not easily manipulated, distracted, or taken advantage of by clients. · Education is a foundational aspect of occupational therapy (OT), and OT would not occur without structure, transfer of knowledge, provision of feedback, and overall leadership. · Because they are skilled at communicating clearly and effectively with clients, clients tend to grasp, learn, and adhere to the activities and tasks of therapy. · Convey to client that they are invested in positive outcomes. · Certain clients who value authority and expert knowledge are more likely to trust in the therapist's expertise if the therapist assumes an instructing-coaching mode.	· Clients with difficulties trusting or relating to health care professionals who assume an attitude of authority may interpret some therapists' behavior as controlling, dominant, or parental. · Because of their strong tendencies to lead the process rather than follow it, some clients become locked into power struggles and arguments with therapists. · Because they are highly invested in client successes or failures, some therapists personalize or assume too much responsibility for therapy outcomes. Negative or less-than-desirable outcomes may have an exaggerated impact on therapists' self-worth and professional identity. Others convey disappointment in otherwise earnest clients who do not perform as expected. · Some therapists who overutilize this mode are too eager to facilitate remediation, teach clients to compensate, or attempt to "fix the problem" rather than just listen and validate.
Problem-solving	· Technically skilled and highly creative. · Focus on biomechanical approaches, cognitive rehabilitation, and use of assistive devices. · Approach interpersonal difficulties by reasoning with clients, engaging in pragmatic problem-solving, or by using other logical and strategic approaches, such as Socratic questioning.	· Due to their high level of focus on the technical aspects of therapy, they are more likely to see significant improvements in occupational performance and participation earlier in the therapy process. · Because they are oriented toward outcomes, they may be more likely to witness and evaluate tangible, direct benefits of their work. · Clients are likely to understand the expectations and limits of the therapeutic relationship and client–therapist boundaries regarding the nature and extent of communication and behavior inside and outside of therapy are likely to be clear. · Clients who are less comfortable with a more emotion-focused approach to the relationship may value and feel more comfortable with the predictability and professionalism conveyed by these therapists.	· Over time, a strong emphasis on the technical aspects of therapy and a lack of emphasis on getting to know clients on a more intimate level as unique individuals may lead some therapists to believe that their work is redundant or repetitive. · Therapists who overemphasize problem-solving approaches may be at risk of assuming an expert stance without attending to the needs of the client. · Therapists may be vulnerable to using technical terms and jargon with clients and non-OT staff. · Therapists who are less comfortable with other modes (e.g., empathizing) may become emotionally and psychologically disengaged from or frustrated with difficult clients who are emotional or interpersonally demanding. · Some therapists over-rely on pragmatic, technical, and mechanical aspects of therapy when communication and empathy are what is needed in a given situation.

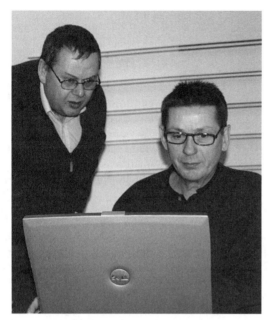

FIGURE 4.2 Advocating mode. Roland Meisel appears serious and assertive when working to locate the right equipment for a client

Strengths of the Advocating Mode

The advocating mode is an important one. If occupational therapists did not advocate for their clients, the clients would be on their own to battle insurance companies, agencies that provide public or private aid, landlords, educational systems, employers, and other powerful organizations. Those who function in the advocating mode go out of their way for their clients to provide them with access to vital resources that ensure physical mobility and access, socialization, equal participation, and appropriate work or educational opportunities. Occupational therapists are most often called on to function in the advocating mode when they recognize the advantages of raising a client's awareness of an injustice or when clients are themselves unable to overcome social and economic barriers without additional resources.

Cautions of the Advocating Mode

As with any other mode, the cautions associated with the advocating mode manifest when the mode is overused or misapplied. Some therapists are prone to overfunction on behalf of a client who is perceived as powerless but who is actually capable of becoming empowered. Conversely, the strong ideological orientation that often characterizes a

---

Box 4.2 Using the Advocating Mode

Virgil[1] is a man in his late twenties with cerebral palsy and moderate learning disabilities who has lived in an institution for most of his life. The managers of his care team at the institution had built a plan that he would move into independent living within the community with staff support to accommodate him. Before I was referred to work with Virgil, his care team from the institution had already located, set up, and obtained funding for his new housing situation. I was referred to provide Virgil with a bath board to facilitate his bathing in the terraced house that was to become his home.

Virgil had been schooled in the notion that his home was suitable to his needs, and he was thrilled about the possibility of moving into a new home. When I met with him within this new environment it was immediately evident to me that the housing arrangement was not acceptable. Fundamentally, the way the house was set up did not facilitate Virgil's independence, maximize his dignity, or provide a safe environment for staff to support him.

Instead of providing the bath board, I felt it was my duty to inform the managers of Virgil's care team and the organization that was to fund his new housing that I had found the proposed accommodations unacceptable. I provided a report that outlined the safety risks that would have been associated with providing a bath board. The report emphasized other shortfalls in the environmental design of the house and outlined the oversights in the overall care plan for Virgil.

The managers took offense at my report and attempted to remove me from the situation. They insisted that Virgil was no longer in need of occupational therapy services. However, I pursued my agenda and held meetings with the funding organization and the managers to explain the rationale behind my position. As a result, the funding organization conducted an independent review and later decided to offer Virgil an alternative accommodation. The housing that Virgil was eventually provided enabled him to move freely about the entire home and gain access to the bath, toilet, and other areas in a much safer and more dignified manner.

— **Jane Melton**

[1]All client names and geographic information have been changed.

---

therapist in the advocating mode may lead some therapists to overestimate a client's desire, ability, and/or resources for autonomy and independence.

Because clients differ in their experience of disability, they respond differently to advocacy efforts that involve consciousness-raising. For some clients, it may be premature to raise their awareness about injustices that they would rather deny or discover in their own time. In addition, because the advocating mode is characterized by an emphasis on removing environmental barriers over reducing impairments, it may unwittingly deprive clients of their preferred emphasis in therapy.

Collaborating Mode

The growing emphasis on client-centered practice in occupational therapy underscores the importance of the *collaborating mode*. Therapists functioning in the collaborating mode make decisions jointly with clients, involve clients in reasoning about therapy, expect clients to participate actively in all aspects of therapy, and are egalitarian in their approach. Therapists functioning in the collaborating mode also solicit ongoing feedback from their clients about the therapy process.

Therapists in the collaborating mode believe that clients are more likely to achieve positive outcomes if they take ownership of the therapy process. They tend to view clients as capable of determining what they need from therapy and selecting occupational therapy goals and tasks that address those needs. In this way, they work to promote

client empowerment, autonomy, independence, and personal choice. When disagreements or other interpersonal difficulties with clients occur, therapists who utilize the collaborating mode encourage clients to use their own judgment (Box 4.3).

Strengths of the Collaborating Mode

The collaborating mode reflects many of the core values of occupational therapy. Specifically, the field places a strong emphasis on promoting client choice, freedom, and autonomy. Therapists who utilize the collaborating mode demonstrate these values by enabling clients to choose activities, have opinions, and participate actively in evaluating the process of therapy and reflecting on their own performance. Use of the collaborating mode is likely to instill confidence in clients because it conveys the idea that the therapist views them as competent in their ability to direct their treatment, choose occupations, and gain greater control in determining the course of their own lives (Fig. 4.3).

Box 4.3 Using the Collaborating Mode

I met Edward, a 17-year-old boy, when he was admitted to the adolescent psychiatric unit for aggression toward staff and peers at his residential placement. At this time his primary diagnoses were conduct disorder, bipolar disorder, and posttraumatic stress disorder. Treatment was initiated with administration of the Adolescent Occupational Self Assessment, an interview developed for this setting based on the Model of Human Occupation (Kielhofner, 2002).

During his initial interview, Edward was cooperative but made no eye contact and gave vague answers to the questions asked about his daily routine. He lacked insight into his aggressive behaviors and took no personal responsibility for his actions. He perceived himself as being alone in the world and was anxious to move to independent living where he could come and go as he pleased. Edward had low self-esteem and a poorly defined sense of self. He was motivated to be successful in the role of worker, friend, boyfriend, family member, and student yet consistently experienced failure in all these roles. Edward also reported on the initial assessment interview that he was having some difficulty managing his affect and regulating his feelings.

Edward had a strong interest in origami and experienced a sense of success and pleasure when engaged in this activity. After a few weeks of interacting with Edward in various ways I felt that I could approach him with an idea that he might share his interest with the other clients on the unit. In an unassuming manner I asked him in the privacy of his own room if he would be interested in teaching his peers how to make some simple origami shapes. I asked him to think about it and made it clear that this was not a required assignment but felt that others might find this activity interesting. The next day I approached him in his room, and he

stated that he would like to teach this to others. I explained that we could co-lead an Interest Exploration group that meets every other Wednesday. I asked him what materials he needed, how much time he needed, and any other supports required. I wanted to empower him and encourage him to take a strong leadership role. We talked about how much time he needed to prepare and scheduled a time for us to meet and plan the group structure.

When the day came for group he was nervous about being in front of his peers, so we had a practice session where he role-played with me about what might occur in his role as a leader. We talked about listening when peers had a question and to be patient if some people had difficulty. I helped him empathize with his peers who might not have done this before and needed more support. I also explained to him that I was there to support him and that I was learning as well. If he needed any help, he could just ask. He agreed that I could help let him know when to slow down his teaching or if people were having difficulty hearing his directions (he had a soft voice and sometimes mumbled his words).

During the group meeting, I watched as his face broke into a shy smile when peers would thank him for sharing his skills and told him how much fun they had. Edward, if only for a brief time, had experienced what if feels to be appreciated, respected and even admired for his abilities. As we processed the group afterward, he shared that he had felt nervous at first but then became more comfortable and asked if we could co-lead another group. I felt that our therapeutic rapport had reached a new level in terms of Edward's willingness to trust me and to allow me to challenge him around developing a more defined sense of self.

— **Stephanie McCammon**

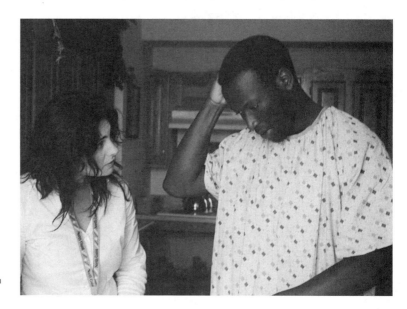

FIGURE 4.3 Collaborating mode. When planning a project, Stephanie McCammon is careful to look to her client for answers

Cautions of the Collaborating Mode

The cautions associated with a collaborative style are subtle and involve overreliance on this style or using it nonjudiciously across all types of therapy clients. The collaborating mode may not be received well by clients accustomed to, and who prefer to, view service providers as experts. Clients inclined to participate in social or cultural networks with hierarchical role structures may not value collaboration in therapy. Such clients may be looking for structured instruction, advice, resources, and ongoing direction.

Therapists who overvalue the collaborating mode may misunderstand or misperceive less-engaged clients as being passive or even apathetic about their therapy, when these clients are merely behaving within their own sociocultural comfort zones. This misperception is likely to be associated with a lack of understanding of the client's narrative, a breakdown in trust, and a lower quality of communication between the client and the therapist. If the therapist does not identify and examine this discrepancy in preferred working styles at a conscious level, she or he may become disappointed in the client or emotionally disengaged.

In some cases, unrestrained or unstructured collaboration may result in diffusion of responsibility or uncertainty regarding who is responsible for which part of the therapy process. Occasionally, it causes confusion about roles in the therapeutic relationship. In addition to these cautions, therapists who overutilize the collaborating mode run the risk of overestimating their clients' strengths and capacities, thereby minimizing the client's need for direction. There are times when clients need more directive therapy to feel a sense of psychological security and emotional stability. Asking clients to participate collaboratively before they are ready, or without grading the collaboration, sometimes causes clients to feel confused, lost, insecure, and/or anxious about the therapy process.

Empathizing Mode

As noted in the first chapter, there is a strong emphasis on empathy in contemporary discussions of occupational therapy. Use of the *empathizing mode* involves bearing witness to and fully understanding a client's physical, psychological, interpersonal, and emotional experience. Therapists who utilize the empathizing mode put a significant amount of time and effort into striving to understand a client's interpersonal needs and perspective as accurately as possible. They are able to notice and respond to the nuances in clients' affect and behavior, and they pay particular attention to clients' emotional experiences during therapy. Generally, they listen carefully, are watchful of what their clients communicate, and adjust their approach accordingly (Fig. 4.4).

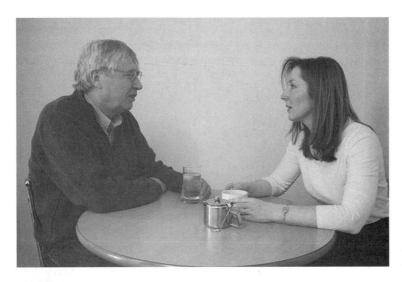

FIGURE 4.4 Empathizing mode. Jane Melton pauses from the usual activities of therapy in an attempt to understand a client's perspective

To ensure that they see things from the perspective of the client, therapists utilizing the empathizing mode periodically summarize what a client has said or make other nonverbal attempts to reflect their understanding of what the client is communicating. This strategy leads a client to either affirm the therapist's accuracy or reassert or reexplain his or her perspective. This process of careful listening/observing inevitably leads to a richer understanding of what is being communicated. During occupational therapy sessions that involve activity, empathizing requires a brief period of intermission from the "doing" aspects of therapy so the therapist can process and convey an understanding of what a client has communicated.

Therapists utilizing the empathizing mode take the time to accept and validate clients' difficult problems and painful emotions. They do not rush to intervene, solve or ameliorate them. Instead, they work slowly and cautiously, emphasizing an accurate reflection of the client's perspective and relying on their continual striving toward understanding to resolve rifts, obstacles, and conflicts that occur during therapy (Box 4.4).

> Therapists utilizing the empathizing mode take the time to accept and validate clients' difficult problems and painful emotions. They do not rush to intervene, solve, or ameliorate them.

Strengths of the Empathizing Mode

Empathy is vital to a functional and trusting therapeutic relationship (Kohut, 1984). Witnessing, validating, actively listening to, and understanding clients' experiences in the absence of judgment facilitates emotional healing and enables clients to organize their thinking independently and gain perspective on their difficulties. Empathizing with clients provides a model for them to learn to empathize with themselves and to self-reflect and gain insight into their emotional reactions and behaviors (Fig. 4.5).

In addition to these strengths, empathy is fundamental to the resolution of conflicts, rifts, and misunderstandings that occur during therapy. Because therapists who utilize the empathizing mode tend to be patient and understanding of negativity when it occurs, they are able to work more effectively with interpersonally challenging clients. Empathizing tends to disarm clients who are reluctant, resistant, critical, or otherwise negativistic in therapy. When therapists utilize empathy, clients are likely to feel responded to, cared about, and respected. They are more likely to achieve open, honest communication with clients. This

---

Box 4.4 Using the Empathizing Mode

Gretta is an 80-year-old woman who has had many life experiences, including an enduring and loving relationship with her husband. Four months before I met her, she experienced a severe stroke. Following her stroke and within weeks of beginning outpatient occupational therapy, her beloved husband died. Gretta had been depending on caretaking from her children and in-home attendants. She was referred to outpatient therapy to increase mobilization and participation in activities of daily living and independent activities of daily living.

Immediately, I recognized that Gretta was in a period of intensive mourning. I could see that this woman was searching for a human connection. She wanted to grieve and talk about her loss. At that time she was less interested in pursuing occupational therapy goals that would address her functional limitations. I knew I would have to wait to begin work on activities of daily living and, instead, focus on what she wanted to talk about: her husband, what he meant to her, how difficult it was to live in his absence, her thoughts about not wanting to burden her children.… I was very conscious about when to talk and when not to talk.… I made sure she knew that I had heard what she said and that I understood all of the difficulties she was facing.… I also made sure she knew that her thoughts and feelings made sense to me and that I accepted them and honored their importance.

For weeks we talked about her current situation, the limitations her stroke caused, how she reacted to it, and how her family reacted. In time, we worked together to create a family situation that would make it easier for everyone to cope with the recent death. I was careful not to mention our discussions or disclose her private thoughts and feelings to her family members. A feeling of mutual trust developed between the two of us. We worked together to manage her stroke and her grieving. As a result, we also made progress toward the original goals of the therapy.

Gretta taught me the importance of having empathy. For her, it was important that I showed an interest in her grieving and that she could tell a person outside her family about her problems and worries. Because Gretta allowed me to support her through empathy, we both saw the improvements in her emotional condition during therapy.

— **Anne Reuter**

---

typically increases trust and results in a more stable therapeutic relationship.

Cautions of the Empathizing Mode

It would seem that a therapist could never empathize too much with clients. However, the empathizing mode is no different than the other modes in that its overuse can cause difficulty. For some clients, overemphasis on the empathizing mode can place emotions too much in the foreground of therapy. Some clients may not be ready to see or hear their emotions reflected back to them. Instead, they may feel more stable and comfortable focus-

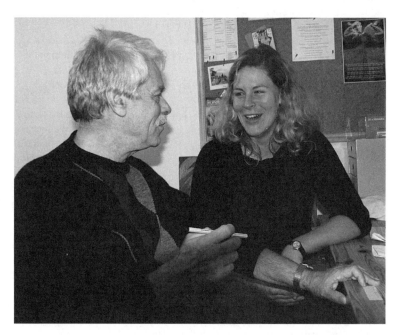

FIGURE 4.5 By sharing a laugh with her client, Anne Reuter reflects her client's value for humor and conveys that she understands the irony of a story he just told

ing on activity and other practical behavioral aspects of occupational therapy. Similarly, if a therapist relies too heavily on empathy, the pacing of treatment is slow, and some of the fundamental tasks of therapy may be delayed or left unaccomplished. For clients who are not yet ready to engage in occupational therapy, this slower pace may be necessary and appropriate. However, therapists who rely too heavily on the empathizing mode may project their own needs for empathy onto the client. As a result, they may misread the client's actual level of need for empathy. Therapists who show their own emotional reactions to what the clients are saying and/or that probe too much for emotional expression from the client are perceived by some clients as overinvolved or psychologically intrusive. These clients may respond by recoiling from what they perceive as too much intimacy or emotional intensity.

Even when a client invites or appears comfortable with the empathizing mode, overutilizing it can overprotect clients. Listening and validating may occur at the expense of questioning or challenging clients to engage in occupation when they are ready. Overreliance on empathy may encourage an inappropriate level of dependence in more vulnerable or isolated clients. In addition, there is a risk that some clients may become confused about the goals of therapy and about the role of the occupational therapist in his or her treatment. In the absence of appropriate boundaries (e.g., time limits, delineation of the limits of the professional relationship) some clients begin to perceive the occupational therapist as a friend and become disappointed, rejected, or abandoned when the therapist does not behave accordingly in other domains. Other risks associated with overreliance on the empathizing mode include the possibility of overidentification with clients, emotional overinvolvement, guilt over the limitations of what a therapist can actually do for clients, and resulting feelings of burnout.

Encouraging Mode

The *encouraging mode* is one in which a therapist works to instill clients with hope, courage, and the will to explore or perform a given activity. Some therapists refer to themselves as "cheerleaders" when functioning in this mode. Therapists who use the encouraging mode frequently use such strategies as compliments, applause, and cheering. They make heartening statements as a means of evoking a desired behavior in a client. They may rejoice and celebrate with clients when they are successful.

Some therapists use such strategies as humor, entertaining gestures or antics, singing or dancing, and demonstrations of involvement to improve their clients' mood, distract them from anxiety or reluctance, and improve their desire to participate in occupations. Generally, therapists who utilize the encouraging mode attempt any clever or creative twist on activity to generate or help sustain a client's interest in occupational engagement (Box 4.5).

Strengths of the Encouraging Mode
There are a number of strengths associated with functioning in the encouraging mode. Therapists who prefer this mode tend to be open and generous in their emotional expression. They project a great deal of positive energy, and they are particularly skilled at conveying their optimism and hope to their clients. They are willing to celebrate and be joyful with their clients. Some therapists functioning in this mode are viewed as playful by their clients, and this playful attitude may be particularly effective with children. Similarly, therapists functioning in the encouraging mode may be particularly capable of reaching clients with more severe developmental and cognitive impairments because they may use forms of communication that convey emotional energy and have multisensory components. Some therapists functioning in the encouraging mode are also skilled at using incentives to elicit participation. Because of their ability to convey their belief in a client's potential for success, these therapists may be more likely than other therapists to elicit participation from clients who are otherwise anxious, demoralized, or reluctant to participate in therapy (Fig. 4.6).

Cautions of the Encouraging Mode
Although there are few cautions associated with providing clients with encouragement, if the encouraging mode is overused clients may become desensitized to its use over time. Some clients grow to expect the therapist to bolster them to such an extent that they have difficulty developing a sense of intrinsic motivation independently of the therapist.

In some circumstances, use of the encouraging mode with the wrong type of client carries a risk of being misinterpreted. Some clients are in an emotional state that does not allow them to hear or internalize compliments, a hopeful scenario, or comments about their strengths and capacities. Certain clients may undervalue or interpret a therapist's efforts to introduce hope, humor, play, or games into the relationship as being insulting, belittling, foolish, or manipulative. For example, a therapist once relayed a story in which she attempted to conduct a therapy group for adults with substance abuse problems that focused on ways to increase positive energy and hope. Her ideas were quickly rejected by the group members.

Box 4.5   Using the Encouraging Mode: Michele Shapiro Finds a Way to Capture a Client's Interest

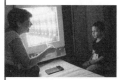

Rachel was a 4-year-old girl who was referred for treatment of selective mutism. She would speak only at home with her mother and father. I decided that the framework of a playgroup of peers her own age would be the optimal medium to increase her desire to speak with others. During the months of treatment, I told her that she would only be accepted into the playgroup on the condition that she would *not* speak in the group. I told her she would be allowed to make animal noises and other sounds but that talking was prohibited. I saw by the stars in her eyes that she liked the idea.

Along with sensory integration techniques, I tied up a big sheet that divided the treatment room into two halves. Among other things, I produced dramatic plays that featured the children in the playgroup as actors. The stage became an enticing place for all the children in the playgroup to show their talents while acting out different scenarios. At first, Rachel would smile and draw during the plays. Slowly, she began to make animal sounds. I showed greater appreciation of her performances when they included characters that made sounds.

After a short time, Rachel decided that sounds did not adequately convey what she wanted to express, and she began to say words. I would respond dramatically by making a fuss and contending that speaking words was not in keeping with the group's rules. Soon, her peers sensed her disappointment about not being permitted to say words. They began to support her by trying to convince me to change the rules so that Rachel could speak during the plays. As a group, we then decided that the new rule for the group would be that everyone, including Rachel, had to use words to communicate. Rachel agreed to this plan and over time she began to speak more fluently in full sentences. She made significant progress at school, too.

I chose to be dramatic and demonstrative in the groups so the playgroup was infused with high emotional valence, and Rachel could easily read my feelings toward her. Through my affect I conveyed that I believed in her, was excited about her participation in the group at any level, and was willing to vigorously support her and meet her at the level at which she wanted to begin work (not speaking). At the same time, I made it clear to her (and to her peers) that I took the group, and its rules, very seriously. Through my emotional tone and enthusiasm, the playgroup became a big deal for Rachel and her peers.

Initially, I deliberately ignored the importance of Rachel's speech to her participation in the playgroup so its emotional and social desirability would become self-apparent over time. Quickly it became clear to Rachel that, without speech, she was limited in the extent and level at which she could interact with her peers to create plays. In addition, speech became desirable to Rachel because its meaning was transformed from an anxiety-provoking activity that others demanded from her into an enticing and taboo behavior in which only she was forbidden to participate. In addition to this particular approach to use of self, the fact that she enjoyed creating plays was motivating for Rachel. Peer pressure from her new similar-aged friends also served as a powerful lever for her full participation in the group.

— **Michele Shapiro**

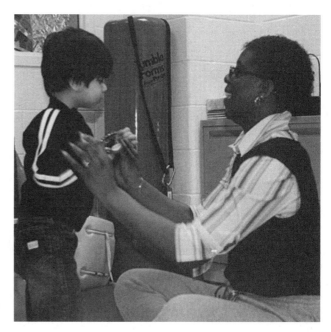

FIGURE 4.6 Encouraging mode. Belinda Anderson enjoys a song and a dance with a client.

Instructing Mode

Therapists who utilize the *instructing mode* emphasize education of clients in therapy and assume a teaching style in their interactions with clients. Therapists who use the instructing mode are skilled at providing clients with detailed descriptions of the objectives and tasks of therapy, providing a clear rationale for the content of therapy, training clients in the performance of specific occupational therapy activities, and providing feedback to clients about the therapy process. They can speak clearly and confidently about any aspect of the therapy process and excel at being structured, active, and directive.

They provide their clients with information, direction, recommendations, and in some circumstances advice. When functioning in the instructing mode, therapists utilize instructional statements and mini-lectures, role-modeling and demonstrations, statements that convey feedback to the client, and a dialogue that involves questions and answers as the primary form of therapy communication. Therapists functioning in the instructing mode are unafraid to state their professional opinion, set limits, provide feedback, or disagree with clients. When certain clients and/or circumstances make it necessary, these therapists are skilled at gentle or finessed approaches to confrontation in order to introduce the need for change. Therapists functioning in this mode may approach disagreements with clients by reexplaining their own point of view, providing more of a rationale for their perspective, explaining consequences of

a poor decision, and/or educating clients further about the value of their approach (Box 4.6).

Strengths of the Instructing Mode

The instructing mode is one of the fundamental modes required for the competent conduct of occupational therapy. Without some degree of structure, transfer of knowledge, provision of feedback, and overall leadership, occupational therapy simply would not occur.

Therapists who utilize this mode tend to be excellent teachers and clear communicators. They empower and inspire their clients by sharing information, noting accomplishments, providing constructive feedback, and training their clients to utilize the tools required for adaptation and participation. They convey caring and hope through their investment in a client's performance and in the positive outcomes of therapy. Therapists who function in the instructing mode tend to be highly organized and systematic in their approach to therapy. They inject a lot of intellectual energy and creativity into the therapy process.

Cautions of the Instructing Mode

As with any of the other modes, cautions emerge when therapists overutilize or inappropriately and indiscriminately apply the instructing mode with clients. Because the instructing mode usually involves focusing on positive outcomes over process, some therapists functioning in this mode may overinvest and thus react more negatively when they cannot get clients to do what they would like them to

---

Box 4.6 Using the Instructing Mode: Kim Eberhardt Responds to a Client's Question About Cookware

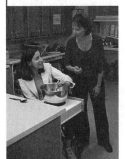

Kay is a 26-year-old woman who was severely injured in a skiing accident. She is paralyzed as a result of a spinal cord injury. Because she also had a hip fracture as a result of the accident, her hospital stay was prolonged. I saw her as an inpatient for a period of 4 months. She is a naturally positive, strong, motivated, internally driven person. She had a creative outlook on occupational therapy and approached her goals in a systematic and self-disciplined manner.

Because Kay was so self-motivated, most of the time I found myself functioning in the collaborating mode when we planned therapy goals and activities. However, there were many times during Kay's therapy when I felt she was asking me to function in the instructing mode. These were times when Kay

requested that I teach her specific skills related to activities of daily living. It was common that Kay would begin our sessions by anticipating that she would need to learn a certain skill, such as handling glasses in a restaurant or learning how to cut her own food.

Another responsibility included in my role as instructor was to bear witness to Kay's self-monitoring of her own performance. To do this, we put a piece of paper on the wall that listed her functional accomplishments for each day of therapy. Our systematic daily monitoring of her progress made it feel like she was in school. I believe this was developmentally familiar to her and it gave her a sense of consistency and control. At first, her accomplishments were small. We would write "I moved my little finger today" or "I rolled to the side by myself." Soon her accomplishments progressed to: "I ate today without Kim dropping any food." By the time Kay left the hospital the wall was covered with documentation of her accomplishments.

— **Kim Eberhardt**

do. Alternatively, they may tend to bolster, overprotect, or overinstruct their clients to prevent them from experiencing failure in therapy. These behaviors can undermine clients' confidence, choice, and autonomy.

Occasionally, clients misunderstand or misinterpret therapists' behavior in the instructing mode as being parental, authoritarian, dominant, controlling, or demanding. Therapists who overutilize this mode may feel obligated to help all clients address their difficulties and may miss the point at which clients want them to simply listen and validate them. As a result, they are occasionally at risk for getting locked into arguments and power struggles with sensitive or vulnerable clients or parents who require a more empathic approach.

Problem-Solving Mode

Individuals who favor the *problem-solving mode* rely heavily on using reason and logic in their relationships with clients. They may be exceptionally talented technical thinkers, or they may have excellent technical abilities. For example, some have the expertise required to create new devices or approaches to treatment. They may have expertise in theory-based interventions, evidence-based practice, complex treatment protocols, splinting, developing or redesigning physical environments to make them accessible, modifying or constructing equipment, or creating other kinds of physical adaptations for clients.

Therapists functioning in the problem-solving mode generally approach the interpersonal aspects of therapy by reasoning or by using other logical approaches, such as strategic questioning aimed at enabling a client to see a wider range of options, consequences, or dimensions of the issue. They often pose strategic questions so clients may consider alternative perspectives. To resolve interpersonal difficulties with clients, therapists functioning in the problem-solving mode are likely to structure the dialogue, outline guidelines for negotiation of differences, or draw on other well-established steps to resolve conflict (Box 4.7).

Box 4.7 Using the Problem-Solving Mode

Madam Bouchard is a 47-year-old woman with schizoaffective disorder. She was admitted to the inpatient unit after a police officer arrested her for driving on the wrong side of traffic on a highway at 5:00 in the morning. She was brought to the hospital because she seemed lost and confused about the incident.

At the beginning of therapy, Madam Bouchard was hypersensitive about the sounds, expressions, and movements made by me and the other therapists on her care team. She would often misinterpret the intentions behind very benign and meaningless body movements as being judgmental, menacing, or threatening. When participating in activities, she fixated on environmental stimuli and on my nonverbal reactions to her rather than concentrating on the activity itself. She often expressed a fear that staff (including me) would keep her in the hospital indefinitely and that we intended to physically harm her. (I discovered that these fears stemmed from an abusive relationship with her husband, and I initiated a social work intervention to address the situation.)

One of the many goals of individual therapy sessions with Madam Bouchard involved reducing her interpersonal anxiety, hypersensitivity, and misinterpretations of nonverbal behaviors during interactions. I arranged a series of structured craft activities with specific steps that would lead to replication of a real-life object (e.g., weaving a basket, painting watercolor according to a model, making a drinking cup out of clay according to a model). These activities allowed Madam Bouchard to orient to reality and center her thinking in the present moment. To address her interpersonal anxieties, I also engaged in other types of craft activities alongside her. I selected my activities based on their potential to force me to move and be physically active during our sessions.

The fact we worked beside each other on a separate activity gave ample opportunity for Madam Bouchard to interpret my gestures and reactions. Once she was emotionally stable and centered in her activity, I would initiate a medium level of physical activity in the room related to completing my craft. Then I would invite her to share her perception of a specific recent situation in which I moved in her presence. If her perception was correct I would affirm its accuracy.

If her perception was incorrect and not based in reality, I used strategic questions to inquire about the basic point of reference that prompted her to arrive at her conclusion. If my questioning did not lead her to recognize that the reality of our here-and-now interaction was different from her internal thoughts and worries, I invited Madam Bouchard to engage in hypothesis testing. I would introduce a set of alternative hypotheses for interpreting my movements and nonverbal reactions during the session. Together, we analyzed each possibility using a problem-solving approach. To make our analysis concrete, I wrote the options down on paper or on a dry-erase board. The objective of this problem-solving exercise was to introduce the possibility of doubt into her misperceptions and to broaden her viewpoint regarding the myriad possible motives behind another person's actions.

This process allowed Madam Bouchard to verbally express and describe her perceptions without fear of judgment. It also allowed her to practice utilizing reasoning as a means of testing the accuracy of her interpretations of other people's social behaviors. Over time, she naturally used problem-solving as a means of coping with her worries and fears concerning her relationships with others.

— **René Bélanger**

Strengths of the Problem-Solving Mode

Therapists functioning in the problem-solving mode are efficient, self-disciplined, straightforward in their communications, and solution-oriented. Because of their high level of focus on the techniques of therapy and on expanding clients' thinking about activity, their work carries an increased potential to result in tangible and direct benefits to clients ready to engage. Owing to the logical and systematic manner in which they choose to communicate, some therapists functioning in the problem-solving mode are more likely to work through interpersonal difficulties with clients in the absence of abundant emotion or drama. Clients uncomfortable with a more emotion-focused approach to the therapeutic relationship may feel more at ease with the structure, predictability, and professionalism conveyed by therapists who use the problem-solving mode. Because of this air of professionalism, all clients who work with problem-solving therapists are more likely to understand the interpersonal boundaries and limitations of the therapeutic relationship (Fig. 4.7).

Cautions of the Problem-Solving Mode

As with other modes, it is impossible for the problem-solving mode to work with all clients in all situations. When therapists function in the problem-solving mode, some are vulnerable to assuming an expert stance or a more challenging approach without paying enough attention to other interpersonal needs the client may bring to the relationship. Some clients find a therapist's adoption of such roles reassuring or enlightening, whereas others interpret the therapist's behavior as too strategic or even intimidating. In addition, therapists in the problem-solving mode may be vulnerable to the unwitting use of technical terms and language in settings where using such language may not be optimal. Some clients and professionals from other disciplines may not understand this language.

In the presence of sensitive, vulnerable, or otherwise interpersonally demanding clients, the interpersonal behavior of problem-solving therapists may be misinterpreted as aloof, judgmental, or distant. Therapists who overutilize the problem-solving mode may be less comfortable with approaches that require more emotionally intense levels of interaction and communication. For example, some therapists replace the need for empathy with overreliance on the more pragmatic technical and mechanical elements of therapy. If this is the case, it leaves the relationship more vulnerable to misunderstandings and other rifts in communication and interaction.

Modes in Perspective

The six therapeutic modes described in this chapter are based on frequently observed interpersonal behaviors that occur in occupational therapy. Although examples of how each of these modes is used in practice are provided, there is no single "typical" manner in which a therapist might enact a mode or a set of modes when working with a client.

Also, the modes were discussed and illustrated in isolation of each other. However, there are countless possibilities for ways in which these modes are combined during therapeutic encounters. Modes may and should be used

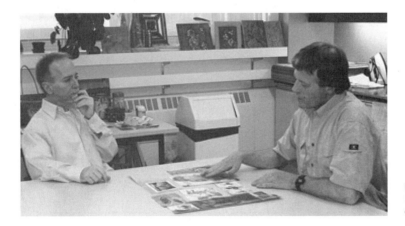

FIGURE 4.7 Problem-solving mode. René Bélanger and his client analyze the past and consider choices for the future

interchangeably provided they do not blend into one another during a single communication. As introduced in Chapter 3, to be most therapeutic a mode must be used purely, without confusion with another mode. Pure use of modes communicates a single message, and it ensures that the therapist is taking responsibility for his or her chosen means of communicating within a given moment. When you wish to shift from one mode to another, you should ensure that there is a strong rationale for the mode shift and that the two modes can be easily distinguishable. For example, when a therapist functioning in the collaborative mode when a client is engaging in a familiar task notes that a client appears to need more structure and guidance when engaging in an unfamiliar task, it may naturally prompt a shift from the collaborating mode to the instructing mode. In this case the therapist may cease turning to the client for input and may instead step in to provide clear instruction, make suggestions along the way, and provide constructive feedback.

Blending modes occurs when a therapist is not clear about her or his intended message and conveys two modes simultaneously within a single moment of communication. For example, when a therapist intends to empathize with a client but, instead, blends the empathizing mode with the instructing mode, he or she sends a mixed message to the client about his or her true thoughts, feelings, and intentions. For example, a therapist locked in a power struggle with a client over his or her alcohol use sends a mixed message by saying in a single breath: "I understand why you want to use alcohol, but I need to educate you on why you shouldn't." This can be confusing for clients, and it weakens the intended message or messages. Ultimately, it may weaken the therapist's influence within the relationship and the client's trust in the process.

Much more can be accomplished interpersonally if a therapist shifts modes more deliberately. In this case, the therapist would take considerable time to listen and understand the client's perspective on alcohol use and then shift into an instructing mode to educate the client only after verifying that the client has received the intended empathic message first. Additional suggestions for ensuring that each of the modes a therapist selects is used purely include:

- Think about what message you believe the client needs to hear at the moment and remain utterly loyal to that message for that moment.
- Occasionally remind yourself why it is therapeutic for the client to hear a given message.

- Take responsibility for what you say or ask of a client, even if you are setting a limit or engaging in something else that feels interpersonally risky. This means that if a message was intended to set a limit or to challenge the client, you should maintain the message even if the client reacts negatively. Therapists should never try to deny or distort the original message based on a client's reaction to it.

Additional examples of ways in which therapists have drawn upon the various therapeutic modes to manage various interpersonal events in practice are included in later chapters.

Therapeutic Style: Using The Modes

As therapists become more experienced, they may begin to notice that they emphasize and draw upon certain modes more often than others when treating clients. Accordingly, they develop a *therapeutic style*, or a skill set that incorporates the therapeutic modes they view as being maximally therapeutic for their clients.

For example, Jane Melton describes herself as having a "natural optimistic belief in people" and as drawing upon her determination, patience, and ability to empathize and listen to clients reflectively as well as her honesty, tact, resilience, and gentleness when providing feedback and working with clients. Although Jane utilizes a number of interpersonal modes and adapts them thoughtfully depending on the unique needs of each client, her self-description indicates that she draws most heavily on her natural hope and optimism, her belief in her clients' capacity for autonomy and independence, her self-discipline as it manifests in the form of patience, her preference for listening and understanding over activity-focusing or rushing into doing, and her overall gentleness of style. Empathizing, collaborating, and encouraging are Jane's primary modes of interaction.

However, we saw earlier in this chapter that she also uses the advocating mode to ensure that her clients receive the entitlements they deserve, such as fully accessible housing. Although Jane mostly uses the empathizing, collaborating, and encouraging modes, she maintains and utilizes additional modes as required by the unique demands of any given client or therapeutic situation. As an experienced therapist, Jane possesses a broad repertoire of therapeutic modes.

Broadening One's Repertoire of Modes: A Central Objective of the Intentional Relationship Model

The broader the repertoire of modes a therapist can draw upon to adjust to clients' various interpersonal presentations and demands, the more likely it is that the therapist can function effectively with even the most resistant and interpersonally difficult clients. Because therapists' personalities are relatively stable, it is a natural inclination for them to invoke modes that fall within their "comfort zone." For example, a person who is reserved, quiet, and mostly other-oriented during most social interactions likely feels more comfortable in the empathizing and collaborative modes (i.e., empathizing with and listening to clients, allowing them to take the lead in therapy, and facilitating their independence, autonomy, and choice). This same therapist may feel less comfortable working with passive clients or those who require a therapist to be more directive, assertive, frank, evaluative, or even appropriately confrontational.

Conversely, a therapist who is extroverted, comfortable asserting her needs in relationships, and self-assured in sharing her knowledge with others may find it relatively easy to be directive, assertive, frank, evaluative, or even confrontational with her clients. This therapist's preferred modes may be the instructing and problem-solving modes. However, a therapist such as this one may unwittingly undermine a client's autonomy and choice; he or she may lack patience, may pace the therapy too quickly, or may be vulnerable to becoming involved in power struggles with clients who behave in resistant or confrontational ways.

Any preferred mode that falls within our comfort zone has a benefit and a downside. Moreover, one's preferred modes do not work for all clients or in all circumstances. To function with as much intentionality in therapeutic relationships as possible, therapists have a responsibility to extend their capacity to function within a wide range of interpersonal modes during therapy. A more extensive repertoire of interpersonal modes allows you to communicate more effectively with a wider range of clients. More specifically, it allows you to respond to clients in ways that more accurately address their interpersonal needs. Accurately identifying each client's preference for therapeutic interaction and responding in ways that meet each client's interpersonal preferences conveys

to our clients that we are willing to interact and work with them in their comfort zones rather than in our own.

Adjusting our own responses to the covert or expressed interpersonal needs of each client is possible only if we possess the capacity to exhibit a wide enough range of interpersonal behaviors in therapy. When we draw on ways of interacting that are inconsistent with our values or that we simply have not learned or practiced as often in social situations, we are immediately forced out of our own interpersonal comfort zones. However, the departure from our own comfort zone is sometimes the only means by which it is possible to enter the interpersonal worlds of our clients.

For example, Michele Shapiro works with pediatric clients, some of whom are nonverbal and severely developmentally disabled. With these low-functioning clients, Michele had for many years been accustomed to assuming a structured and goal-directed approach to therapy. Once she broadened her approach to include careful vigilance toward her clients needs and nondirective strategies, Michele recognized that she was more able to engage a wider range of her clients in therapy. During our interview, Michele disclosed:

> Years ago when I worked with learning disabled kids, I remember sometimes feeling that I must try to "control" the child's behavior. Now I prefer working with a child who has special needs and is out of control. When I do my detective work and decipher the base of the sensory problem, then it makes me feel good. In the past I needed to see things happening to know I was successful—today a child's smile makes me feel that the session was successful.

Locating One's Comfort Zone of Preferred Modes

A central objective of the intentional relationship model (IRM) is to identify one's current "comfort zone" of interpersonal behavior during therapy. As you develop as a therapist, it is similarly important to practice broadening that comfort zone to include increasingly unfamiliar and unutilized interpersonal styles, or modes. The beginning of the chapter asked you to complete the Self-Assessment of Modes Questionnaire located in the Activities section (Exercise 4.1). Now, you should use those responses to fill out the Personal Modes Profile that follows in Exercise 4.1. Doing so will indicate your preferred therapeutic modes and their relative strength. Following this, you should identify less familiar modes that might strengthen your relationships with clients or allow you to practice more successfully with a broader range of client personalities in Exercise 4.2.

Therapeutic Style and Personality: Striving Toward Integration

The idea of developing a therapeutic style and using modes can be misunderstood as lacking a sense of genuineness. However, this conclusion emanates from a misunderstanding of the role of genuineness in therapy. The genuine therapist is one who sincerely wants and makes an effort to do what is best for the client. Genuineness is not simply being yourself. It is being the best person you can be, given the client's needs.

That said, it is nonetheless important for therapists to strive toward and integrate their therapeutic style and their more innate personalities. The closer one's core personality is to one's therapeutic style, the more likely it is that a therapist feels able to interact therapeutically with clients in ways that feel natural. Thus, although it is important to broaden one's repertoire of therapeutic modes, it is equally important to develop a therapeutic style that feels true and is generally consistent with one's personality.

To a certain extent, every therapist must practice a degree of interpersonal self-discipline. That is, you must exercise restraint regarding the extent to which you reveal all aspects of your personality to clients. The Occupational Therapy Code of Ethics (AOTA, 2005) and occupational therapy's core values statement (AOTA, 1993) reinforce that it is in the best interest of clients to conduct therapy with prudence and circumspection. This sometimes includes controlling one's interpersonal impulses and always avoiding interactions with clients that may be perceived as exploitive or emotionally harmful. Any experienced therapist knows that at certain moments during therapy practice, particularly with more challenging clients, it takes impulse control and significant restraint to draw only on the aspects of one's personality that have the potential to be therapeutic. It is impossible to appreciate all clients equally, and there are moments when we may wish to show clients we find more difficult how we really feel about them, but our values, ethics, and better judgment prevent us from doing this.

As therapists develop expertise in the therapeutic use of self, they find that they do not have to work as hard as

they did before to exercise this capacity for circumspection and self-restraint. As therapists become more experienced in the use of self, the act of interacting therapeutically comes to feel natural. This sense of naturalness comes from knowing the benefits and limits of one's natural modes and developing comfort utilizing the modes that were not, at first, as easy to use. In addition, therapists often feel they can function more seamlessly with certain types of clients and in settings that match their natural inclinations, using certain modes rather than others. For example, a therapist once shared that she enjoys working with young children because she can freely draw on the encouraging mode without fear of judgment if she happens to overuse the mode with a given client. Similarly, another therapist once told me that she prefers working in physical rehabilitation settings because she enjoys functioning in the role of teacher in that much of her job involves demonstrating certain tasks and instructing clients to relearn important daily living skills.

More-experienced therapists often see little difference between their therapeutic styles and the ways they typically behave with friends and family. Even though they may feel more relaxed and spontaneous in their relationships with clients, therapists for whom there is little difference between their therapeutic styles and their everyday personalities tend to make fewer interpersonal oversights with their clients; they tend to say and do the appropriate things at the right times. For example, when they provide feedback to a client that might be difficult to hear, it is well timed—consistent with their general way of relating—and presented with great sensitivity and tact. Therapists whose therapeutic style matches their personality generally feel they do not have to exercise considerable emotional restraint and extensive tactical thinking during therapy.

Vardit Kindler provides a succinct description of this match. She describes her therapeutic style and her personality as relatively indistinguishable.

> My general style of relating is very informal. I accept everyone as an equal. I look at people's strengths without being overly critical. This is my style of relating both inside and outside therapy. — Vardit Kindler

Similarly, Carmen-Gloria de las Heras explains:

> I flow easily between the two. I keep my way of being. I am spontaneous and generous. I am firm when I have to be, but I keep my fundamental belief in people. I am myself with clients as I am with everyone else. — Carmen-Gloria de las Heras

This ability to integrate and see an increasing number of parallels between one's therapeutic personality and one's personality outside of therapy, combined with the ability to draw on a wide repertoire of interpersonal behaviors as appropriate for any given interaction, may be associated with decreased feelings of burnout and frustration. Having a therapeutic style that feels consistent with one's day-to-day personality is referred to as an ***integrated*** use of self.

 KEY TERMS

Integrated use of self: having a therapeutic style that feels consistent with one's day-to-day personality is referred to as integrated use of self.

References

American Occupational Therapy Association (AOTA) (2005). *Occupational therapy code of ethics.* Bethesda, MD: AOTA. Retrieved from http://www.aota.org/ on October 1, 2005.

American Occupational Therapy Association (1993). Core values and attitudes of occupational therapy practice. *American Journal of Occupational Therapy, 47,* 1085–1086.

Beck, A. T., Freeman, A., & Davis, D. D. (1990). *Cognitive therapy of personality disorders.* New York: Guilford Press.

Carlson, N. R. (1998). *Physiology of behavior* (6th ed.). Boston: Allyn & Bacon.

Kagan, J. (2000). Temperament. In A. E. Kazdin (Ed.), *Encyclopedia of psychology* (Vol 8, pp. 34–37). Washington, DC: American Psychological Association.

Kohut, H. (1984). *How does analysis cure?* Chicago: University of Chicago Press.

Summary: No Therapist is Perfect

The "cautions" section under each of the interpersonal modes reveals one of the hidden secrets of therapeutic use of self—that no therapist is perfect. There is no way to escape the caveats and downsides that go along with any therapeutic mode or set of modes. One key to intentional use of self is to familiarize oneself with the caveats to each of the modes that are part of one's therapeutic style. The more you develop an ability to draw on as many modes as necessary and appropriate for a given client, the more likely you are to avoid overutilizing one style at the expense of using a more appropriate or more indicated style for that client.

ACTIVITIES FOR LEARNING AND REFLECTION

Self-Assessment of Modes Questionnaire

As noted earlier in this chapter, it is important that you complete this assessment before reading the rest of the chapter. It will reduce any inclination you may have to go back and change your responses based on the contents of this chapter and increase the likelihood you will achieve more accurate insight into your therapeutic style.

This assessment is designed to allow you to identify whether you have a dominant way or central set of ways of responding to various interpersonal issues that arise in therapy. Please do not think too hard about the responses and respond with your first impulse as if you were facing the situations described in real-time practice. All responses represent plausible therapeutic actions, and there are no incorrect responses. It is essential that you check *only one* response for each question. It is recognized that your actual response may depend on information that is not available in the case description. The point of this questionnaire is not to ascertain a correct response but to ascertain the one that is most comfortable for you at first impulse. When you respond, you should choose the response that would be the easiest, most natural, or most comfortable for you in that situation.

1. Daniel, a client with schizophrenia, just began a supportive employment program. He indicated that with the stress of working he is starting to have increased auditory hallucinations, and he is worried that his supervisor will notice that something is wrong and he won't be able to keep his job. He is following his psychiatrist's recommendation to increase his medication. What is the *first* thing that you would do?
   a. ___ Review with Daniel strategies he might use to manage his hallucinations on the job.
   b. ___ Ask Daniel what he thinks he will need to do in order to continue to work.
   c. ___ Work with Daniel to list and evaluate options for how he might cope with these circumstances.
   d. ___ Point out to Daniel that he has certain rights to accommodation in the workplace and offer to help him negotiate for what he needs.
   e. ___ Acknowledge how difficult it is to begin a new job and at the same time have his symptoms increase.

2. A young client's insurance company denies a wheelchair that the client had his heart set on. The client shows that he is emotionally upset. What is the *first* thing that you would do?
   a. ___ Tell the client that there is always a way to work the system to get the right equipment.
   b. ___ Tell the client you see how upset he is and tell him he has a right to be upset.
   c. ___ Help the client look at alternatives, other wheelchairs, other possible ways of funding.
   d. ___ Ask the client what he thinks should be done about it.
   e. ___ Offer to call the insurance company, file a complaint, and ask for a review.

3. An elderly client becomes tearful over the difficulty that she is having making a toilet transfer and indicates that she is worried that she is going to end up in a nursing home and won't be able to return to her home that she has lived in for 30 years. Assuming that the client does have the ability to eventually learn the transfer, which would be your *first* course of action?

   a. ____ Comment on how difficult a situation she feels that she is in and offer to stop the activity to talk about it.

   b. ____ Show her how to do it so that she can see that she can master it, counting on the likelihood that this will help her feel better.

   c. ____ Reassure the client that with sufficient practice she will be able to learn to make the transfer.

   d. ____ Tell her that there are organizations out there who will see to it that she is not put in a nursing home against her will.

   e. ____ Encourage the client to think about other options to entering a nursing home, such as recruiting a full-time personal assistant if she ultimately can't learn the transfer.

4. Carrie, a 12-year-old client with cerebral palsy, tells you she is sad about something one of her peers said about her at school today in reference to her disability. She tells you that she is tired of being different and that she just wants to fit in like everyone else. What would be your *first* response?

   a. ____ Tell Carrie you can see how sad she is about this comment and encourage her to tell you more about it.

   b. ____ Tell Carrie not to worry about it and that you know there are lots of students who like her. Remind her of something positive a classmate said about her a couple weeks ago.

   c. ____ Tell Carrie you have confidence she can handle this and ask her what she thinks she ought to do.

   d. ____ Tell Carrie you are going to call the teacher and recommend that the class have a lecture to raise her classmates' awareness of disabled people and their experiences and rights.

5. Rod is a 48-year-old client with an orthopedic injury and a major depressive episode that began following a break-up of a long-term relationship 1 year ago. Rod tells you that he feels very isolated and doubts anyone would ever want to date him. What would be your *first* response?

   a. ____ Reassure Rod that there are many people in the world who would likely want to date him.

   b. ____ Educate Rod that the feelings he is having stem from his underlying depression.

   c. ____ Work with Rod on building social skills to help him feel more confident in social/dating situations.

   d. ____ Provide Rod with suggestions or resources where he can meet people.

   e. ____ Ask Rod if he would like to work on outlining options for meeting people as one of his therapy goals.

6. Julie, your 60-year-old client with multiple sclerosis, chose to raise her children as a stay-at-home-mom rather than work during most of her life. Recently, her illness has become more severe, and you have been working with her on energy conservation strategies. While you are in the process of fitting her with a motorized wheelchair, she tells you that she is envious of your health and your ability to be able to do something meaningful with your life. How would you be inclined to respond?

   a. ____ Support Julie to review options for ways she might find more meaning in her current occupational roles.

   b. ____ Reassure Julie that mothering is, in itself, a very meaningful occupation and that the choices she made were the right ones at the time.

c. ___ Ask Julie if she would like to switch the focus of therapy to considering what might be meaningful occupations for her.

d. ___ Convey concern in your emotional expression and make your best effort to summarize how she must be feeling.

e. ___ Tell Julie that, if it is something that is important to her, with the right equipment, accommodations, and accessibility, she would be able to engage in work that was meaningful to her despite the severity of her symptoms.

7. You have been seeing Jennifer, a 16-year-old client with low average intellectual functioning and who has had symptoms of autistic spectrum disorder since she was 10 years old. Over time, you have noticed that Jennifer has difficulty saying "no" to things that she does not want to do. Instead, she simply does something else or does not follow through. For the past few weeks, you have noticed an unusual pattern develop where she occasionally goes to the local video game machines (next door to the rehabilitation center) during the times you and she usually meet for therapy. The new pattern does not make sense to you because you thought she was enjoying therapy. What would you be your first inclination?

a. ___ Remind Jennifer of the importance of attending therapy rather than playing video games.

b. ___ Ask Jennifer about the reasons behind her recent decision to go to the video arcade instead of attending therapy.

c. ___ The next time Jennifer doesn't show up for therapy, go to the video arcade and see if she'll allow you to play some games with her. Use that as a launching pad for discussion about her recent attendance problems.

d. ___ Encourage Jennifer to develop a schedule that will allow her enough time to play video games and attend therapy.

e. ___ View Jennifer's desire to play video games as an indirect communication that she may not need therapy or find it as useful as she did in the past. Discuss this possibility with Jennifer and show that you are open to taking a break if she wishes.

8. You are seeing Janice, a gifted and accomplished young woman, to facilitate management of symptoms of depression as well as chronic fatigue. Over the past five sessions, you have noticed an interpersonal pattern develop in which she poses a dilemma, asks for your advice, and then explains why what you have advised would not work. At this point you are perplexed and possibly a bit frustrated. The next time she poses an unsolvable dilemma, what would be your first course of action?

a. ___ Tell Janice that you see that she is facing an insolvable dilemma and you are feeling just as frustrated about her problems as she is.

b. ___ Show her that she can solve smaller problems by selecting and assigning an activity that you know she does very well.

c. ___ Share with her that you are confident in her abilities even if she is not.

d. ___ Provide options for seeing the situation from different perspectives.

e. ___ Interpret Janice's tendency to be critical of your recommendations as reflecting an underlying desire to cope with her symptoms more independently. Work with her to increase her feelings of empowerment.

9. Adam, a 65-year-old client, has been referred to OT following a stroke that resulted in cognitive difficulties and deep paralysis of the left side. Because he identified gardening as one of his favorite leisure activities, the OT asks him to plant some seeds in a pot as if he were working outdoors in his garden. The therapist provides soil, a shovel, seeds, and a watering can. The client, who appears very confident in his ability, sprinkles the seeds at the very bottom of the

pot, covers them with too much soil, and forgets the water. You tell Adam that he did not plant the seeds correctly. He appears irritated with you and comments that you do not know very much about gardening. The neurology report in Adam's chart indicates that he exhibits a profound lack of awareness of the impairments that have resulted from his stroke. What would be your *first* response?

a. ___ Explain to Adam in more detail what he did wrong, educate him about his problems with awareness, and attempt to teach him how to plant the seeds correctly.

b. ___ Accept Adam's comment and tell him that you can see that this activity has been frustrating.

c. ___ Ask Adam about other activities he does well and see if there is an opportunity for him to try those so he might have an experience of competence.

d. ___ Describe to Adam how your opinion of how the seeds should have been planted differs from his opinion and ask him if he is able to see that your approach would be effective.

e. ___ Accept Adam's comment and ask for his input about next steps for therapy.

10. Claire, a 19-year-old woman, has been working with the therapist for the past 2 months following a spinal cord injury that occurred in a motor vehicle accident. Until now, she has been an exceptional client—following all of your recommendations and giving 110% for each session. One day she exhibits an abrupt change in her usual approach to therapy. She appears deeply sad and begins to question the utility and point of therapy. She reports that she has just realized that, no matter how much therapy she receives, she will never be able to walk again. How do you respond?

a. ___ Ask Claire questions to help her clarify or evaluate her thinking about her abrupt change in approach.

b. ___ Educate Claire that her reaction makes sense in terms of stages of adjustment to spinal cord injury.

c. ___ Remind Claire that no one knows the extent or nature of the gains she might be able to make in the next 6 to 12 months of therapy.

d. ___ Just be present with Claire in her new state of mind, let her know you can see that she is struggling and see where she takes the therapy over time.

e. ___ Suggest to Claire that it would be a good idea to join a peer support group because she would benefit from learning how other people with her type of impairment lead productive lives.

11. Christine, a 28-year-old woman with Down's syndrome and borderline intellectual functioning, is one of the OT's clients at a residential facility. The therapist has known her for approximately 2 years, and they have a strong relationship. A new staff member has arrived at the facility and has singled out Christine as a problem resident. The OT can see how this rift has occurred because the staff member tends to be rather authoritarian, and the OT knows that Christine can be resistive during times when she feels she is being ordered around and told what to do. One day soon after, Christine approaches the OT in an emotional state and tells the OT that the staff member has been mean to her. Following further inquiry, you discover that the staff member reminded Christine, for a third time, that it was her turn to do dishes. When Christine responded "I'll get to it," the staff member changed her tone of voice and commented that perhaps Christine would lose some weight if she "got to it" more quickly. What would be your *first* course of action?

a. ___ Tell Christine that you are going to investigate what happened and that you will do everything you can to make sure that this staff member does not treat her badly again.

b. ___ Tell Christine that she can't behave in her usual resistive way with this staff member and teach her alternative ways to respond to the staff person's directions so she can learn to be more self-protective around this individual.

c. ___ Encourage Christine to raise the issue with the staff member and to ask the staff member why she is treating her badly.

d. ___ Ask Christine what she thinks she wants to do about it.

e. ___ Tell Christine that it makes sense she is upset, and that these kinds of comments are mean and inappropriate.

12. David is a 2½-year-old boy with speech and fine motor delays and behavioral problems. His behavior at home (and in the clinic) is highly oppositional and defiant. He demands his own way and often throws major tantrums when his mother takes him shopping, attempts to groom and bathe him, or attempts to put him to bed at night. During his first clinic visit, David's mother would not leave him alone with the therapist. During the assessment, David was observed to be destructive with toys and to throw them at his mother and at the therapist. He is not in day care and refuses to stay with anyone except his mother. Before the therapist can accomplish anything in OT, the therapist realizes that his behavior problems must be addressed. To this end, the therapist approaches David's mother and outlines some behavioral modification objectives, one of which includes practicing time-outs every time David becomes destructive and throws a tantrum. After trying other more empathically based approaches, the therapist decides that it is time to use behavior modification and to teach mom to do the same. The therapist explains that David will receive three warnings, and after the third warning he will be asked to sit in a padded chair in the corner of the room. The therapist explains that if he does not respond, she will ask his mother to carry him to the chair and to hold him in the chair if he tries to leave. Mother agrees to this plan. However, the first time David throws a tantrum, the therapist exhausts the warnings and coaches mother to carry him to the chair, David begins to cry, and the mother refuses to follow through. The therapist asks the mother why she did not follow through, and the mother reports that she couldn't stand to hear him cry that way and did not want to harm her baby. Assuming you are a therapist who believes in this method for addressing more extreme and difficult-to-treat behavioral issues like these, what would be your *first* inclination?

a. ___ Ask the mother to tell you what specifically about putting David into a time-out would be harmful to him.

b. ___ Reassure the mother that she will not be harming David by putting him in a time-out and provide her with words of encouragement to try it again.

c. ___ Remind the mother that she is not harming David by putting him in time-out and that the consequences of not putting David in time-out will be much worse over time.

d. ___ Tell the mother that you can see how she would worry that the time-out was painful for him and tell her that a lot of mothers get nervous when their children cry during time-out.

e. ___ Ask the mother what you can do to make the time-out procedure easier for David and easier for her to follow-through with.

13. The OT has been working with Beth, a woman with tetraplegia following a high-level spinal cord injury, for the past 6 months. Only 1 month prior to her injury, Beth's mother died of cancer. Beth has very little family support and has felt lonely and isolated. The therapist has formed a strong bond with Beth over the course of therapy. After a long search, the therapist's partner has finally found a dream job in Europe, and the couple has decided to move. The therapist will no longer be able to provide therapy for Beth and will be moving within the month. Upon learning this news, Beth accepts it but becomes silent and less engaged for the remainder of the session. She becomes increasingly withdrawn during the subsequent sessions until it reaches a point that it begins to interfere with her performance on rehabilitation-oriented therapy activities. As the therapist, what would be your *first* inclination?

a. ___ Tell Beth you have noticed that she has become increasingly withdrawn and ask her to tell you why.

b. ___ Encourage Beth to reflect upon the accomplishments she has already made in therapy and advise her not to allow your leaving to interrupt her progress.

c. ___ Tell Beth that you recognize that your leaving will be disruptive to her therapy and ask her how she might prefer to spend your last few sessions together.

d. ___ Realize that Beth has disengaged and do your best to connect Beth with the person who will be replacing you so as to provide a smooth transition.

14. A client's insurance company has just notified the OT that the client will only be allotted five additional sessions of OT. Due to the extent of the client's impairment, it is clear to the OT that the client will need at least 20 additional sessions. The OT and referring physician make numerous attempts to extend the duration of treatment without success. The client cannot afford to pay for the sessions independently, and he is clearly worried and frustrated upon learning that he will no longer be able to receive any more OT. What would be the *first* thing you would do in responding to the client?

a. ___ Tell the client you intend to report the insurance company to the National Association of Insurance Commissioners and assist the client in obtaining legal assistance.

b. ___ Tell the client that you share his concern and frustration about this situation and show your concern through your facial expression or tone of voice.

c. ___ Present the client with a series of options and recommendations for treatment alternatives and assist the client in choosing the optimal course of action.

d. ___ Teach the client occupational therapy activities that he can perform at home alone and some that he can try with the assistance of a caregiver.

e. ___ Tell the client that you are hopeful and confident that he will be able to continue to practice what he has already learned and that most clients are able to transfer what they have learned in therapy into their home environments.

15. Amy, a 26-year-old woman who recently had to have both legs amputated because of severe injuries sustained in a motor vehicle accident, tells the OT that she is worried about her return to work. The therapist then learns she is less concerned about job performance and more concerned about how her coworkers will react to her. Thus far, Amy has not allowed anyone to visit her outside of her immediate family because she fears their reactions to her physical appearance. After time passes and Amy begins to heal, the therapist suggests a graded approach to desensitize her to the reactions of others. For the first step, the therapist will accompany Amy to a museum or to another public place of her choosing; and as Amy becomes more comfortable around others, they will slowly progress toward allowing people she knows to see her. Amy confides that she is dreading to go anywhere in public, and she does not even want to encounter people she does not know outside of the hospital. She explains that she does not want to see expressions of sympathy or horror on people's faces. Amy very much wants to return to work but is immobilized by these concerns. What of these strategies would you be *most inclined* to try *first* in your attempt to assist Amy in managing her concerns and get her to try going into public?

a. ___ Highlight Amy's strengths in coping with her amputations and tell her you are confident that if she can face people in the hospital you know she can face people at a museum.

b. ___ Tell Amy that she should not be concerned with how others react to her. Advise her that if folks have difficulty with her appearance then the problem is with others and not with her.

c. ___ Provide Amy with a rationale for your graded approach to desensitizing her to the reactions of others and explain the psychological and behavioral principles behind what you are doing.

d. ___ Ask Amy if she can think of any strategies she might use to overcome her fears.

16. An OT is conducting group therapy on an inpatient psychiatric unit. There are four members in the group, one of whom is Bill, a 45-year-old man who is receiving treatment for severe depression. The topic of the day's group is leisure, and the therapist begins the group by asking clients to identify leisure activities they have enjoyed at any time in their lives. The client complies and says he likes running but then asks the therapist why he has chosen to discuss leisure. The client then suggests that the group talk about whether they have ever attempted suicide. The client contends that this would be a more relevant topic for a group about depression. At that point two of the three other group members chime in and say that this would be a better thing to discuss for today's group. The remaining group member remains silent but does not appear to object. In responding to the group members, what would be your *first* inclination?

a. ___ Allow the group to make suicide the topic of the day and ask Bill if he would like to lead the discussion.

b. ___ Allow the group to make suicide the topic of the day and ask the members who would like to begin.

c. ___ Encourage group members to stick with the original topic of leisure and educate them why it is likely to be more therapeutic to discuss leisure as opposed to suicide.

d. ___ Provide group members with options for devoting some of the group time to a conversation about suicide and the remaining time to a conversation about leisure.

17. Lizzie, a 54-year-old woman with multiple sclerosis is consulting an occupational therapist to learn energy conservation strategies. From week to week, her affect appears to change markedly from being grateful for your efforts and complimentary of your approach to being rejecting or critical of your approach. Lizzie's behavior seems to be related to the severity of her physical symptoms and to the level of her mobility difficulties that week or day. She appears to lack insight and seems unaware of this pattern. The next time Lizzie rejects your suggestion or becomes critical of your approach, how would you be most inclined to respond?

a. ___ Mention to Lizzie that you have noticed that her mood tends to change when she is having a harder time with symptoms and mobility. Assist Lizzie in understanding her reaction to therapy in terms of whether she is having a good day or a bad day in terms of physical symptoms.

b. ___ Mention to Lizzie that you have noticed that her mood tends to change when she is having a harder time with symptoms and mobility. Invite Lizzie in joining you to consider options of how she might still benefit from therapy even on her bad days.

c. ___ Provide Lizzie with feedback that she tends to come across as being critical on her bad days and educate her about alternative ways of getting her needs met in therapy on the bad days.

d. ___ Ask Lizzie for more feedback on why she is having difficulty with your approach and ask her for suggestions about how you can better accommodate her when she is having difficulty.

e. ___ Anticipate that Lizzie is having a bad day and provide her with more support and encouragement on that day.

18. Adam, a 34-year-old client, has been seeing the OT for 2 months following a hand injury. At one session, Adam mentions that he hasn't gotten as much movement back in his hand as he had expected. He adds that during his first session with you you had reassured him that he would regain more movement. You respond by asking Adam if he has been practicing his exercises regularly. Adam returns an angry look and with irritation in his voice tells the therapist

that he has been following through with all of the therapy recommendations since the first day of treatment. In responding to Adam, what would be your first inclination?

a. ___ Educate Adam that a certain percentage of individuals continue to have limitations, even if they have followed through with all of the therapy recommendations. Make suggestions about other approaches he might try.

b. ___ Tell Adam you understand that his lack of return on movement was not his fault and apologize for anything you might have said that could have implied that he would get more functioning back than he already has. Seek to understand Adam's perspective.

c. ___ Tell Adam you are hopeful that he will continue to regain movement over time and encourage him to continue practicing the recommended exercises at home.

d. ___ Apologize for giving the message that Adam's only option was to reduce his impairment and work with him to locate assistive devices and information about the kinds of accommodations he can request so that he can continue functioning in the maximum ways possible.

e. ___ Ask Adam for his input and feedback about what he feels he is missing from the therapy.

19. Don, a 49-year-old client with a traumatic brain injury, tells the therapist that he witnessed a verbally angry client in the waiting room accusing the secretary of incorrect billing. Apparently when the secretary did not give him the answer he wanted, the angry client walked out of the office and slammed the door behind him. Don appears shocked and unnerved by having witnessed the incident. Since his injury, Don has become very sensitive to stress and to sensory stimulation, and he prefers social isolation and quiet environments. As his therapist, what would be your initial response to Don?

a. ___ Use the incident as a teachable moment and educate Don that part of his reaction to the event might be explained by the fact that he is more sensitive to stress and stimulation because of his brain injury.

b. ___ Reassure Don that he is safe and that he is going to be ok now that the situation is over.

c. ___ Tell Don that you can see how the event would have been upsetting to witness.

d. ___ Tell Don you will raise the issue with administration and take additional steps to ensure that the waiting room is as safe and neutral an environment as possible.

e. ___ Ask Don if he would like to make management of his hypersensitivity a goal in therapy.

20. Justin is a 10-year-old boy being seen by a school-based OT for academic difficulties attributable to attention-deficit hyperactivity disorder. The therapist has noticed that when she upgrades an assignment to make it slightly more challenging for Justin, he reacts immediately by saying he doesn't get it. It is clear to the therapist that Justin is capable of doing the slightly upgraded assignments, but he gives up before even attempting them. The therapist figures out that Justin claims he does not understand as soon as the therapist tells him they are going to try something new or slightly more challenging. Without fail, during the next session the therapist presents Justin with a slightly upgraded assignment and Justin claims he does not understand it. As the therapist, what would be your first response?

a. ___ Point out to Justin that you have noticed that he tends to react to anything new by saying that he does not understand. Tell him that a more accurate thing to say would be that he is worried about trying something new.

b. ___ Tell Justin that you are wondering if it's possible that he is worried about trying something new and that instead of saying he is worried he says he doesn't understand.

c. ___ Tell Justin that you know he can complete the assignment and encourage him to just give it a try.

d. ___ Ask Justin what about the assignment makes him think that he won't be able to do it.

e. ___ Point out to Justin that you have noticed that he tends to react to anything new by say-ing that he does not understand. Ask him what would be most helpful for you to do for him the next time you give him something new to work on.

A scoring key and interpretation map for this assessment are presented on the following pages. So you will have a better understanding of the strengths and limitations of each mode, it is recommended that you read this chapter before scoring your self-assessment.

Scoring for Exercise 4.1: Determining Your Therapeutic Style

To determine your therapeutic style (i.e., the modes you are more or less inclined to use) you should first record your responses to the Self-Assessment of Modes Questionnaire on the Modes Scoring Key by circling the response you chose for each question. Then, add up the number of times you chose responses corresponding to each mode and record them at the bottom of each col-umn. The total possible number of responses for each mode is 16. You may calculate your percent-age score for each mode by dividing the total number of responses for each mode by 16 and then by multiplying by 100. The higher your score for each mode, the more comfortable you may feel with using the mode.

You can plot your profile on the Therapeutic Style Form by darkening each area in the arrows that fall inside the concentric circle that corresponds to your mode scores. This will provide a visual representation of the therapeutic style you are most likely to use during therapy.

Modes Scoring Key					
Advocating	**Collaborating**	**Empathizing**	**Encouraging**	**Instructing**	**Problem-solving**
1-d	1-b	1-e	—	1-a	1-c
2-e	2-d	2-b	2-a	—	2-c
3-d	—	3-a	3-c	3-b	3-e
4-d	4-c	4-a	4-b	—	—
5-d	5-e	—	5-a	5-b	5-c
6-e	6-c	6-d	6-b	—	6-a
7-e	7-b	7-c	—	7-a	7-d
8-e	—	8-a	8-c	8-b	8-d
—	9-e	9-b	9-c	9-a	9-d
10-e	—	10-d	10-c	10-b	10-a
11-a	11-d	11-e	—	11-b	11-c
—	12-e	12-d	12-b	12-c	12-a
13-d	13-c	—	13-b	—	13-a
14-a	—	14-b	14-e	14-d	14-c
15-b	15-d	—	15-a	15-c	—
16-a	16-b	—	—	16-c	16-d
—	17-d	17-a	17-e	17-c	17-b
18-d	18-e	18-b	18-c	18-a	—
19-d	19-e	19-c	19-b	19-a	—
—	20-e	20-b	20-c	20-a	20-d
Advocating Total:____/16 Percent: ___%	Collaborating Total:____/16 Percent: ___%	Empathizing Total:____/16 Percent: ___%	Encouraging Total:____/16 Percent: ___%	Instructing Total:____/16 Percent: ___%	Problem-solving Total:____/16 Percent: ___%

Examining your Therapeutic Style

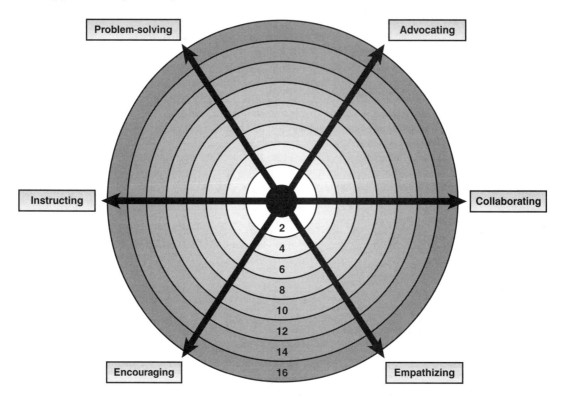

The therapeutic style form indicates the relative amount of comfort you have with each mode. In the end, however, you should reflect on and plan your own therapeutic style. A good beginning is to think about:

• Your natural modes and their strengths and cautions
• The modes you want to incorporate into your therapeutic style (including the modes with which you may wish to become more comfortable and proficient)

Your Natural Modes and Their Strengths and Cautions

By examining your Therapeutic Style Form and reflecting on the descriptions of the modes provided in this chapter, you should first decide for yourself the extent to which you are comfortable with each mode. To facilitate this process, you can use the table below to think carefully about the six modes and decide your degree of comfort with each of them.

My natural/preferred mode(s)	
Mode(s) I can use when I need to	
Mode(s) with which I am less comfortable/less able to use	

Next go back and review Table 4–1, looking at the potential strengths of your preferred mode(s). Each person uses a given mode in different ways, so the actual strengths of your use of a mode depend on how you typically use it. So, reflecting on *the particular way that you use your preferred mode(s)*, list five key strengths of your therapeutic style.

1.
2.
3.
4.
5.

Next, examine the cautions of your preferred mode(s) and consider to which of the potential pitfalls of the mode(s) you might be prone. Based on that self-examination, list five key areas of caution for yourself.

1.
2.
3.
4.
5.

Modes You Want to Incorporate Into Your Therapeutic Style

Now, examine the strengths of the modes that are *not* your preferred modes (either those you listed as "Mode(s) I can use when I need to" or "Mode(s) with which I am less comfortable/less able to use"). Consider whether the strengths of these modes are a good counterbalance to the liabilities of your preferred modes. Based on this consideration, identify the mode(s) you wish to use more naturally and regularly. Record them here.

If the mode(s) you wish to incorporate into your therapeutic style fall in the category of "Mode(s) I can use when I need to," you may wish to make plans for the situations in which you want to practice these modes and monitor your use of them. Record your thoughts here.

If the mode(s) you wish to incorporate into your therapeutic style fall in the category of "Mode(s) with which I am less comfortable/less able to use, you may wish to seek supervision, training, or other kinds of support that would help you develop the ability and comfort with using that mode.

CHAPTER 5

KNOWING OUR CLIENTS:
Understanding Interpersonal Characteristics

Occupational therapists strive to know their clients from multiple perspectives. The field emphasizes the importance of comprehending a client's impairment, performance capacity, occupational functioning and lifestyle, and occupational history. Knowledge of the client's interpersonal characteristics is not typically in the forefront. Such information is most often gained as a by-product of the interactions that occur as part of the overall therapy process.

Nonetheless, actively and reflectively seeking to know and understand each client's interpersonal characteristics is essential to establishing an optimal therapeutic relationship. According to the Intentional Relationship

Model (IRM), the therapist must work to develop a tailored relationship in which the client feels comfortable. This relationship requires a therapist to act intentionally guided by knowledge of the interpersonal characteristics of the client (Fig. 5.1).

Interpersonal Characteristics

Interpersonal characteristics are client emotions, behaviors, and reactions that occur during interactions between the client and therapist and that emanate from the client's

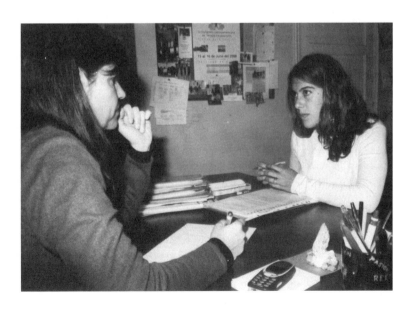

FIGURE 5.1 During an initial meeting, Carmen-Gloria de Las Heras works to get to know a client's personality

immediate circumstances and the client's underlying personality traits. When clients' interpersonal behaviors are inconsistent with how they typically interact with others and are largely linked to some external stressful circumstance, they are referred to as *situational*. By contrast, emotions, behaviors, and reactions that mostly emanate from underlying traits of the client are referred to as *enduring* interpersonal characteristics. This chapter provides guidance in understanding both situational and enduring interpersonal characteristics.

The rationale for differentiating these two categories of client characteristics is to highlight the difference between acute, common interpersonal reactions to impairment-related or medical situations and those interpersonal behaviors that are part of a client's personality and occur generally across a wide range of situations. Both types of client characteristics must be responded to therapeutically, but the nature and extent of the response vary depending on whether a client's interpersonal behavior is situational or enduring. The same skills, modes, and reasoning approaches offered by IRM should be used with both categories of client characteristics, although they may vary in terms of emphasis, duration, and intensity. For example, one's response to a client who is apprehensive about an immediate medical crisis but otherwise self-confident and relaxed may be different than one's response to a client who is chronically apprehensive about any new task or activity that is presented.

Situational Interpersonal Characteristics

Situational interpersonal characteristics are emotions, behaviors, and reactions that are context-specific and inconsistent with how the client typically interacts. Situational characteristics call for the therapist's attention when a client's interpersonal behavior is viewed as unusual in that it suddenly causes the therapist to experience sorrow, worry, stress, or frustration in reaction to the client. In practice settings, these characteristics may be linked to a stressful experience associated with an acute medical crisis or other impairment-related circumstance. For example, many clients who encounter occupational therapists as a result of a new, recurring, or exacerbated impairment/illness are more vulnerable to experiencing a variety of feelings associated with loss. Moreover, the impairments and circumstances that bring clients into occupational therapy affect many aspects of life, including daily routines, the level of independence regarding physical and cognitive functioning, employment, friendships, intimate relations, parenting, and emotional well-being. The circumstance of impairment may involve fatigue, pain, or discomfort; economic expense; stigmatizing attitudes of others; social and environmental obstacles to full participation and equal access; stressful interactions with the health care system; and uncertainty about the future. These experiences can lead to feelings of disorientation or confusion, helplessness, isolation, abandonment, stigma, despair, and anxiety in even the most resilient, resourceful, well-adapted, and interpersonally oriented individuals (Johnson & Webster, 2002; Moorey & Greer, 2002).

The stresses associated with impairments and other difficult circumstances also affect the way clients relate to therapists. Clients may, at some point during their therapy, experience or express any of the following emotional reactions, beliefs, or behaviors.

- Experience physical or emotional discomfort
- Feel overwhelmed or shocked
- Feel isolated or misunderstood
- Feel sadness, grief, or acute awareness of loss
- Feel helpless, subjugated, or powerless (e.g., relinquishing control or responsibility)
- Feel irritable or angry (e.g., having limited patience, limited motivation for therapy, and high expectations for outcomes)
- Have a heightened sensitivity to negativity
- Feel nervous, preoccupied, or tense
- Face or anticipate social judgment, stigma, and discrimination (including concerns about body image and sexuality)
- Contemplate mortality and meaning
- Be withdrawn or highly emotional
- Feel insecure and need increased support
- Seek information or be confused about treatment

Individuals react to circumstances associated with their impairments with tremendous variability. In addition, some clients vacillate among a wide range of these interpersonal characteristics depending on the situation, other circumstances and resources in their lives, and/or the particular state of mind in which they find themselves at the time. Recognizing that many of these characteristics are normative reactions to stress and responding appropriately to this heterogeneity in and among clients is vital to an optimal therapeutic relationship.

Enduring Interpersonal Characteristics

Enduring interpersonal characteristics can be defined as emotions, behaviors, and reactions that are consistent across time and circumstance and that emanate primarily from the client's underlying personality. Generally, they are evident in clients' interactions regardless of the circumstances or context. Enduring interpersonal characteristics include such things as a client's preferred style of communicating, capacity for trust, need for control, and usual way of responding to change, challenge, or frustration.

Recognizing that many of these characteristics are normative reactions to stress and responding appropriately to this heterogeneity in and among clients is vital to an optimal therapeutic relationship.

regardless of situation or context. By becoming aware of these categories of interpersonal variability, a therapist can become more attuned to each client's unique interpersonal characteristics. In the Activities section of this chapter, a brief rating scale is presented that enables you to evaluate how clients vary on each of these dimensions. This scale is a helpful tool when learning to observe and reflect on clients. Additionally, exercises are provided to familiarize you with these characteristics and facilitate reflection about characteristics you might find difficult to manage in practice situations.

Challenging interpersonal emotions, reactions, and behaviors are discussed in the sections that follow. Importantly, these discussions refrain from proposing simple solutions. This is because the optimal solution always requires a reflective intentional process in which the therapist:

- Recognizes the emotion, reaction or behavior
- Seeks to understand its source
- Consciously and reflectively considers options for how to interact with the client
- Closely monitors the client's response to the therapist's action

These steps are essential to guide and monitor a use of self tailored to the client's unique interpersonal characteristics.

General guidance in how to select interpersonal strategies that optimize the therapeutic relationship can be found in the use of modes discussed in Chapter 4. Consequently, after presenting the categories of interpersonal characteristics, there is a discussion of the therapeutic modes that are most likely to be successful with different interpersonal characteristics.

Categories of Interpersonal Characteristics

Therapists encounter a wide range of interpersonal characteristics within and among clients. This section identifies 12 categories of interpersonal characteristics within which clients may vary. They include:

- Communication style
- Capacity for trust
- Need for control
- Capacity to assert needs
- Response to change and challenge
- Affect
- Predisposition to giving feedback
- Capacity to receive feedback
- Response to human diversity
- Orientation toward relating
- Preference for touch
- Capacity for reciprocity

On some occasions, variability in client characteristics may be attributable to the circumstances taking place in therapy. In many cases, however, this variation is the result of true differences between people in terms of personality, or the interpersonal characteristics that endure

Communication Style

Communication style refers to clients' approaches to a formally spoken or signed language. Style of communication includes clients' preferred amount, nature, and pacing of the interaction that occurs during therapy. Communication style is the function of many diverse factors, including:

- The client's natural predisposition toward interacting and communicating with others
- How a client might be thinking or feeling toward the therapist
- The client's social or cultural background
- Neurological impairments (e.g., a traumatic brain injury or stroke)
- Symptoms of a psychiatric disorder (e.g., a mood or psychotic disorder)
- Effect of intoxication with a substance (e.g., alcohol or drugs)
- Transient feelings about the situation

It is important to recognize the nature of a client's communication and reflectively consider its possible sources (Fig. 5.2).

If a client's communication is unusual or cumbersome, it may be an early sign of some reaction to the process of therapy and/or challenging dynamics in the relationship. For example, if a client is capable of language but refuses to communicate, it may reflect a disagreement over goals, disappointment over the outcome of particular efforts, and/or questioning the efficacy of therapy. Clients who are reluctant or who require extensive questioning and encouragement may be unsure of their own abilities for a task or ambivalent about the utility of participating in a therapy task. Such behavior may, instead, reflect a long-standing pattern of shyness or interpersonal discomfort or some uncertainty about the degree to which the therapist can be trusted. Alternatively, the reluctance may be a reaction to the topic of conversation or to the nature of the questions being asked. The quality of any therapeutic relationship is linked to the extent to which a therapist can objectively recognize, understand, and respond to the client's communication style.

Capacity for Trust

Within the therapeutic relationship, trust is built over time. However, a client who is particularly cautious or who has

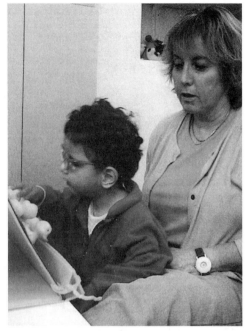

FIGURE 5.2 Vardit Kindler cues into the multidimensional aspects of communication when working with a nonverbal client

difficulties with trust can present challenges to the therapeutic relationship. Such caution or difficulties may be evident in clients' nonverbal cues, conversation, or choices during therapy. For instance, a client may ask questions that reflect concern about the adequacy, ultimate effectiveness, appropriateness, or safety of the therapist's approach or recommendation. A client may be reluctant to engage in the tasks of therapy or fail to provide the therapist with important information or feedback (Fig. 5.3).

Other clients may engage in certain patterns of behavior that indicate the client is having difficulty with trust. For example, a client may make repeated special requests to test a therapist's loyalty or commitment. A client may ask the thera-

> The quality of any therapeutic relationship is linked to the extent to which a therapist can objectively recognize, understand, and respond to the client's communication style.

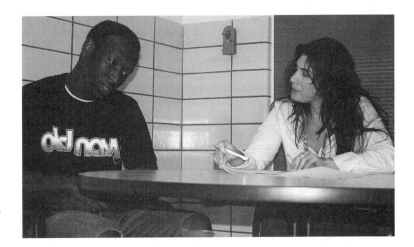

FIGURE 5.3 Stephanie McCammon puts herself in touch with a client's difficulties with trust

pist personal questions that have the potential to reveal vulnerabilities, or the client may refrain from disclosing relevant information unless the therapist self-discloses a personal vulnerability. When a client withholds information or fails to provide the therapist with helpful feedback, it may reflect preoccupation with being judged or concern about the way the therapist might react to or handle the information to be provided.

Sometimes difficulties with trust merely indicate that more work needs to be done to build a therapeutic alliance. At other times, clients are reacting to something the thera-

pist said or did that made them uncomfortable. Sometimes, something about the therapist (e.g., age, sex, personality, or ethnicity) may make it difficult for a client to feel trust. When this is the case, the therapist needs to locate and address the source of the discomfort or distrust. Some clients behave in a similarly cautious or distrustful manner toward family and friends as well as other professionals. In this case, the client's difficulties with trust are more likely to be deeply rooted in past experiences. In this instance, the therapist must be even more vigilant and responsive to the client's interpersonal behavior (Fig. 5.4).

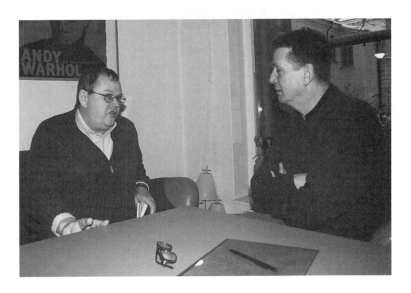

FIGURE 5.4 Roland Meisel realizes that work is needed to build a trusting alliance with his client

Need for Control

Occupational therapists strive to empower their clients by providing them with as much choice and control over their lives as possible. The degree to which a client attempts to assume control over what is said and done during therapy inevitably affects the way in which the therapeutic relationship evolves over time. Despite the field's value for promoting clients' autonomy, there are times when a client's needs related to control can interfere with the therapy process (Fig. 5.5).

Difficulties with control typically manifest in terms of degree. Some individuals have an unusually high need for control in relationships with others, whereas others may relinquish control altogether, behaving in passive or indifferent ways. During therapy, a number of behaviors indicate that a client has an unusually high need to control the interpersonal aspects of the session. These behaviors can include but are not limited to:

- Attempting to dominate or manipulate
- Resisting advice or suggestions while at the same time not being able to provide feedback or alternative suggestions
- Showering the therapist with compliments or indirect feedback strategically designed to influence the therapist's behavior
- Making excessive demands

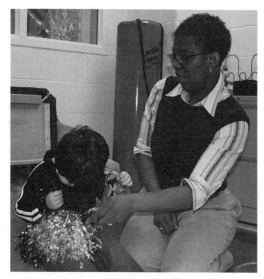

FIGURE 5.5 Understanding a client's need for control is an important aspect of Belinda Anderson's use of self

- Failing to respond to limits or boundaries
- Making strong statements about how health providers "should" behave
- Providing examples of how other health care providers have done a better job
- Comparing the therapist to other health care providers in a way that idealizes the other providers (and by implication devalues the therapist)
- Providing feedback that is excessive or highly critical in nature
- Seeking assistance or opinions and then rejecting them
- Otherwise having unusually high expectations of the therapist

A client who relinquishes control can also complicate the therapeutic relationship and disrupt the natural flow of therapy. The following behaviors may indicate that a client has abdicated control in the therapeutic relationship.

- Failing to generate ideas or give input on goals and objectives for therapy
- Behaving in an emotionally indifferent or passive way during therapy
- Seeks a high level of structure and direction from the therapist
- Demonstrating a high level of approval-seeking or other signs of emotional dependence on the therapist

Therapists need not attend to issues of control in the therapeutic relationship when clients share an appropriate level of control with the therapist given their cultural background and the situation of therapy. However, when a client demonstrates an unusually high or low level of need for control that negatively affects the therapy process, the therapist is faced with several choices about how to respond. How a therapist reacts determines the extent to which control issues lead to rifts and misunderstandings in the relationship. Because control issues have a high potential to disrupt the therapeutic relationship, therapists must practice a high level of interpersonal self-discipline when choosing how to respond (Fig. 5.6).

Capacity to Assert Needs

Clients often need assistance, information, resources, emotional support, structure, and other things the therapist can provide. When it comes to asserting such needs within the therapeutic relationship, some clients are easy to read whereas others leave a therapist guessing. Asserting needs requires clients to be able to discuss what they want from the therapist openly and directly. For example, if a client

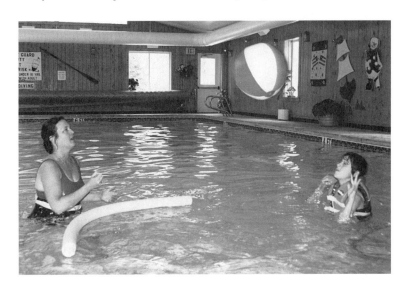

FIGURE 5.6 Kathryn Loukas and a client share taking control during therapy

wants the therapist to challenge him to work harder on days when his motivation is low, the client makes statements such as, "I'm feeling low—I need you to push me today." Conversely, if a client is discussing an occupational dilemma with the therapist and wants the therapist to listen rather than make suggestions, a client provides feedback such as, "I just need you to hear me right now" or "Please listen to what I have to say."

Other clients may provide the therapist with nonverbal cues that point toward their needs. If these cues are clearly interpretable and provided in a context the therapist can understand, they can be just as effective as verbal statements. For example, an adolescent client may roll her eyes if she feels that the therapist is behaving in an overprotective way during the therapy session. If this is the client's usual response when the therapist becomes overprotective and if the feedback has been discussed or otherwise explicitly verified before, the nonverbal cue may be all that is required to convey her needs from the relationship at that moment.

From time to time, clients have difficulty expressing their needs within the therapeutic relationship. The following behaviors may indicate that a client is struggling to assert his or her interpersonal needs:

- Not recruiting assistance or asking for support in a situation when it obviously is needed
- Rarely or never providing the therapist with verbal or nonverbal cues that point to interpersonal needs or to the therapist's failure to address those needs

- Asserting needs in an indirect manner by dropping hints (e.g., "I like people who listen more than they talk"), presenting a need for assistance or feedback vaguely (e.g., "I'm not sure if this brace is on right." "I guess I did that right."), or asking casual questions that suggest a need to discuss something important (e.g., "Do many of your clients have sexual difficulties?")
- Asserting needs by allowing problems to emerge or making mistakes (e.g., going ahead with a step in a task that the client does not know how to do, rather then asking for guidance)
- Making passive statements that cause the therapist to worry outside of therapy (e.g., "It worked here, but I don't know what will happen when I get home")
- Making jokes or offhand comments that may contain an insinuation (e.g., "You make it sound easy")

When clients do not assert their needs directly, it can be easy for a therapist to fail to meet those needs, particularly if she or he is not aware of the client's difficulties in this area (Fig. 5.7).

An equally challenging situation can arise when clients are excessive or demanding when asserting their needs. When clients recruit assistance in situations when it is clearly not necessary, it may indicate that they are nervous or upset about a recent event and are attempting to soothe themselves. Clients who are repeatedly excessive in their demands for support or assistance are more likely to be exhibiting an enduring interpersonal characteristic.

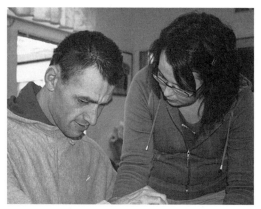

FIGURE 5.7 Kristin Alfredsson Ågren encourages and coaches a client on how to assert needs while at the day center

Some examples of behaviors that suggest a client is excessively asserting needs are:

• Recruiting assistance in situations when it is clearly not necessary
• Being emotionally demanding of the therapist (e.g., becomes angry or critical if the therapist does not respond in a way that is perceived by the client as sensitive or supportive enough)
• Appearing indifferent to the therapist's efforts or forgetting what the therapist has already done to support his or her needs
• Failing to respect the therapist's time
• Failing to respond to limits or social cues (e.g., does not move to leave when the session time is over)

These and similar behaviors can cause therapists to have negative reactions. One natural reaction is for a therapist to feel inadequate and guilty when working with such clients. Over time, some therapists may begin to feel resentful of these clients, and they may dread working with them. If therapists are not vigilant about a client's difficulties with appropriate needs assertion, the likelihood that misunderstandings and rifts will occur increases.

Response to Change and Challenge

Clients often come to occupational therapy during difficult periods marked by a significant challenge and/or change. Moreover, clients who are long-term participants in therapy are periodically faced with significant challenges. Some clients have the internal strengths and coping mechanisms to weather the changes and challenges associated with therapy. Some have extensive social support networks that bolster their ability to manage change and challenges (Fig. 5.8).

Other clients, however, without the same internal and/or external resources have more difficulty managing the stress associated with change and significant challenges. Some clients have difficulty with even minor change and challenges. For example, some more sensitive clients may experience difficulty with changes in the therapy schedule, in the way the therapy room is arranged, or in the way the therapist looks or behaves on a given day.

At some point during the therapy process, most clients encounter some difficulty coping and adjusting to change and challenges. This is particularly true during long-term therapy relationships when challenges and frustrations are inevitable over time. When clients have difficulty with change and challenges, they may exhibit any of the following behaviors in anticipation of therapy activities or events.

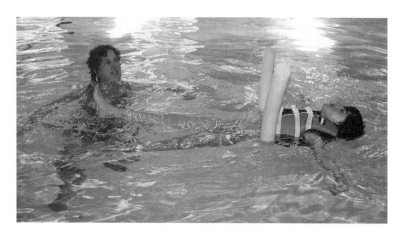

FIGURE 5.8 Kathryn Loukas encourages a client while she bravely takes on a challenge in swimming

- Expressing worry, anxiety, or fear about the task or activity
- Becoming easily demoralized or self-doubting
- Withdrawing or shutting down emotionally
- Giving up before the activity or shortly after beginning it
- Avoiding therapy tasks or activities altogether
- Underestimating performance capacity (e.g., saying "I can't do it")
- Becoming easily irritated or angry
- Challenging the therapist when presented with an activity or task

If such difficulties with change are not acknowledged and addressed, they are likely to be repeated and interfere with progress in therapy.

✳Affect

Clients' affect not only reveals information about their thoughts and feelings, it influences the thoughts and emotions experienced by the therapist in reaction to the client (Fig. 5.9).

Clients vary in terms of the degree to which they express emotion during therapy. Some clients express their feelings more freely, frequently, or intensely than others. High emotionality may be accompanied by periods of emotional numbness or void. Clients who vacillate between extremes of high intensity and low intensity may be having difficulty regulating or controlling their emotional states. Emotion regulation difficulties may reflect natural reactions to acute crisis situations. However if these difficulties are chronic, they suggest the presence of a mood disorder (e.g., bipolar disorder), a neurological disorder (e.g., traumatic brain injury), side effects of medications or other substances (e.g., alcohol intoxication), or a personality disorder (e.g., borderline personality disorder). Any of the following behaviors may indicate that a client is having emotion regulation difficulties.

- Exhibiting a wide range of intense emotions within a short period of time (e.g., ranging from showing devastation and tears to gregariousness and laughter within a matter of minutes)
- Exhibiting behavioral impulsivity or poor judgment
- Having difficulty controlling emotional reactions (e.g., inconsolable sobbing or uncontrolled rage)

If a client's emotion regulation difficulties are chronic and remain unaddressed, they eventually disrupt the process of therapy.

Emotion regulation difficulties are not the only affective issues that can challenge the therapeutic relationship. There are other clients who fail to show an appropriate level of emotion during therapy and appear chronically emotionally numb or void. When circumstances arise that would otherwise prompt an emotional reaction in a person, such clients may appear stoical, displaying constricted or blunted affect. There are a number of potential explanations for a client's absence of emotion. They include, but are not limited to, a neurological condition (e.g., stroke), a developmental disorder (e.g., autism), a psychiatric disorder (e.g., melancholic depression or negative symptoms of schizophrenia), or a personality disorder (e.g., avoidant or schizoid personality disorder).

In other cases, absence of emotion may be a natural aspect of a client's personality, coping style, and/or cultural identity. Whatever the explanation for a person's absence of affect, it is important that its source be recognized so the therapist does not personalize or misinterpret it in such a way that could have negative implications for the therapeutic relationship.

Another circumstance in which a client's affect can influence the therapeutic relationship is when a client demonstrates an inappropriate emotional response to a given situation. For example, the client may laugh inap-

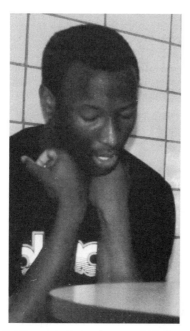

FIGURE 5.9 Clients vary in the extent to which they express emotion during therapy

propriately during group therapy when another client is discussing something painful or serious. Another example is a client who bursts into tears for no apparent reason or suddenly becomes nervous or agitated. In many cases, inappropriate affect suggests that a client may be uncomfortable or anxious and may not know how to respond. However, when a client's inappropriate affect seems unrelated to stress or social discomfort, it may indicate that a client is responding to internal stimuli or experiencing a psychotic process.

When a client's emotional reactions are consistent with the external events in his or her life or match the interpersonal circumstances occurring within the therapeutic relationship, they typically enhance communication, natural relating, and understanding between client and therapist. However, clients who differ from therapists in the way they convey emotion may at first seem overwhelming to therapists, particularly if the therapists lack experience managing diverse emotional reactions and styles or if they themselves have difficulty managing their own emotional reactions. Because emotional styles are deeply embedded aspects of psychological functioning, therapists must make an earnest attempt to truly understand the client from an empathic perspective. Such effort also helps the therapist attenuate any personal reactions to the client's affect. As therapists attempt to understand their clients' emotional reactions (or lack thereof), they maximize the likelihood that the clients themselves will achieve more self-understanding of their own reactions. Information on managing emotional intensity as it relates to sadness, anger, and anxiety is provided in Chapter 9.

Predisposition to Giving Feedback

Therapists rely on feedback from their clients so they can adjust their strategies to maximize the likelihood of positive outcomes. However, clients differ in the degree to which they are comfortable with and predisposed toward appropriately providing this essential feedback. Clients who are comfortable giving feedback provide it in a straightforward manner without angry affect. When clients are comfortable providing feedback, they are able to provide it regardless of whether it is solicited or unsolicited, and they are confident about what they are saying. Some clients exercise tact, sensitivity, or diplomacy when providing feedback (Fig. 5.10).

Some clients have difficulty providing feedback; these difficulties can manifest in the following ways.

- Never providing unsolicited feedback (whether positive or negative)
- When feedback is solicited, client maintaining only a neutral stance (e.g., "everything is fine" or "it's ok")
- Providing unsolicited positive feedback but failing to provide negative feedback
- Providing feedback in a protective manner (e.g., provides feedback only if solicited or prefaces negative feedback with a compliment)
- Presenting negative feedback in an indirect manner (e.g., uses language that is abstract, general, or otherwise vague; dropping hints; asking a casual question; making a negative statement and then recanting with "just joking")
- Providing negative feedback in a reluctant manner (e.g., confirming the therapist's guess that something is wrong)

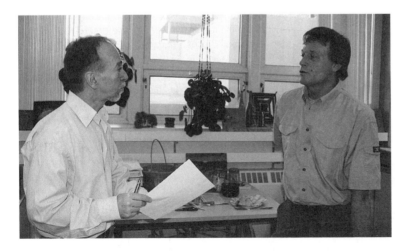

FIGURE 5.10 René Bélanger listens while a client spontaneously shares his impression of an assessment

Clients' difficulty providing feedback may stem from unawareness of the utility of feedback, cultural norms, viewing the health provider as an authority figure, perceived vulnerability of the therapist, or fear that the therapist might become angry or react negatively. In some instances, a client's difficulties with feedback stems from a lack of open communication or lack of trust or a therapist's failure to indicate the importance of feedback. For instance, a client who provides negative feedback to a therapist who does not respond with validation and an attempt to correct the problem will be reluctant to provide feedback in the future.

Another way in which feedback can become problematic within the therapeutic relationship is when clients provide feedback in a way that is excessive or overly negativistic. The following are examples that characterize this approach to feedback provision:

- Negative feedback is accompanied by an angry affect or tone of voice.
- The nature of the feedback is overly critical or harsh.
- Negative feedback is frequent or excessive.
- Negative feedback is used to gain control of the therapy or otherwise subjugate the therapist.

Therapists who leave this kind of behavior unaddressed are likely to experience feelings of anger or dread at the thought of continuing therapy with the client.

Capacity to Receive Feedback

Occupational therapy involves providing clients with ongoing feedback. A therapist may provide a client with feedback on issues such as:

- The nature or consequences of an impairment
- Ability for, or quality of, the performance of an activity
- Level of interest or curiosity to pursue an occupation
- Occupational history or habit patterns
- Current or future occupational choices
- Follow-through on treatment recommendations
- Goal attainment

When an occupational therapist provides positive feedback, it typically takes the form of praise, encouragement, or approval (e.g., "You are doing well so far" or "Did you notice it took you only 5 minutes to button your shirt today?"). Constructive feedback serves to give the client critical information to assure or support safety, learning, positive choices, and reflection. In some instances, feedback involves informing a client that he

or she has disappointed the therapist somehow (e.g., "I trusted you were telling me the truth when you told me you have not been falling lately").

A client's capacity to receive feedback from the therapist is just as important as his or her capacity to provide the therapist with feedback. Negative feedback can be difficult for almost any client to hear. Some clients are uncomfortable even when receiving positive feedback. This is because feedback always conveys some degree of judgment. For example, informing some clients that they have improved leads them to wonder just how poor their performance was before. There are some circumstances in which a client's response to feedback may be isolated to a specific situation. However, the way clients respond to feedback about one aspect of therapy can be an initial indication of how they are likely to respond to feedback about other aspects (Fig. 5.11).

Clients who willingly receive feedback find it helpful and actively respond to it with questions and/or efforts to make a correction. Client difficulties receiving feedback may be evident in any of the following behaviors.

- Dismissing, ignoring, or minimizing the significance of the feedback
- Becoming self-critical or deflated
- Becoming irritable, visibly angry, or verbally hostile
- Becoming passive-aggressive (disengages, fails to follow through, or changes behavior in some other maladaptive way)
- Being defensive (argues for own point of view or challenges therapist)

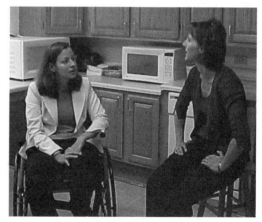

FIGURE 5.11 A client is receptive and interested in Kim Eberhardt's opinion about future directions for therapy

These or other negative reactions to feedback may signal an underlying vulnerability. A client may be feeling doubtful or powerless about the task itself or be facing more pervasive feelings of low self-esteem or helplessness.

Irrespective of its source, a client's negative reaction is likely to affect the therapist emotionally. This is particularly likely if the therapist has put a great deal of thought and care into the decision to convey the feedback. In these situations, the therapist must determine whether a client's negative response to the feedback is part of an enduring pattern of sensitivity to feedback, a temporary reaction specific to the task, or a product of the way in which the therapist delivered the feedback (e.g., timing, word choice, affect). Additional information about providing clients with feedback, strategies to maximize the likelihood that it will be received positively, and suggestions for repairing feedback-related rifts within the relationship is presented in Chapters 8 and 13.

Response to Human Diversity

Human diversity is a term that encompasses a wide range of differences that distinguish individuals from one another. In occupational therapy the differences that may be most relevant to the client–therapist relationship include, but are not limited to, differences in:

- Sex
- Race
- Ethnicity
- Age and developmental level
- Religious orientation
- Political orientation
- Cultural values and belief systems
- National origin
- Disability status
- Educational status
- Economic status
- Marital status
- Parental status
- Intellectual capacity
- Sexual orientation

Accepting others' differences and working to understand their perspectives can be challenging, especially if these differences pose threats to trust, communication, or resource acquisition. Some of these differences test a client's comfort zone more than others. For example, for a highly religious and conservative client, a therapist who appears to be secular and liberal may be uncomfortable.

Therapists inevitably differ from their clients in any number of ways. Depending on the circumstances and the nature of the differences that exist, issues related to human diversity can become significant within the client–therapist relationship. Differences between client and therapist can result in either positive or negative outcomes. It is largely the responsibility of the therapist to manage issues related to diversity (Fig. 5.12).

Achieving acceptance and respect for diversity is not easy, and some clients have difficulty attaining this ideal. Difficulty accepting and respecting a therapist's differences may be intensified if a client is already stressed or made vulnerable by issues related to his or her impairment situation. Clients may manifest difficulties with human diversity in a variety of ways; for example, a client may:

- Question the therapist about his or her personal characteristics (e.g., "Do you have children of your own?" Do you attend church?)
- Make statements or proclamations about the inability to work with certain types of therapists (e.g., "I can't see myself working with a therapist under the age of 30")
- Make indirect statements indicating discomfort with people in general of a certain age, religion, ethnicity, and so on

Clients' difficulty with differences may reflect an underlying concern that the therapist will not be able to understand them on some fundamental level. In some cases, difficulties with diversity may stem from a client's history of negative experience. In other cases, difficulties with diversity have their origins in an individual's

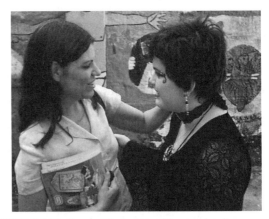

FIGURE 5.12 Carmen-Gloria de Las Heras and a client embrace their mutual differences at Reencuentros

immutable ideology, world view, personal convictions, or limited experience. More information about managing issues related to human diversity is provided in Chapter 9.

Orientation Toward Relating

Clients differ widely in what they want from their therapists. For example, most clients who disclose difficult experiences feel comfortable if the therapist shows some emotional reaction in his or her response (provided the response is somewhat attenuated and the therapist maintains appropriate control over his or her emotions). However, some clients become anxious if the therapist shows any emotion in his or her response. Such clients prefer to tell their stories in a dispassionate way, and they do not wish to share any accompanying emotions with the therapist. They prefer their therapists to say the appropriate thing in response but not to convey an emotional response through words or affect. Showing emotion with such clients may provoke worrying that they have shocked or overwhelmed the therapist. Some clients feel smothered or otherwise uncomfortable with a therapist's level of emotion and thus withdraw.

Still other clients feel emotionally abandoned if the therapist does not show an emotional response. Such clients may express anger or concern if the therapist does not react with emotionally demonstrated care and concern. Such clients may desire such closeness or emotional inti-

macy that they are never satisfied with the therapist's efforts to care and show concern. These clients may show signs of dissatisfaction with the usual professional boundaries that characterize the client–therapist relationship. For example, they may disclose details about their lives or experience that are unnecessary or make the therapist feel uncomfortable, or they may invite the therapist to engage in activities that would be more appropriate for a friendship or other type of personal relationship (Fig. 5.13).

Some clients are focused strictly on the business of therapy. They desire a more formal, dispassionate relationship characterized by a high degree of structure and an emphasis on the tasks of therapy. Such clients avoid discussing personal problems or sharing their feelings with their therapists. If they are asked about such issues, they are likely to avoid the topic or provide a brief, emotionless response.

These differences exist not only among clients but also within individual clients. The same client may prefer different levels of connection with the therapist depending on the length and stage of the therapeutic relationship and on the issues being faced.

Preference for Touch

In occupational therapy, touch has been characterized as having an important potential to support and enable clients (Huss, 1977). At the same time, tactile defensiveness, alo-

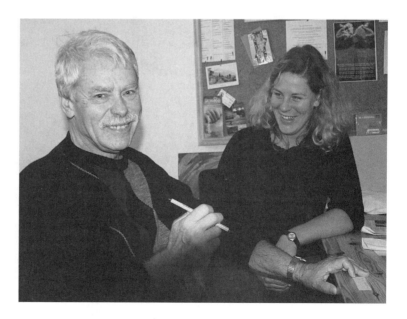

FIGURE 5.13 Anne Reuter recognizes a client's preference to relate on a more personal level

dynia (a condition in which a person experiences pain from stimuli that are not normally painful), and other symptoms and sensitivities associated with being touched may represent major reasons why clients are being evaluated and treated by an occupational therapist. Many approaches to occupational therapy require therapists to touch clients in a wide range of places, with various levels of pressure and intensity and using many different objects, technologies, or assistive devices. Consequently, clients' preference for touch must be carefully considered (Fig. 5.14).

In some instances, a client's preferences for touch correspond closely with their orientation to relating. In other cases, the two may be disparate; a client may be much more comfortable talking than touching (or vice versa). Failing to recognize and respect a client's difficulty can negatively affect trust and comfort within the therapeutic relationship.

The degree of preference for touch can be observed in any of the following behaviors.

- Physically shrinks away from or shows emotional signs of discomfort with any form of touch, even when it is solely mechanical or technical in nature
- Tolerates touch only when it is mechanical or technical in nature; shows discomfort with social forms of touching

- Responds positively to any form of touch initiated by the therapist
- Initiates or seeks out caring touch from the therapist

Clients may have difficulty receiving touch initiated by a therapist for any number of reasons. These reasons may include but are not limited to:

- A person's upbringing or cultural background
- Bodily pain or other physical symptoms that prevent touch from being enjoyable
- Tactile defensiveness or other sensory processing difficulties
- A posttraumatic reaction associated with prior experiences of physical, sexual, or emotional trauma (e.g., childhood physical or sexual abuse, domestic violence, rape, assault, and/or emotional abuse during childhood or adulthood)
- History of deprivation or neglect (e.g., deprived of touch during infancy and/or childhood or emotionally neglected by a parental figure)
- Feelings of sexual attraction toward the therapist

Some clients are conscious and knowledgeable about why they have an aversion to touch. Some even have the presence of mind to discuss these issues with the therapist upfront (e.g., "I can't stand it when people approach me from behind. If you are going to touch me, I need to see

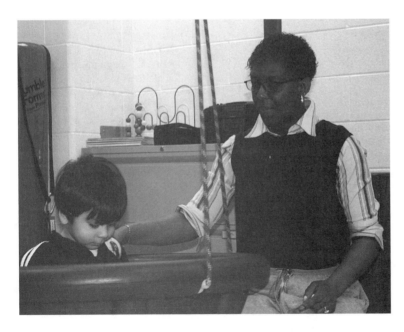

FIGURE 5.14 Belinda Anderson approaches touch carefully when working on sensory issues with a cautious client

you in front of me first"). However, many clients are unaware of or unable to discuss the reasons behind their difficulties with touch. Thus, it is important for therapists to be aware that a client may be covertly uncomfortable or disturbed when subjected to touch. Maintaining appropriate boundaries with clients requires becoming knowledgeable about and respecting a client's preference.

Capacity for Reciprocity

Within the occupational therapy literature, writers have emphasized the importance of giving and sharing between client and therapist (Ayres-Rosa & Hasselkus, 1996; Prochnau, Liu, & Boman, 2003). A person is drawn to the field of occupational therapy because of the opportunities for developing meaningful relationships with clients. At the same time, therapists learn the importance of treating all clients equally and maintaining a stance of objectivity and neutrality toward clients.

Nonetheless, even when therapists are effective at controlling their reactions to clients on a behavioral level, it is impossible to avoid feelings about clients. Some therapists have emotional reactions to clients because they remind them of an acquaintance or family member. Other therapists are moved by clients who appear vulnerable and are receptive to support. Still other therapists have strong reactions to clients who are resilient, independent, and willful. In sum, each therapist has a personal disposition to react differently to different types of client. A client's capacity for reciprocity is one of the most general and ubiquitous qualities that affects the development of a mutually gratifying relationship between client and therapist (Fig. 5.15).

The capacity for reciprocity has been linked to an individual's ability to relate to others in a psychologically healthy and developmentally appropriate way (Kohut, 1984; Seidler, 1999). Individuals with a limited capacity for reciprocity may have a tendency to be self-oriented rather than other-oriented in their interactions with others. Their psychological development may have been arrested for any number of reasons, and this is likely to be evident in their interpersonal behavior—particularly when under stress or in long-term relationships that require a substantial amount of give and take. A client's capacity for reciprocity may be reflected in a wide range of interpersonal behaviors. These behaviors include but are not limited to:

- When a disagreement occurs the client is capable of understanding the therapist's point of view
- Express gratitude to the therapist when appropriate and in a way that feels comfortable to the therapist
- Ability to show tolerance or patience if a therapist is particularly preoccupied or overwhelmed on a given day
- Ability to forgive the therapist for a minor oversight or mistake
- Ability to show empathy toward the therapist (e.g., to sense that the therapist may be having a difficult day and to ask about it or show concern rather than take it personally)
- Occasionally show interest in the therapist as a human being by asking questions the therapist is comfortable answering

Clients who are able to engage in reciprocal relationships with therapists are more likely to experience positive treatment outcomes (Wilczek, Barber, Gustavsson, Asberg, & Weinryb, 2004). However, it is important for therapists to provide the same level of care to clients regardless of the client's capacity for reciprocity. Being aware of and having insight into your reaction to clients can help ensure that all clients are treated equally, regardless of their individual capacities for reciprocity.

Approaching the Therapeutic Relationship in Light of Client Interpersonal Characteristics

The previous sections described and explained 12 categories of interpersonal characteristics. The point of these

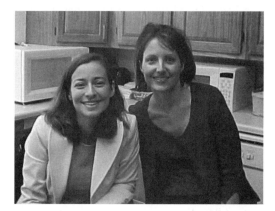

FIGURE 5.15 Some clients have a unique ability to share themselves with therapists in a way that feels mutually gratifying

discussions was to draw attention to the many ways these characteristics have the potential to influence the therapeutic relationship. Importantly, understanding and effectively responding to a client's unique interpersonal characteristics within the therapeutic relationship involves:

• Recognizing and empathically understanding the client's unique interpersonal characteristics
• Being aware of how those interpersonal characteristics affect the client's reactions to the therapy process and to yourself as the therapist
• Reflectively observing the client's personal reactions within the therapeutic relationship
• Maintaining a reflective consciousness of your own reactions to the client's interpersonal characteristics within the therapeutic relationship
• Managing your own behavior to support an optimal therapeutic relationship

The last of these tasks is closely related to how one selects and uses the therapeutic modes, which is discussed in Chapters 4, 7, and 12.

Using Therapeutic Modes in Response to Client Characteristics

Knowledge of a client's unique interpersonal characteristics[1] should inform one's selection and use of the specific therapeutic modes. Therapists should seek to use those modes that are most likely to coincide with the client's preferred or more comfortable way of being treated during therapy. The necessity of selecting and using modes that match a client's interpersonal characteristics is underscored by Principle 7 of IRM: *the client defines a successful relationship* (emphasized in Chapter 3). This principle acknowledges that clients differ in terms of the kind of relationship they seek with their therapists. For example, whereas some clients prefer a therapist who creates a warm, unconditionally accepting, emotionally gratifying

atmosphere in therapy, other clients desire a highly structured relationship that feels more professional in nature.

Table 5.1 summarizes general guidelines for selecting a therapeutic mode according to a client's unique interpersonal characteristics. The table is a general guideline for how to match a mode to the dominant way in which the client behaves within each category. It is important to recognize that you should select the mode that would be most comfortable for the client given where the client is at the present time. Modes should not be selected based on where you would like the client to be or to where you would like to see the client evolve. By matching your mode to clients' characteristics, you are responding to their interpersonal needs of the moment. Doing so optimizes the possibility for positive therapeutic communication and relationship building.

With many clients, therapists find that they can select modes that are consistent with the natural interpersonal tendencies or comfort zone. In such cases, interpersonal relating occurs effortlessly, especially once a therapist is adept at recognizing and responding to the most common client interpersonal characteristics. However, when clients' characteristics present interpersonal challenges, the level of intentionality in the use of modes must be high. This circumstance may occur when you find a particular client more challenging or when certain events in therapy challenge what is for the most part an easy therapeutic relationship. In such instances, a therapist who can step back and think about what modes might be helpful (perhaps those not as familiar or comfortable) and would be more likely to result in success with the client.

It is important to bear in mind that clients often change over time in terms of what they are seeking from the therapeutic relationship. A client may change in terms of what he or she wants from the therapeutic relationship for any number of reasons, including stress associated with the occurrence of an interpersonal event during therapy, stress unrelated to the therapy process, personal growth, or some other developmental process. These situations call for the therapist to initiate a mode shift in which use of a former mode is replaced by use of a different mode (Box 5.1).

Finally, it must be recognized that there are no hard-and-fast rules about what makes human interactions successful or unsuccessful. Thus, the process of matching modes to interpersonal characteristics must be done consciously and reflectively. The matching of modes to characteristics provided in Table 5.1 should be treated as general guidelines, not as an explicit recipe for success within the therapeutic relationship.

---

[1]This chapter does not elaborate on the additional complexities involved in clients diagnosed as having Axis I or Axis II psychiatric disorders. When therapists are providing services to clients with these psychiatric disorders, it is important to have an awareness of the diagnoses and how best to respond to them in the context of therapy.

Table 5.1 Interpersonal Modes Most Comfortable for Clients Based on Their Characteristics

Parameter	Advocating	Collaborating	Empathizing	Encouraging	Instructing	Problem-solving
Communication style	Any communication difficulty	Talks excessively	Any communication difficulty	May be effective if client is reluctant		
Capacity for trust	Distrustful of others but not therapist		Highly distrustful or distrusts therapist	Distrustful of others but not therapist		
Need for control		High to moderate need for control	High to moderate need for control		Indifferent or relinquishes control	
General relating with providers			Ambivalent, uncomfortable	High need for closeness	Openly hostile or high need for closeness	
Response to change, challenge, or frustration			Any difficulty with change (fearful, demoralized, angry)	Fearful or demoralized	Fearful	
Capacity to receive feedback			Dismisses, self-critical, or angry			
Predisposition to give feedback			Provides indirectly or overly critical	Does not provide feedback	Does not provide feedback	
Affect regulation			Any difficulty with affect		Any difficulty with affect	Absent/blunted affect
Preference for social contact		High level of social contact	Overly discriminative		Isolative	Isolative
Capacity to assert needs			Any difficulty with needs assertion	Does not assert needs	Does not assert needs	
Respect for human diversity			Any difficulty with human diversity			
Preference for structure/direction	Never or seldom attempts	Prefers a semi-structured approach	Resists or minimally tolerates		Prefers a high level of structure	Prefers a high level of structure
Recruiting assistance			Any difficulty with assistance	Recruits too much assistance	Recruits too much assistance	
Preference for autonomy			Any difficulty with autonomy		Any difficulty with autonomy	
Emotional intensity	Avoids emotional intensity		Able to show and/or receive		Avoids emotional intensity	Avoids emotional intensity
Preference for touch						

Cells are left blank if the mode is either not applicable or not particularly optimal for a given characteristic.

> ### Box 5.1 Mode Shifts
>
> In my work with Kayla,[2] I step into and out of different interpersonal modes depending on what she needs at the time. Most of the time, I utilize the collaborating mode in that I encourage her to have a lot of choice in terms of therapy goals and activities. In addition, I give her a lot of control during therapy activities. However, Kayla is the type of client who plunges full force into any activity that we do. If I notice that she is approaching a physical activity in such a way that it puts her at risk for injury, I draw upon the instructing mode to stop her and explain to her what I see. I do this frequently because I know that a part of Kayla very much appreciates my stepping into the instructing mode and guiding her during physical activity. Still, there are other times when it is clear that Kayla wants to discuss something personal with me and prefers that I simply listen to what she is saying. It is during these times when I draw upon the empathizing mode to convey to Kayla that I understand where she is coming from and respect her thoughts and feelings about the issue.
>
> — Kate Loukas

Key Terms

Interpersonal characteristics	Client emotions, behaviors, and reactions that occur in interactions between the client and therapist and that emanate from underlying client personality traits and from the client's circumstances
Situational interpersonal characteristics	Client emotions, behaviors, and reactions that are context-specific and linked to the experience of an acute medical or impairment-related circumstance or some other external stressor
Enduring interpersonal characteristics	Emotions, behaviors, and reactions that emanate primarily from the client's underlying personality

[2]All client names and geographic information have been changed.

References

Ayres-Rosa, S., & Hasselkus, B. R. (1996). Connecting with patients: The personal experience of professional helping. *The Occupational Therapy Journal of Research, 16,* 245–260.

Huss, A. J. (1977) Touch with care or a caring touch? *American Journal of Occupational Therapy, 31,* 11–18.

Johnson, C., & Webster, D. (2002). *Recrafting a life: Solutions for chronic pain and illness.* New York: Brunner-Routledge.

Kohut, H. (1984). *How does analysis cure?* Chicago: University of Chicago Press.

Moorey, S., & Greer, S. (2002). *Cognitive behavior therapy for people with cancer.* Oxford, UK: Oxford University Press.

Prochnau, C., Liu, L., & Boman, J. (2003). Personal–professional connections in palliative care occupational therapy. *American Journal of Occupational Therapy, 57,* 196–204.

Seidler, G. H. (1999) Destructive narcissism and the obliteration of subject-object separation: Various manifestations of an underlying psychodynamic configuration. *British Journal of Psychotherapy, 15,* 291–305.

Wilczek, A., Barber, J. P., Gustavsson, J. P., Asberg, M., & Weinryb, R. M. (2004) Change after long-term psychoanalytic psychotherapy. *Journal of the American Psychoanalytic Association, 52,* 1163–1184.

ACTIVITIES FOR LEARNING AND REFLECTION

Please see Exercises 5.1 and 5.2 on DavisPlus at http://davisplus.fadavis.com/landing–page.cfm?publication_id=2129.

CHAPTER 6

CHALLENGES TO CLIENT–THERAPIST RELATIONSHIPS:
The Inevitable Interpersonal Events of Therapy

During any single therapy session, several critically important events have the potential to influence the therapeutic relationship and, ultimately, the overall course of therapy. These *interpersonal events* are naturally occurring communications, reactions, processes, tasks, or general circumstances that take place within the context of the client–therapist interaction. They can be distinguished from all other therapy events in that they are emotionally charged and ripe with both threat and opportunity.

That is, these events may produce feelings such as disappointment, despair, worry, or anger. On the other hand, if addressed appropriately by the occupational therapist, these events may lead to positive outcomes that involve feelings such as gratification, fulfillment, satisfaction, or intimacy.

Because interpersonal events are inherently emotional and sometimes even threatening, therapists and clients alike can be tempted occasionally to repress, ignore, or minimize their significance. However, therapists should watch for these events and openly discuss them with their clients. If approached carefully, having a dialogue about a painful or difficult interpersonal circumstance strengthens the therapeutic relationship. Depending on the event and the message that is conveyed, such dialogue may also serve to improve the client's emotional well-being and self-esteem (Kohut, 1984). If these events are ignored, minimized, or responded to without significant care and thought, they have the potential to threaten both the therapeutic relationship and the client's occupational engagement. These adverse consequences are particularly likely to occur when a therapist repeatedly fails to address interpersonal events appropriately (Fig. 6.1).

Chapter 2 presented therapists' stories about particularly challenging moments of therapy. Each was an example of an interpersonal event. Additionally, Chapter 3 briefly defined interpersonal events in light of the intentional relationship model (IRM). This chapter extends those discussions, describing and giving examples of the major categories of interpersonal events that occupational therapists report as most common. These descriptions and the corresponding examples are designed to help you anticipate and recognize these events as well as understand their implications for the therapeutic relationship. Later chapters of this book illustrate how many of the examples described in this chapter were ultimately responded to and resolved by the therapists.

The 11 categories of interpersonal events are:

- Expression of strong emotion
- Intimate self-disclosures
- Power dilemmas
- Nonverbal cues
- Crisis points
- Resistance and reluctance
- Boundary testing
- Empathic breaks

> Interpersonal events are ripe with both threat and opportunity.

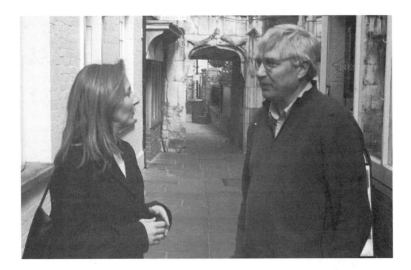

FIGURE 6.1 Jane Melton raises the possibility that an interpersonal event might have occurred

• Emotionally charged therapy tasks and situations
• Limitations of therapy
• Contextual inconsistencies

The focus of this chapter is to characterize these events and their potential impact. Subsequent chapters provide guidelines for responding to them.

Expression of Strong Emotion

Clients often become emotional during occupational therapy. *Expressions of strong emotion* are external displays of internal feelings that are shown with a level of intensity beyond usual cultural norms for interaction. These emotional expressions may be positive or negative. They occur because clients:

• Bring their private emotional states with them into therapy
• Express emotion in reaction to a task or activity of therapy
• Have an emotional reaction to something the therapist says or does

Regardless of their source, clients' expressions of strong emotion should always be viewed as significant interpersonal events. Box 6.1 provides an instance of a client who expressed strong emotion in therapy.

Clients who feel strong emotions and are not able to (or inclined to) attenuate them may exhibit the following behaviors.

• Laughing hard, loudly, or for a prolonged period
• Talking loudly (or signing demonstratively)
• Using language that is laden with emotional expression and/or terms
• Becoming tearful, crying, or sobbing
• Making angry statements, cursing, using angry gestures, or physically expressing anger through aggression

---

Box 6.1 Expression of Strong Emotion

Peter[1] is a businessman in his mid-thirties. I treated him in an inpatient rehabilitation setting for occupational issues related to paraplegia, which he acquired as a complication of a medical procedure. At the time of his procedure, he was happily engaged and very successful in his work as an accountant. He experienced the paralysis as devastating, and it placed a significant strain on his relationship with his fiancé. In therapy, he began to describe feelings of alienation and separation from his fiancé. He felt her behavior toward him had changed, and he wondered if she would still be willing to marry him given that his paralysis was likely to be permanent. When he would describe these feelings, he would often appear intensely anxious, and sometimes he would be so profoundly sad and distressed that he would weep. Peter stands out in my mind as one of the most intensely emotional clients I have ever worked with.

— **Kim Eberhardt**

---

[1]All client names and geographic information have been changed.

• Appearing nervous, panicked, agitated, or anxious as evidenced by the pitch or tremor of the voice, facial expression, fidgeting or wringing hands, shaking, trembling, or pacing

Unless they have lost emotional control entirely, individuals always exercise some degree of choice in deciding whether to reveal their most profound, entrenched, or perhaps untold feelings to others. When clients express strong emotions in the presence of a therapist, it conveys that they are sharing something significant with the therapist. Such emotional displays are a form of communication that invites the therapist to pause, take notice, and respond appropriately.

Intimate Self Disclosures

Intimate self disclosures are statements or stories that reveal something unobservable, private, or sensitive about the person making the disclosure. They can assume the form of:

• Information or stories about oneself
• Information or stories about close others

Clients usually do not make disclosures unless they believe that the therapist is worthy of having such information and responding to it in a gratifying way. Hence, they require careful responses. For instance, clients may perceive that the therapist has not responded appropriately if the therapist:

• Underreacts or conveys no response
• Overreacts or appears overwhelmed by the information
• Makes statements that minimize the significance of the information
• Asks follow-up questions the client perceives as undermining, judgmental, or dubious
• Provides unsolicited advice that does not convey full understanding of the complexity of the situation

Box 6.2 provides an example of a client's self-disclosure. Appropriate responses to self-disclosures can be powerfully affirming, supportive, or validating for a client. Responding in ways the client finds satisfying strengthens the therapeutic relationship and may result in greater self-knowledge or confidence on the part of the client, resulting in feelings of empowerment or new wisdom. If managed carefully, intimate self-disclosures can also result in mutual feelings of closeness and understanding between client and therapist. If managed poorly, they

---

Box 6.2 An Intimate Self-Disclosure

During rehabilitation, Jake, a male client in his thirties, used a variety of coping methods to get through and be productive. Some of these included putting things off (denial) and a lot of humor, and for about 4 months he behaved as one of the most resilient, disciplined, and industrious patients with whom I had ever worked. I had a lurking feeling that these coping strategies were ultimately going to give way to a lot of intense feelings of insecurity, self-doubt, and maybe even despair. But I never dared to interrupt Jake's natural ways of coping, given that they were working very well for him. Eventually, Jake did approach me on his own. In his own language he told me that he was having nightmares and other difficulties anticipating what life would be like when he left the hospital. During this conversation he expressed several concerns about masculinity, intimacy, rejoining the workforce, and about how his children would perceive him as a parent. He told me he had been worried about these issues for a long time but only now felt comfortable discussing them.

— Kim Eberhardt

---

can spawn numerous unintended consequences that may involve feelings of abandonment, shame, self-doubt, distrust, or betrayal.

Power Dilemmas

In occupational therapy, every client–therapist relationship is characterized by an undeniable difference in power between the client and therapist (Pinderhughes, 1989). Within the treatment relationship, therapists typically hold more power because they are the gatekeepers of knowledge, information, and other resources that can influence the client's functioning or quality of life in some way. In addition, many clients face some form of discrimination, stigma, and restricted access because of their impairments. This can contribute to their awareness of injustices that exist at a more global level. For these and other reasons, the negotiation of power between client and therapist can be central to the treatment relationship.

Power dilemmas are tensions that arise in the therapeutic relationship because of clients' innate feelings about issues of power, the inherent situation of therapy, the therapist's behavior, and/or other circumstances that underscore clients' lack or loss of power over aspects of their lives. An example of a power dilemma is provided in Box 6.3.

Box 6.3 A Power Dilemma

Nickolas was a young adult with a diagnosis of bipolar illness. At the time of the referral, he was living alone with financial support from his family. His therapy was provided as part of a multidisciplinary package. The referral was for support to enable Nickolas to make healthy meals. The duration of treatment was over 2 years with, on average, a session per fortnight [every other week] provided either at his home or within his community environment.

While observing his interactions with service providers, I noticed that Nickolas responded very negatively to any goals that others tried to impose on him to make him conform to societal norms. Anytime his providers attempted to impose these kinds of values on him, Nickolas would dig his heels in further and behave according to his own preferences. This behavior was not unique to me or to the discipline of occupational therapy; he enacted it with all of his service providers. His priorities for occupations were framed strongly around his passion for playing the drums, whereas his family and service providers were expecting him to form routines around domestic tasks like meal preparation, grooming, housekeeping, maintaining order, and setting daily schedules involving a balance of work, leisure, and rest. Nickolas did not perceive his living situation as chaotic but everyone else around him (including me!) did. Thus, he became quickly involved in power struggles with everyone around him.

— **Jane Melton**

Dilemmas that involve power are particularly likely to occur in circumstances such as the following.

- The client's experience of impairment has suddenly or chronically resulted in a loss/lack of personal power.
- The client is feeling compelled by circumstances or others to participate in therapy (e.g., therapy is required by the school system or the client's employer, is urged by family members, or is necessitated by a traumatic event).
- The circumstance of therapy places the therapist in a position of authority (e.g., the therapist makes recommendations about the client's ability to work or the type of living situation the client can manage).
- The client has a history of difficult experiences with authority figures or people who assume a position of authority.
- There is an obvious or significant disparity between the therapist's knowledge, resources, abilities, or advantages and the client's own.
- There is a difference between what the therapist strongly believes is in the best interest of the client and what the client wants.

- The therapist does or says something that takes advantage of knowledge or authority in an attempt to persuade or influence the client's attitude or behavior.

Dilemmas related to power are common in occupational therapy and might be reflected in the following client behaviors.

- Passivity
- Resistance
- Directly confronting or challenging the therapist
- Attempting to control or manipulate the therapist

When managed thoughtfully, power dilemmas can ultimately lead the client to experience increased feelings of autonomy or to have new insight about negotiating issues related to power. If managed less thoughtfully, power dilemmas can perpetuate feelings of inferiority, powerlessness, or resentment and can lead to increasing tension or conflict within the relationship.

Nonverbal Cues

Nonverbal cues are communications that do not involve the use of formal language. They include but are not limited to:

- Facial expressions
- Movement patterns
- Body posture
- Body position (the way we hold our arms and legs while sitting or standing)
- Aspects of gait (unique features involved in the way we walk)
- Proxemics (the amount of physical space put between ourselves and others while interacting)
- Tone of voice
- Eye contact
- Touch
- Clothing selection and style
- Other aspects of physical appearance (hair style, makeup)

Because they may be subtle and fleeting, and may vary according to cultural background, nonverbal cues are often subject to multiple interpretations. However, if perceived and accurately understood, these cues may provide critical information about a client's thoughts or feelings. An example of a nonverbal communication is presented in Box 6.4.

Box 6.4 A Nonverbal Cue

Eynat was a child with Rett syndrome and moderate developmental disability. She had lost the ability for verbal communication and would only communicate with her eyes. She had no functional hand use (only stereotypic hand movements). Eynat was referred for occupational therapy so she could learn to eat with utensils within the classroom environment.

Eynat's teachers and other service providers described her as being known to cry and scream without reason. My initial goal within the framework of the class was to teach her to eat with utensils. When I first attempted to work with her on eating skills, she cried and screamed the entire time. At that point I knew my primary goal was no longer to get her to eat with utensils but, instead, to find the way to her heart. The only way to do this was by watching her nonverbal communications and cues.

I learned from observation that Eynat cried less when the class was quiet. When she was offered food and she could choose, she would become interested in eating. She preferred me to whisper into her ear than speaking out aloud. In addition, I learned that she responded better when I would look at her from a very close distance, almost nose to nose rather than regular distance. All of these communications enabled me to reach a point where Eynat knew who I was and acknowledged me as a working partner and ally.

— **Michele Shapiro**

Any nonverbal cue may play an important role in the therapeutic relationship. For example, a therapist and client may share the same taste in clothing style, and this source of commonality may lead the client to believe that the therapist may be better able to understand his or her perspective. Alternatively, a watchful therapist notices that a client is revealing her anxiety through her tentative body movements and preoccupied facial expression. These and other nonverbal behaviors offer therapists timely opportunities to comment on what they are observing in order to promote increased communication, sharing, or problem-solving with clients. In sum, a nonverbal communication or cue from a client can function within therapy as a:

- Positive cornerstone of the relationship
- Key precipitant for communication between client and therapist
- Means of enriching your knowledge of a client
- Means of gathering or conveying feedback
- Harbinger of a problem in the relationship
- Source of a problem in the relationship (if nonverbal behavior is misperceived or misinterpreted)

Crisis Points

Crisis points are unanticipated, stressful events that cause clients to become distracted and/or that temporarily interfere with clients' ability for occupational engagement. Although crisis points occur in everyone's life, they are likely to occur with greater frequency in the lives of occupational therapy clients because of their health or impairment status and the changes and challenges that often accompany these conditions. An example of a crisis point that occurred during the author's work with a client is presented in Box 6.5.

Points of crisis may include but are not limited to:

- A change in the client's health status (e.g., client develops pneumonia, infection, a serious pressure sore, a new injury or experiences an increase in pain, nausea, fatigue, or other symptoms)
- A change in the client's functional capacity (e.g., muscle strength, endurance, range of motion, coordination, cognitive functioning)
- A change in the client's psychological state (e.g., mood, level of arousal)
- Death or serious emotional or physical illness of the client's friend, partner, or family member
- Breakup, separation, divorce, or other loss of an intimate relationship

---

Box 6.5 A Crisis Point

Virgil was a man in his mid-twenties with a diagnosis of Sjögren's syndrome, an autoimmune disease. Virgil also abused alcohol. When able, he spent his time doing odd jobs as a painter and handyman, playing and watching sports on television, and socializing with others at a local bar. He referred himself for therapy in order to establish more consistency in his work schedule and to overcome social anxieties related to explaining his limitations to potential friends, employers, and coworkers. A secondary goal of therapy, which was therapist-initiated, was to reduce his alcohol intake.

The crisis point came approximately 8 weeks into the course of therapy when Virgil was involved in a serious car accident. It had happened one evening when he had become highly intoxicated and then attempted to drive himself home from a bar. While driving under the influence, he blacked out, drifted into oncoming traffic, and was involved in a head-on collision. He and the other driver were both injured.

— **Renee Taylor**

- Conflict or loss of a close friend
- Issues related to pregnancy or to the birth of a child
- Difficulties related to employment or loss of employment
- Other serious economic difficulties
- Educational difficulties
- Legal difficulties or stress related to illegal actions (e.g., client is facing a conviction for driving under the influence of drugs or alcohol)
- Assault or theft (e.g., burglary takes place at client's home while client is in the hospital)

If clients remain in therapy during a crisis point, therapists must be prepared to respond and adapt the treatment relationship to accommodate the client's reactions when they occur.

Resistance and Reluctance

This section discusses two types of interpersonal events that share some common features, but that should be distinguished from each other (Egan, 2001). *Resistance* is a client's passive or active refusal to participate in some or all aspects of therapy for reasons linked to the therapeutic relationship. The following client behaviors are examples of resistance.

- Direct refusal to do something
- Challenging, questioning, or confronting the therapist
- Passive forms of refusal (e.g., actively ignoring the therapist's recommendations; being uncommunicative or unresponsive; efforts to refuse, skip, avoid, underperform, or fail to follow-through with the tasks and recommendations of therapy)

Client resistance may be difficult for therapists to understand because it typically does not serve the client's best interests. Resistance may be attributable to such factors as:

- Issues within the client–therapist relationship (e.g., a client perceives that the therapist is forcing an agenda or experiences an empathic break)
- Difficulties the client is having with others outside of therapy that are being reenacted with the therapist during therapy
- Misunderstanding or disagreeing with the aims and/or methods of therapy

In some cases, client resistance is attributable to a combination of situations. For example, some clients are predisposed to becoming resistant within the therapeutic relationship because they have difficulty getting their needs met in other relationships. Thus, when a circumstance arises during therapy that contradicts the clients' wishes or presents some other kind of dilemma, it may trigger them to behave in a resistant manner.

Reluctance is disinclination toward some aspect of therapy for reasons outside the therapeutic relationship. Reluctance differs from resistance in that it is easy to understand (makes sense to the therapist), and the therapist is able to see how it serves the client's best interest. Reluctance typically manifests in terms of increased anxious questioning, passivity, or lack of follow-through on a given task or activity. It is not rooted in the therapeutic relationship. Instead, reluctance may be explained by:

- Symptom escalation (e.g., client too fatigued today)
- The task perceived as too difficult or demanding
- Preexisting attitudes about health care (mistrust of the process)
- Low self-esteem, depression, feeling overwhelmed

Regardless of their nature and source, resistance and reluctance must both be understood as indicators that a client is not comfortable with the therapy process. An example of resistance is provided in Box 6.6.

Boundary Testing

A boundary is an interpersonal framework in which the client–therapist relationship occurs. Boundaries help clients know what to expect and what not to expect from the therapist. They define the limitations of the relationship and ensure that it remains professional and ethical. They enable the client to know that the therapists will not attempt to exploit, manipulate, or use the relationship as a means of getting their own needs met. At the same time, boundaries protect the therapist from becoming overwhelmed by the emotional needs and personal demands of clients. Occasionally, clients test the boundaries of the therapeutic relationship. *Boundary testing* is a client behavior that violates or that asks the therapist to act in ways that are outside the defined therapeutic relationship. Box 6.7 provides a case example of boundary testing. The following are some additional examples of boundary testing.

- Asking the therapist to reveal personal information
- Making personal observations or unsolicited comments about the therapist

- Giving the therapist an expensive or exorbitant gift
- Contacting the therapist at nonscheduled times
- Bartering or offering to perform services for the therapist
- Inviting the therapist to participate in a dual relationship (e.g., going into business together)
- Inviting the therapist for a personal get-together or to attend a personal event
- Touching or hugging the therapist without the therapist's invitation or permission

When clients test the boundaries of the therapeutic relationship, it can be stressful for therapists to decide when and how to set limits without jeopardizing rapport.

Some clients naturally test the limits of the therapeutic relationship. They are likely to be unaware that what they are doing is inappropriate or uncomfortable for the therapist. These clients may test boundaries in order to feel they can more easily relate to and trust the therapist with their difficulties. This way of approaching professional relationships may be consistent with their cultural values.

Other clients may test boundaries because they are confused about the nature of their relationship with the therapist. These clients usually have difficulty figuring out what the limitations are in their other relationships, and they may also offend friends or family by saying or doing things that are unsolicited and feel imposing, intrusive, or smothering. A final group of clients may intentionally test the boundaries of the therapeutic relationship to control or intimidate the therapist. Generally, this group of clients exhibits other interpersonal difficulties during therapy and require extensive limit setting.

Empathic Breaks

As therapists and as people we are not perfect. We all have certain blind spots that make us less sensitive toward the needs of others than we would like. Moreover, what one person might perceive as completely acceptable may be a negative interpersonal behavior to another person. This makes it inevitable that the actions (or failure to act) of even the most sensitive and caring therapist occasionally and unwittingly leads to a client's hurt feelings. Empathic breaks are thus natural occurrences during therapy.

An *empathic break* occurs when a therapist fails to notice or understand a communication from a client or initiates a communication or behavior that is perceived by the client as hurtful or insensitive. Box 6.8 presents an example of a client who perceived an empathic break.

Clients may experience empathic breaks for any of the following reasons.

- A client perceives that a therapist has demanded too much.
- A client perceives that the therapist is being too directive or not directive enough.
- There is a disruption of therapy due to therapist illness, vacation, pregnancy, or other reason for cancellation.
- The therapist is forced to enforce professional boundaries (time limits or other restraints).
- A client perceives a therapist's question or comment as hurtful, offensive, intrusive, or emotionally difficult to face.
- A client and therapist differ in their opinions concerning the aim of therapy (e.g., a client insists on a goal that the therapist believes is not attainable, or the therapist recommends a goal that the client rejects).

- A client perceives that the therapist did not respond or listen in the way the client wanted.

Some clients experience our actions (or failure to act) as neglectful, hurtful, or offensive, but they may not be able to talk about it directly. Instead, they dismiss their feelings and act them out by disengaging from the relationship, minimizing the importance of therapy, becoming passive or irritable, missing the next appointment, or making an indirectly hostile comment toward the therapist. Therapists who are vigilant regarding the possibility that an empathic break has occurred realize it shortly thereafter by cueing in to these kinds of behaviors. Information about how to resolve empathic breaks can be found in Chapter 13.

Emotionally Charged Therapy Tasks and Situations

Occupational therapy sometimes involves *emotionally charged therapy tasks and situations* that are activities or circumstances that can lead clients to become overwhelmed or experience uncomfortable emotional reactions such as embarrassment, humiliation, or shame. Box 6.9

Box 6.8 Empathic Break

Madam Roucharlamange was a woman in her mid-fifties with few economic resources and few sources of social support. Her diagnoses included mild cognitive impairment, depression, borderline personality disorder, and alcohol dependence. She was also entrenched in a problematic marriage that involved physical abuse by her husband. I saw her for 7 weeks on the inpatient psychiatric unit. Once we understood that her depressive symptoms and drinking binges were linked to her marital situation, we began a course of therapy that aimed to validate her memories and improve linkages between her lost memories and her specific problems. We also worked with her on improving her attention span and increasing her ability to endure low levels of work. After Madam Roucharlamange achieved these goals, we observed that her confidence had improved. She told us that she was ready for a new type of life and motivated to take more responsibility in taking steps to secure employment. At that time she also began to question her relationship with her alcoholic and violent partner. To this end, we decided to initiate an occupational therapy assessment that offered a more precise measurement of her true performance capacity.

Despite the fact that her cognitive skills, motivation, and problem-solving abilities had improved, she continued to have

numerous deficits. We recommended the Assessment of Motor and Process Skills (AMPS) to assess her effort, efficiency, safety, and independence in daily living tasks and routines. Specifically, we hoped that the AMPS would reveal the specific areas she would need to improve in order to ensure more independent functioning. The emphatic break occurred at the beginning of this second step of the therapy process. Madam Roucharlamange agreed to be assessed with AMPS, but the results revealed numerous problem areas. She had difficulty in 14 of 21 process skills assessed. Because it is standard practice on the unit and I assumed my therapeutic relationship with Madam Roucharlamange was solid enough, I allowed myself to share these findings with her.

Shortly thereafter she had a very negative reaction and demanded to stop her inpatient treatment and return home to her abusive partner. After some time had passed, she decided to remain on the unit. She openly expressed her dissatisfaction about the results of the AMPS with her psychiatrist, her psychiatric nurses, and her social worker but not directly with me. Instead, she decided to stop attending occupational therapy without warning me.

— **René Bélanger**

> ### Box 6.9 Emotionally Charged Therapy Tasks and Situations
>
> Howard is a 6-year-old boy who is one of nine children in a family where all of the boys and one of the girls have learning difficulties of various sorts. Howard was referred for therapy by his teacher; his mother was aware of his problems but made the decision not to enroll him in a special education facility. When I first started working with Howard he was very introverted. He made no eye contact, and he would not talk to me. Instead, he was very active in moving aimlessly around the room. It was also extremely difficult for him to be the focus of attention. As soon as he was presented with an assessment activity his immediate reaction was, "I can't do it." He refused to do most activities for fear of failure. Furthermore, each time he actually did try to do something with a resultant failure, his mother and two sisters who accompanied him to the therapy sessions would start to laugh. It was reported that this pattern of behavior also happened at home.
>
> **— Vardit Kindler**

provides an example of a client who repeatedly experienced feelings of shame and humiliation when attempting the activities of occupational therapy.

The following are some additional examples of emotionally charged therapy tasks and situations.

- Learning a new skill, craft, or activity that produces frustration or apprehensiveness
- Failing when attempting to perform a once-valued activity
- Losing control of a bodily function during therapy
- Relearning fundamental self-care tasks, such as dressing, bathing, toileting, bathing, grooming, and eating
- Discomfort associated with awareness of being observed or evaluated by the therapist in terms of strengths and deficits
- Entering a public setting for the first time to travel, shop, eat, or use the toilet

Although these situations represent much of what occupational therapists are accustomed to doing, clients may experience the situations as novel and, in many cases, uncomfortable. This is particularly likely when clients have had past experiences of shame and humiliation in their families or peer groups. When therapists are mindful of this possibility, they are more likely to respond empathically by taking more time to process a situation with a client, normalize his or her feelings, provide reassurance, or prepare the client to anticipate difficulties and reactions.

Limitations of Therapy

Even the most generous of relationships have limitations. *Limitations of therapy* refer to restrictions on the available or possible services, time, resources, or therapist actions. Box 6.10 presents an example of a typical limitation of therapy.

In occupational therapy, relationships with clients are limited by a number of parameters. These may include limitations imposed by:

- Payment or insurance issues (e.g., client or client's insurance company does not provide enough funding for the client to receive the services, assistive technologies, or other resources that are necessary)
- Temporal horizon, or the amount of time allotted for each therapy session or for the entire course of treatment (e.g., number of sessions or an ending date) and when and if progress will be assessed
- The location, size, configuration, temperature, lighting, noise level, and odor of the room or space available for therapy not being optimal
- The amount and nature of the resources (e.g., equipment, supplies, toys) available for therapy
- Role definitions and policies that restrict what the therapist is able to do with/for a client
- Mismatches between client and therapist in terms of life experience and general wisdom, personality, or other aspects of human diversity (e.g., client and therapist

> ### Box 6.10 Limitations of Therapy
>
> The most significant limitation I face in practice involves inadequate insurance. Many insurance companies in the United States are inadequate and unresponsive when it comes to providing clients with necessary funding for care, and this example is one of the worst. Bill was an electrician in his early twenties. He fell when working and acquired a high-level spinal cord injury. He had no movement whatsoever. His employer's insurance would only allow him to stay in the hospital for 1 month. I notified him and his family of this injustice immediately. For the next month, we made every appeal possible to extend his stay. At the same time I made a concerted effort to educate him and his family, prepare him for the transition home, and provide him with numerous referrals for outpatient care and other in-home resources within the community. In the end we lost the battle with the insurance company, and he was released from the hospital much earlier than most clients with his type of injury.
>
> **— Kim Eberhardt**

differ in terms of cultural background, age, or religious orientation)

Certain types of limitations, if managed successfully, can have positive outcomes or serve a protective purpose within the therapeutic relationship. For example, therapists who uphold the professional role or policies of the institution prevent clients from becoming confused about the type of relationship possible and the general guidelines of interaction that will be upheld within that relationship. Similarly, limitations in time allotted for therapy can sometimes work to a client's advantage. Some courses of treatment involve one session, a few days, several weeks, or possibly years. Some are open-ended, and others have a fixed start and end date. Some therapy sessions last 30 minutes and others 2 hours. If clients are made aware of the time limitations (e.g., that therapy involves an initiation date, interim dates when progress is assessed, and an eventual termination), it is more likely that they will be proactive in deciding how to best use the time allotted for their course of therapy.

Although these necessary and unavoidable limitations may result in some positive outcomes, in many cases the limitations imposed by therapy lead to feelings of frustration, worry, or guilt. This is particularly likely when a therapist or client is aware that the limitations have interfered with a crucial achievement or outcome in therapy. Therapists may be particularly sensitive to the limitations of therapy because they may be more aware of inequities in resource allocation or other aspects of care that their clients are missing. The limitations of therapy must be made as explicit as possible to clients, and the associated challenges to the therapy process must be managed carefully as they occur.

Contextual Inconsistencies

Similar to limitations, contextual inconsistencies may pose challenges to the natural flow and routine of therapy, particularly if a client is sensitive or vulnerable to such changes. *Contextual inconsistencies* are any aspect of a client's interpersonal or physical environment that changes during the course of therapy. An example is provided in Box 6.11.

Some clients are affected by changes from day to day or from week to week in any of the following contexts.

- Number of other clients, staff, or visitors in the milieu (in the waiting room or in the clinic)
- Clients, staff, or visitors who are new or unknown to the client

---

Box 6.11 Contextual Inconsistencies

In the process of writing this book, I was a catalyst for a number of contextual inconsistencies that affected the clients and the therapists being photographed and observed. In one instance, a client elected to continue working on his scrapbook activity instead of requesting a shoulder massage, which is usually what occurred during the second half of each of his therapy sessions. In several instances, clients asked their therapists a number of seemingly irrelevant questions about me. Because all of the therapists had prepared their clients well in advance for the observation and photography, this appeared to be an attempt to reduce the natural tension that accompanies having an unfamiliar person watch and photograph an otherwise private interaction. On other occasions, clients talked at length with their therapists following the observation. Some therapists reported that experiencing the observation together brought them closer together or revealed undisclosed thoughts and feelings about their work together. Some clients reportedly felt that the fact that they had been chosen by their therapists to be featured in the book was a privilege and that it said something positive about the therapist's regard for them. In no circumstance did I receive any negative feedback from the therapists or clients about their participation in the book. This may have been attributable to the skill with which the therapists managed this particular interpersonal event within the therapy process.

— **Renee Taylor**

- The way the therapist looks or behaves
- Other therapeutic or medical activities taking place in the milieu
- Temperature, noise level, or smell of the milieu
- The room in which therapy takes place
- The configuration of the therapy room or space
- The length of treatment, funding, or resources available
- Presence versus absence of friends or family members in the therapy context
- Presence versus absence of other professionals (e.g., other members of the rehabilitation team)

When a contextual inconsistency occurs during therapy, it is usually advisable to check in with the client to determine its impact. Some clients welcome such inconsistencies, whereas others perceive them as distracting or upsetting. If a therapist predicts that a client may become affected by an inconsistency, there are steps that can be taken to acknowledge the change and minimize its impact (Fig. 6.2).

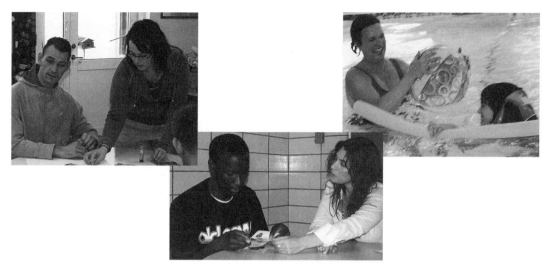

FIGURE 6.2 Therapists regularly face an array of interpersonal events in everyday practice

Summary

This chapter features 11 commonly occurring interpersonal events that have the potential to challenge or pressure the therapeutic relationship. Certainly, any other type of event that occurs during therapy that alters or interrupts the usual flow of therapy or evokes an emotional response in the client or the therapist should also be regarded as having interpersonal implications. Although many of the events described presented the potential for a negative interpersonal outcome, not all interpersonal events should be construed as negative occurrences. As the last example illustrated, some events are unusual because they are uncharacteristically positive occurrences, which rarely occur in professional relationships.

When inevitable interpersonal events of therapy occur, how they are interpreted by the client is a product of the circumstances of therapy and the client's unique set of inter-

personal characteristics. Clients react only to events that carry a unique significance in their own minds. Chapter 5 discussed client characteristics that may predispose clients to react more strongly to certain interpersonal events.

Subsequent chapters of this book demonstrate that when clients are affected by these events the therapist's response is what ultimately determines the interpersonal outcome. Detailed guidance on positive ways that therapists can deal with the interpersonal events of therapy are provided in subsequent chapters.

The Activities section of this chapter presents exercises that allow you to reflect upon and test your ability to identify interpersonal events during therapy. Doing these exercises and carrying out similar efforts in your fieldwork experience or practice will increase your ability to be vigilant toward the possibility of such events, to recognize them when they occur, and to be watchful for clients' reactions to them.

References

Egan, G. (2001). *The skilled helper*. Florence, KY: Wadsworth.

Kohut, H. (1984). *How does analysis cure?* Chicago: University of Chicago Press.

Pinderhughes, E. (1989). *Understanding race, ethnicity, and power: The key to efficacy in clinical practice.* New York: Free Press.

ACTIVITIES FOR LEARNING AND REFLECTION

The exercises included in this section are designed to increase your recognition of and vigilance toward interpersonal events. Exercise 6.1 requires no previous experience in occupational therapy. Exercises 6.2 through 6.4 are designed for readers with more experience in a service role; they require you to reflect upon past experiences in volunteer or therapeutic roles.

EXERCISE 6.1

Identifying Inevitable Interpersonal Events During Therapy

The aim of this exercise is to achieve a foundational ability to identify and label commonly occurring interpersonal events during therapy. List the interpersonal event or events that have occurred in the following scenarios in the space below each case. Keep in mind that any scenario may contain more than a single interpersonal event. The answers to this exercise are presented at the end of the exercise.

Mike

Mike, a clever and proud 15-year-old client with bipolar disorder, has relocated to your area and you are now assigned as his new OT. His mother requests that you work with him on becoming more independent in his self-care and hygiene. When you meet Mike, it is evident from his appearance and odor that he does not practice adequate hygiene. It is also clear that you do not know how to manage the issue with Mike. His mother mentions that every time she raises the issue he becomes defensive and tells her she is overreacting. You are faced with a situation in which you must discuss these issues with Mike, who seems disinterested and unaware of his hygiene problems.

Judy

Judy, a 45-year-old woman, has been working with you for the past 2 months following a spinal cord injury that occurred in a motorcycle accident. Since she began rehabilitation, she has exhibited a take-charge attitude about her therapy and has participated actively in choosing and pursuing goals for rehabilitation. One day she receives news that a close friend and member of her biking group suddenly died of a heart attack. She appears stunned. From that moment on, she discontinues all communication with you, exhibits a masque-like expression, and stops working on any of her therapy goals.

Stefanie

Stefanie is an 85-year-old nursing home resident with mild dementia, a visual impairment, and pernicious anemia. Earlier in the week, she requested to go on a community outing with the other residents, but her doctor refused to give her medical clearance due to concerns about an upper respiratory infection from which she was recovering. As an alternative, you encourage her to accompany you to the cafeteria to play bingo, a game you know she enjoys. She tells you that she doesn't want to play this week and asks if she can participate in the art therapy group instead. Although art is not an activity in which Stefanie has ever expressed an interest and she does not

know the art therapist, just before the group begins you get special permission from the art therapist and allow Stefanie to join the art therapy group. However, instead of participating in the
group, you find her wandering in the corridor. When you ask her why she is not in the group, she
tells you she is disinterested. When you encourage her to come back to play bingo, she refuses.

Gloria

Gloria is a three-year-old girl with auditory and visual-processing difficulties as well as motor
planning difficulties. After she and her mother sat in traffic for an hour, she arrived at the session
sobbing and crying. Her mother reported that Gloria was probably crying because she sensed how
stressful it was for her mother to sit that long in traffic and arrive late to therapy. As Gloria's therapist, it takes you 5 minutes before you can soothe and distract her enough to get her interested in
therapy.

Glenn

For the past 6 months, you have been working with Glenn on self-care issues following a stroke.
Because Glenn has no family support and few friends, you have become his only source of emotional support, and he has developed a strong bond with you. However, you have decided to take a
leave of absence from the outpatient center to pursue further training to support your own professional development. You know that Glenn is not yet ready to discontinue therapy, and you also
know that he may have difficulty forming a bond with a new therapist at first. Still, you have to tell
him that you will be leaving in approximately 2 months. When you tell him of this anticipated
change, he wishes the best for you and tells you that you deserve to further your career. He says he
is ok with the news because you have given him 2 months to prepare for it. However, during the
session you observe that he is visibly trembling.

Bob

You are working in an inpatient unit. Bob, one of your clients, is a 36-year-old man with severe
injuries to his wrists and left leg from a car accident. On occasion you have noticed that his wife
appears exceptionally worried about him, and yet there is some tension in the relationship. During
one of your sessions, you raise a question about sources of support following discharge; after some
discussion Bob confides in you that although he hasn't yet told his wife he had been planning to raise
the issue of divorce with his wife prior to his accident.

Alice

Alice is a woman in her early sixties who has lupus and a secondary depressive disorder. You are
leading a group on stress reduction for individuals with chronic illness, and the topic of conversation focuses on occupations that reduce stress. Toward the beginning of the session, Alice looks
sullen and sits with her eyes cast downward. When it comes time for you to encourage her to provide input, she reports that she has nothing to contribute. Another group member jumps in and
attempts to coax Alice by suggesting she tell the group about her past career as a veterinarian.
Alice responds by telling the group member that she has no business making that suggestion and
continues not to make eye contact with anyone.

Doris

Doris is a 54-year-old woman with poststroke hemiplegia and unilateral neglect who has been
attending therapy for several weeks. From week to week, Doris's affect appears to vacillate from
being relatively flat to being irritable and at times angry.

Esther and Angie

Esther and her four-year-old daughter Angie who has an autistic spectrum disorder have been seeing you weekly for 2 months. Before that, Esther and Angie had been working with a more experienced therapist who had since left the clinic. One session, Esther expresses disappointment in Angie's lack of progress. You respond by asking Esther if she has been following through with the play activities for Angie that you have been recommending as homework. Esther returns an angry look.

Clark

Clark, an elderly client with a developmental disability and diabetes, is pacing the hallways appearing upset and gesturing with his arms. Earlier that morning, he arrived at the day center to find that the sensory room in the basement that he normally enjoys visiting first thing in the morning has been closed off and disassembled due to a flood. When the therapist tries to explain what happened and comfort him, Clark asks if he can have some cake, a food he knows his doctor has prohibited because of his diabetes.

Nick

It is the therapist's third session with an 8-year-old child, Nick, who has an autistic spectrum disorder. The therapist has identified a number of sensory problems in the child. She explains them to the mother and confidently recommends a sensory diet for the child. As the OT begins to describe what would be involved, the child's mother who is about 10 years older than the therapist, gives the therapist a nervous and incredulous look and asks, "Have you ever done this on your kids?" and then chuckles nervously and says, "Assuming that you have kids?"

George

A client's insurance company has just notified the OT that George will be allotted only five additional OT sessions. Due to the extent of George's impairment, it is clear to the OT that the client needs at least 20 more sessions. The OT and referring physician make numerous attempts to extend the duration of treatment without success.

Mercedes

Mercedes is an 11-year-old girl undergoing hippotherapy to address attention and concentration difficulties associated with attention-deficit hyperactivity disorder. The therapist, who has been working with Mercedes for several weeks, has noticed that Mercedes has exceptional balance on the horse and good athletic ability. The hippotherapist has noticed that every time she suggests that Mercedes try to make her horse trot she reports that she is afraid she will fall. After the lesson, Mercedes makes apologetic statements about herself such as, "I know I am a wimp for not being able to trot."

Answers to Exercise 6.1

Mike:	An emotionally charged therapy situation
Judy:	Crisis point; expression of strong emotion
Stefanie:	Power dilemma; resistance; boundary testing
Gloria:	Expression of strong emotion
Glenn:	Limitations of therapy; nonverbal cue
Bob:	Intimate self-disclosure
Alice:	Nonverbal cues; power dilemma
Doris:	Expression of strong emotion

Esther and Angie:	Empathic break; nonverbal cue
Clark:	Expression of strong emotion; contextual inconsistencies; boundary testing
Nick:	Limitations of therapy; power dilemma; reluctance
George:	Limitations of therapy
Mercedes:	Reluctance; intimate self-disclosure

EXERCISE 6.2

Recollection

The aim of this exercise is to increase your awareness of the many ways that interpersonal events manifest and affect therapy and your therapeutic relationship with clients. Based on your experience as a therapist, in fieldwork, or in volunteer or other experiences in which you worked with clients, list in the form below (you can make additional copies) as many possible examples of interpersonal events. Think about how these events ultimately affected the process and outcomes of therapy and/or your relationship with the person involved. Keep in mind that the event can have either a positive or a negative effect.

Briefly Describe the Event	Label the Event	Describe Its Impact on Therapy/Your Relationship

EXERCISE 6.3

Deciphering a Difficult Therapeutic Relationship

The aim of this exercise is to learn to use awareness of interpersonal events to understand how a difficult therapeutic relationship can ensue and be affected by those interpersonal events. Think about a past or present therapy experience in which one of the following was the case.

• You feel very uncomfortable with the client.
• The client is noncompliant, unhappy with therapy, or difficult to work with in some way.
• You had to terminate working with the client or find another therapist to work with the client.
• The client terminated therapy against your or others' advice.
• There was a difficult period when working with the client.
• There was an unnecessarily bad or undesirable outcome to therapy that was linked in some way to the client's behavior and/or your relationship to the client.

When you identify the client who fits one of these situations, describe as many interpersonal events as you can that influenced the therapy process and therapeutic relationship. Describe and label each event and its impact in the table below.

Briefly Describe the Event	Label the Event	Describe Its Impact on Therapy/Your Relationship

EXERCISE 6.4

Deciphering a Positive Therapeutic Relationship

The aim of this exercise is to learn to use awareness of interpersonal events to understand how a positive therapeutic relationship can ensue and be affected by those interpersonal events. Think about a past or present therapy experience in which there was a positive outcome and a good therapeutic relationship. Describe as many interpersonal events as you can that positively influenced the therapy process and therapeutic relationship. Describe and label each event and its impact in the table below.

Briefly Describe the Event	Label the Event	Describe Its Impact on Therapy/Your Relationship

CHAPTER 7

NAVIGATING THE CHALLENGES:
Therapeutic Responding and Interpersonal Reasoning

Occupational therapy involves a complex and dynamic relationship between client and therapist. Along the way, it is likely that certain interpersonal events and/or negative interpersonal characteristics of clients will test the therapist's emotional resolve and challenge his or her ability to apply the usual models and techniques of occupational therapy. Deciding on an optimal response to such challenges is an important skill in the development of your therapeutic use of self. Consistent with the underlying principles of the Intentional Relationship Model (IRM), the process of *therapeutic responding* encourages therapists to be systematic and self-disciplined when deciding what to say, do, and express to clients when faced with a sensitive or negative situation.

Therapeutic responding can be differentiated from nontherapeutic responding in terms of the emotional reaction that the response is likely to produce in the client. Therapeutic responses result in clients feeling understood and supported. By contrast, nontherapeutic responses inevitably lead clients to feel devalued, hurt, judged, defensive, belittled, neglected, or emotionally abandoned. Despite their negative consequences for clients, it is easy for therapists to fall into the trap of nontherapeutic responding, particularly when clients behave in undesirable ways. We are all human and prone to react according to habit or in what we think are self-protective ways when provoked. When others do not behave as we expect, it is natural for us to feel disappointed or hurt. Sometimes we are able to express these feelings in a way that is easy to receive and understand. Other times, we allow our impulses to give way to these feelings, and we act in ways that undermine our relationships. If these feelings are par-

ticularly strong, it is easy for them to test our interpersonal self-discipline and penetrate our therapeutic demeanor.

Sometimes it is not even necessary for a client to say or do anything to cause us to respond in a nontherapeutic way. There are days when we are stressed for no reason or when we are troubled by events in our personal lives outside of therapy. Under these circumstances, it is difficult to hide the fact that we are preoccupied, distracted, or otherwise upset from our clients. Table 7.1 presents examples and descriptions of responses that carry a greater potential to be nontherapeutic if timed inappropriately or conveyed within the wrong context.

Although there are no definitive rules that differentiate therapeutic from nontherapeutic responses, this chapter describes a reasoning process and corresponding types of responses (which are linked to the therapeutic modes) that maximize the likelihood that therapists' responses will be perceived by clients as therapeutic. Therapeutic responding involves three components: an overarching process of interpersonal reasoning and two additional sets of interpersonal capacities—mode use and interpersonal skill level. The process of interpersonal reasoning provides a framework within which therapists can decide on the appropriate selection and application of the therapeutic modes and their associated interpersonal skills. The definition of therapeutic responding is summarized in Figure 7.1.

The IRM encourages therapists to learn to engage in a continuous process of interpersonal reasoning when deciding how to interact with clients at an interpersonal level. Briefly defined in Chapter 3, *interpersonal reasoning* is

(text continued on page 138)

Table 7.1 Responses that Carry a Potential to be Nontherapeutic*

Parental Responses: Particularly when conveyed to school-aged children, adolescents, or adults, parental responses have the potential to be experienced as infantilizing or overprotective. They subtly undermine the client's sense of competence. Although they convey caring, they also have the potential to convey the therapist's uncertainty about the client's judgment or performance capacity. Examples of parental responses include saying things such as, "I am sorry you are having a flare-up ... you have to take good care of yourself"; speaking in a sing-song or ebullient tone of voice; addressing clients using phrases such as "honey" or "sweetie"; or making statements that are supportive but at the same time highlight an age or power differential (e.g., "I'm so proud of you!").

Defensive Responses: Defensive responses are characterized by timing, tone of voice, and choice of language. Defensive responses explain, reiterate, or justify the therapist's position or actions and are usually articulated immediately after the feedback is provided. These responses do not involve time to pause for reflection or attempts to clarify the issue or seek understanding. A defensive response is most likely to occur in reaction to feedback that is perceived by the therapist as critical or inaccurate. Although defensive responses may allow the therapist to clarify his or her intention or position, unless they are accompanied by attempts to understand and validate the client's position, they are limited in the extent to which they are effective in moving the relationship forward.

Patronizing Responses: Patronizing responses involve language that conveys an eagerness to help, complement, or support, but the underlying tone of voice or overall context in which the response is communicated communicates a position of superiority. These responses are sometimes experienced by the client as condescending or belittling, particularly if the client has low self-esteem, feels vulnerable, or is sensitive about his or her position, characteristics, or situation.

Cliché Responses: Cliché responses are trite or overused expressions. Because they lack freshness and clarity, they may imply that the therapist has not thought very carefully about what he or she is saying. Cliché responses may be perceived by clients as minimizing or dismissive. Examples of cliché responses include statements such as "chin up," "every cloud has a silver lining," "you can't win 'em all," "count your blessings," or "it could be worse." Sometimes a client uses a cliché to describe what he or she is experiencing. In that instance, it is more likely that the therapist can repeat the same cliché in the future to convey his or her understanding of the client's viewpoint without negative implications.

Minimizing Responses: Minimizing responses are statements that intend to reduce the magnitude or significance of what a client has said. Although they can be helpful in that they offer a new perspective, they imply that the therapist perceives the client as overreacting or exaggerating what he or she is experiencing. Because they introduce a different viewpoint on the client's experience, they are experienced by some clients as invalidating or judgmental, particularly when clients are not in a position to entertain alternative perspectives on their own experience. Sometimes optimizing responses (i.e., efforts to inspire hope or promote an optimistic outlook) can be misperceived by clients as minimizing if they are not timed correctly. Examples of minimizing responses include statements such as "it's not as bad as it seems," "you'll get over it," "c'mon it wasn't *that* bad, was it," or "you're making it sound like I'm asking you to climb Mt. Everest."

Responses That Prematurely Optimize: Responses that prematurely optimize are well-intended but poorly timed. They represent efforts to instill hope or assist a client in achieving a more optimistic outlook. If they are not timed correctly, these responses can be misperceived by clients as unrealistic, cheerleader-like, minimizing, or dismissive. This is most likely to occur when a client is not yet ready to assume a hopeful outlook, attempt a given task, or achieve a certain goal. Although premature efforts to instill hope in a hopeless client reflect poor emotional resonance, therapists who attempt to instill hope in clients do not cause significant harm to the therapeutic relationship. Examples of responses that prematurely optimize include providing praise or complements in an excessive manner or for relatively minor accomplishments, insisting that a client can do something before he or she feels ready, or telling a client he or she is going to be ok when he or she is not yet ready to hear or believe it.

Dismissive Responses: Dismissive responses are typically curt or flippant statements. They imply an attitude of indifference or a lack of concern or caring about what the client is attempting to communicate. Sometimes they occur when a client is talking excessively or dwelling too much on a single issue, and the therapist does not make an intentional effort to provide the client with direct feedback. Accordingly, dismissive responses may serve as "warning signs" that suggest a therapist is feeling frustrated or mildly irritated with a client. Examples of dismissive responses include phrases such as "we can talk about that next time," "why don't you take something (medication) for that," or ignoring or quickly rejecting a useless suggestion or incorrect opinion made by a client.

Withholding Responses: Withholding responses are subtle and are usually identifiable only within the context of a given interaction. Withholding responses are perceived by clients as denying access to the therapist's true feelings, thoughts, or opinions. Withholding responses are most likely to occur when a therapist feels the need to exercise emotional restraint or to maintain or set a limit or professional boundary. In many cases, withholding responses are early warning signs that the client is testing too many boundaries. Accordingly, they may be necessary to preserve a tone of emotional stability and safety within the relationship. The ensuring empathic break that occurs as a result of the emotional withholding may be unavoidable, but if managed correctly this necessary limit setting can facilitate emotional development in the client and within the relationship. However, in some cases withholding responses emerge from a therapist's overcautiousness, discomfort, or underlying anxiety about becoming emotionally involved with a client—even within the boundaries of the professional relationship. Novice therapists who feel a need to protect themselves and those who tend to interpret rules of conduct literally are at highest risk of emotional withholding with clients. Withholding responses can be nonverbal and reflected in a therapist's lack of emotional expression, or they can be verbal and reflected by statements that carry insufficient content or detail.

Evaluative Responses: Evaluative responses can take the form of compliments or judgments. They occur when a therapist questions, doubts, or provides an unsolicited opinion in response to an activity a client has performed or to something a client has communicated. Evaluative responses are fundamental to occupational therapy. They are consistent with an occupational therapist's duty to provide clients with important feedback and instruction on a range of topics, including safety, accessibility, assistive technology, reasonable accommodation, occupational tasks, or activities. Although many clients perceive such feedback as helpful, when timed inappropriately evaluative responses are perceived by some clients as undermining or judgmental, particularly when they are looking for someone to just listen rather than question their perspective or provide an unsolicited opinion. An example of an evaluative response is: "I'm sorry to hear you are more fatigued than usual. Are you overdoing it again?"

Confused Responses: Confused responses reflect poor listening and convey that the therapist is not clear about what the client has just said. Instead of admitting their confusion or responding with a request for the client to clarify the communication, therapists who make confused responses convey a lack of effort and caring. Confused responses are most likely to occur when therapists are fatigued, preoccupied with other thoughts, or not listening fully because of underlying negative feelings toward the client.

Responses That Exaggerate: Responses that exaggerate transform a client's actions or communications into something more significant than what the client perceives them to be. Therapists are at risk of exaggerating what a client has said or done when they attempt to break through a client's denial or tendency to minimize a difficulty. An example of an exaggerating response is when a client describes a difficulty (e.g., "my mood changes sometimes"), and the therapist uses more powerful language when rearticulating it (e.g., "tell me more about your mood swings").

Responses That Compare: Comparative responses occur when therapists use other clients or individuals as reference points. Often this is done when a therapist intends to highlight an achievement, instill hope, or encourage a client to attempt an activity or task. Although this sometimes has a therapeutic effect by making the client feel he or she is special or exceptional, it may backfire or come across as insincere to skeptical or self-doubting clients. For example, self-doubting clients may wonder to themselves whether the therapist makes similar comparisons with all clients or if they will be compared against some other client one day and come up short. Comparative responses are at greater risk of backfiring when therapists use them to encourage reluctant clients (e.g., "I have seen other clients do this, and I know you can too," "Clients with much more severe limitations than yours have achieved this goal," or "Your roommate, Jacob, has been through more than you'll ever know"). Although such responses may be enlightening or inspiring for some clients, other clients may feel that they are not measuring up to existing standards.

*Please note that many of these responses also carry a potential to have therapeutic effects if timed appropriately or conveyed within certain contexts of interaction.

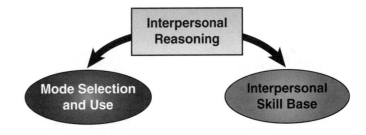

FIGURE 7.1 Three components of therapeutic responding

the process by which a therapist monitors the interpersonal events of therapy, the client's unique interpersonal characteristics, and her or his own behavior in a reflective way to maximize the likelihood that the therapeutic relationship will be successful and supportive of the client's engagement in occupation. It is a stepwise process by which a therapist decides what to say, do, or express in reaction to the client. It includes thinking carefully about a client's characteristics and considering whether there are any negative characteristics that have the potential to incite a nontherapeutic response. It also involves developing mental vigilance toward the interpersonal aspects of therapy in anticipation that a dilemma might occur, and it offers a means of reviewing and evaluating options for responding.

Implied is that the therapist is essentially monitoring the functioning of the therapeutic relationship on an ongoing basis in order to decide what to do about evolving events and key changes.

Interpersonal reasoning is particularly useful when a therapist faces a sensitive or vulnerable client with difficult interpersonal characteristics and/or when an interpersonal dilemma presents itself in therapy. A full description of the steps of interpersonal reasoning and examples of its application in practice are provided in the following sections (Fig. 7.2).

> Implied is that the therapist is essentially monitoring the functioning of the therapeutic relationship on an ongoing basis in order to decide what to do about evolving events and key changes.

Six Steps of Interpersonal Reasoning

Interpersonal reasoning involves six steps.

1. Anticipate
2. Identify and cope
3. Determine if a mode shift is required
4. Choose a response mode or mode sequence
5. Draw upon any relevant interpersonal skills associated with the mode(s)
6. Gather feedback

Step 1: Anticipate

The first step of interpersonal reasoning involves upholding an expectation that an interpersonal event or other behavior on the part of the client is likely to occur that will incite a reaction in the therapist and test, challenge, or threaten the therapeutic relationship. Therapists should be prepared for the possibility that more than one of these events or behaviors may occur even within a single therapy session, depending on the presenting problems, the level of interpersonal complexity involved in the interaction, or circum-

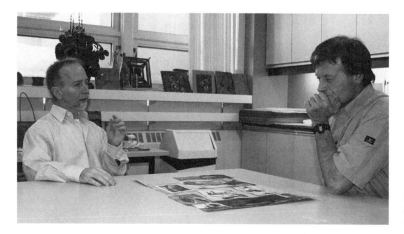

FIGURE 7.2 René Bélanger uses interpersonal reasoning and selects an appropriate mode in response to a client's disclosure

stances in the environment. Early in the therapy process, you should become as familiar as possible with the interpersonal characteristics of the client using the rating scale provided in Chapter 5. When familiarizing yourself with a client, you should pay particular attention to any negative characteristics about the client that, in a nonvigilant moment, have the potential to produce an interpersonal event and/or incite a nontherapeutic response. In addition, you should be familiar with the myriad of other possible interpersonal events that might occur to interrupt the rhythm and flow of therapy. The events that have been found to occur with most frequency were described in Chapter 6.

An example from my own practice is used to illustrate the type of vigilance this process requires.

> Vera[1] was an adolescent client living in a group home for foster children. During one session, I noticed that Vera appeared particularly unhappy. I initiated a conversation with her that involved a lot of empathizing on my part. In the back of my mind, I noted the intensity of Vera's affect that day (an interpersonal characteristic) and, knowing Vera's tendency to assert her interpersonal needs in a rather demanding way when she is feeling down or insecure (a second interpersonal characteristic), I prepared myself emotionally and intellectually for the possibility that some type of interpersonal event might occur.

Step 2: Identify and Cope

The next step of interpersonal responding involves accurately identifying the interpersonal event or events that have occurred. This is best accomplished by labeling the event (either silently to oneself or aloud so the client can hear) and searching for a reaction in the client. In most cases, the IRM recommends that therapists comment on or label the event directly and inquire about the client's interpretation of the event (if the client's reaction is not otherwise obvious).

For example, as predicted, my conversation with Vera culminated in an interpersonal event (i.e., Vera asked if she could come live with me instead of living at the group home). At that point, I made a mental note that a boundary violation had occurred and I employed some coping skills to help me collect my thoughts and formulate an intentional response.

Because they have the potential to test the relationship and interrupt the flow of therapy, these events are easy to ignore or deny. Some therapists, particularly novice therapists, may be prone to thinking that inquiring about or

responding to such events will make the situation worse or waste valuable therapy time. Others may be under the impression that if they do not do anything to respond to such an event, the client will forget about it over time or its significance for the relationship will otherwise dissipate. What these therapists fail to acknowledge is the high likelihood that the event, if left unresolved, may repeat itself in the future or its perceived impact may intensify with time. If the event is precipitated by a client's negative interpersonal characteristic or behavior, it is highly likely that, if unaddressed, it will manifest more than once within the relationship. Whatever the cause, leaving interpersonal events unaddressed is likely to erode the therapeutic relationship over time.

There are some exceptions. For example, there are some occasions when a client may not experience a reaction to the event or regard it as significant. Unless a similar event occurs again, in these circumstances it is recommended that the therapist assess whether he or she would be burdening the client with some personal reaction to the event that the client does not share. Similarly, a therapist may judge that certain clients are in too vulnerable a position to be able to cope with a direct and open discussion about certain events. For example, when Anne Reuter set a limit on Mr. Klein's attempts to hug her (see Chapter 2), she decided that setting a nonverbal limit was enough of a response to the boundary testing. Given Mr. Klein's extended history of loss and rejection, discussion of the event, at least at that stage in the treatment relationship, would have been overkill. While being careful not to overprotect the client, in these situations therapists who can afford the luxury of a longer treatment relationship should respond as empathically as possible and wait until a similar event or a more opportune time for direct discussion and processing.

Once a therapist is able to acknowledge that an interpersonal event has occurred, the next task is for the therapist to cope with this realization. For some therapists, coping involves altering their thinking about the event in order to normalize it or put it into perspective. What is most important is that the therapist's coping counteracts avoidance and denial and leads to suppression of nontherapeutic responses. To cope, the following strategies may be helpful.

- Taking a deep breath
- Normalizing the event and regarding it as a given part of therapy
- If the event was precipitated by something you said or did, reminding yourself that your intentions were honest or that you alone did not cause the event

---

[1]All client names and geographic information have been changed.

• Reminding yourself that other clients might have reacted differently to this event
• Reminding yourself that the client will survive the event (even if the client appears let down or devastated at the moment)
• Avoiding doing what is easiest, comfortable, or habitual (e.g., denying or avoiding discussion of the issue)

The second aspect of effective coping involves having enough self-awareness to know which categories of client characteristics tend to evoke negative feelings and, if necessary, learning to control any impulses toward nontherapeutic responding. (For examples of responses that have the potential to be interpreted as nontherapeutic, see Table 7.1). Vera's request to live with me did not evoke negative feelings in me; but when she does things that cause me to feel embarrassed and disrespected (e.g., mocking me in front of other group members), she does provoke my impulses toward nontherapeutic responding.

When feeling a negative impulse toward a client, it is often helpful to remind oneself which of the client's characteristics may be inciting that impulse and to place those negative client characteristics within a larger context. For example, a therapist might remind oneself that a given client's tendency to become demanding and controlling when she is anxious likely stems from preexisting psychological vulnerabilities and/or a negative experience in her past. In Vera's case, I remind myself that Vera tends to mock me when she feels I am not paying enough attention to her in a group setting and that this behavior stems from a long childhood history of emotional abuse and physical neglect. Collectively, the therapists interviewed for this book identified the following negative client characteristics as being among the most difficult to manage in therapy.

• Expressions of irritability, anger, or rage
• Acts that reveal hostility, disrespect, or dislike toward the therapist
• Other difficulties with emotional expression or emotion regulation
• Client criticism that is experienced as excessive or overly negativistic
• Assertion of needs in a demanding or excessive manner
• Refusal or reluctance to communicate
• Efforts to control or manipulate the therapist by behaving or relating in an inconsistent manner (e.g., client idealizes the therapist one moment and then devalues the therapist the next).
• Deceptive, indirect, or passive-aggressive behaviors

These and other difficult client characteristics were described in more detail in Chapter 5.

Therapists who know themselves well enough to be able to identify which characteristics are most likely to trigger an impulse toward nontherapeutic responding are most effective at controlling that impulse. This ability is enhanced by two additional abilities: (1) situating the client's characteristics in a broader social and environmental context; and (2) thereby not interpreting the client's interpersonal behavior as a personal offense (even when the client's offensive behavior emerges within the context of the therapeutic interaction).

Step 3: Determine if a Mode Shift is Required

As described briefly in Chapter 3, a *mode shift* is an intentional change in the way a therapist relates to a client. Mode shifts assume that a therapist is already interacting with a client within the framework of one of the six therapeutic modes (i.e., advocating, collaborating, empathizing, encouraging, instructing, or problem-solving), and a change from one mode to another is required. Mode shifts are frequently required in response to an interpersonal event or to some other change in the client's interpersonal behavior. For example, during our discussion in which Vera shared her unhappiness about living in the group home, she asked me if she could come live with me instead. Remaining within the empathizing mode, I empathized with Vera's unhappiness and questioned her about the reasons for wanting to live with me. However, Vera refused to process her feelings with me and demanded that I answer either "yes" or "no." At that point I decided that a different type of action was required to protect Vera from continuing to push the boundaries and to prevent myself from reacting to her behavior in a nontherapeutic manner. I decided to shift into the instructing mode to send Vera a stronger message about the limitations to our professional relationship. Thus, I explained why it would be neither appropriate nor realistic for her to live with me. The following are additional examples of circumstances in which a mode shift would likely be required.

• A client provides the therapist with feedback that she wants to feel more independent in performing self-care activities within the milieu. In this case, a therapist who was previously relying heavily on the instructing mode might switch to the collaborating mode in an effort to promote client decision-making and autonomy.

- An otherwise enthusiastic client is reluctant to engage in an activity that the therapist knows would be possible for the client to do. The therapist attempts to reassure the client, but the client remains apprehensive. In this case, a therapist might change from the encouraging mode to an empathizing mode so she can better understand the client's reaction.
- A client appears overwhelmed during a discussion about goal setting. When asked to provide input, he becomes more anxious and tells the therapist that he has no idea where to begin. At this point, a therapist might switch from the collaborating mode into an instructing mode, counting on the likelihood that the client's anxiety is reduced by the introduction of structure and guidance.
- A client appears disengaged from therapy and generally hopeless. Although she does not appear to mind the therapist's use of the empathizing mode to better understand her perspective, the client remains stagnant in terms of progress toward goals. In this instance, the therapist might switch to the encouraging mode in an attempt to instill hope and entice the client into engaging in a previously cherished activity.
- A client reveals that she did not complete the assigned activity at home because the assignment required a partner. The client discloses that she could not think of anyone on whom she might rely to assist her. In this instance, a therapist might shift from the problem-solving mode into an empathizing mode, as the client has just made an important and rather sensitive self-disclosure about her lack of connection with others.

These are just a few of numerous possible therapeutic situations in which a mode shift would be appropriate. When considering whether a mode shift is necessary, you should consider the exact nature of the interpersonal event and the unique constellation of client interpersonal characteristics. In some cases, an interpersonal event may occur, but the therapist and client do not deem it as particularly significant or consequential for the relationship. In other cases, an interpersonal event may occur, but a mode shift is not appropriate because a therapist is already interacting in a mode that is perceived as therapeutic by the client. For example, a therapist who is already using the instructing and encouraging modes with an anxious and disorganized client would likely continue using those modes if an event such as a contextual change occurred that made the client feel even more unstable.

In other cases, a client's personality requires that a therapist use a single mode as consistently as possible. For example, there are certain clients who want to have as much control over the therapy process as possible and require therapists to do nothing else but listen, strive to understand their dilemmas, and support their desires (even if they do not serve the client's best interest). These clients prefer consistent use of the empathizing mode. Other clients, including other health care professionals and other types of individuals with extensive knowledge, may want to engage in a collaborative or problem-solving relationship with the therapist and may feel insulted when the therapist attempts to use the instructing mode. Clients who are anxious or appear to be seeking direction are likely to relax when a therapist relies heavily on the instructing mode to structure and guide the activities of therapy. Clients who prefer a single mode or a more limited range of modes are easy to identify because they appear less comfortable and are less likely to engage in therapy when therapists use other modes.

Even if a client tends to prefer a single or more limited range of modes, there are still occasions when a mode shift is necessary. Without practice, mode shifts are not easy to accomplish. They require the therapist to possess the following capacities.

- Knowledge of the therapeutic modes and how they differ
- The ability to correctly label your own use of modes during live interactions
- An acknowledgement that not all modes are equally therapeutic at all times for all clients
- An openness to learning to communicate in ways that are unfamiliar, uncharacteristic, or less comfortable
- Capacity to relate effectively with a wide range of personality styles
- Knowledge of which modes are likely to work best given a client's interpersonal characteristics
- Knowledge of which modes are likely to work best given the interpersonal event that is occurring
- Capacity to match the primary mode or modes chosen for a client to the implicit and unspoken expectations and preferences of the client and to the circumstances that are occurring during therapy or in the therapeutic milieu at any given time
- Capacity to identify when a mode shift might be required based on an empathic awareness of the potential interpersonal events of therapy and needs of the client at any given time

Another guideline to bear in mind when shifting modes is the importance that the new mode is communicated to the client accurately in its pure form. In some cases, it may be important to inform a client that you are shifting to a different mode of communication and explain why. For example, a therapist shifting from the instructing to the empathizing mode might say something like: "It seems to me I may be asking you to do something you are not comfortable with yet, so I'm going to pause for a moment and just check in with you to see why this is not working for us." Similarly, if a therapist shifts modes too rapidly it may also lead to confusion or weakening of the communication, depending on the cognitive level and emotional maturity of the particular client. In circumstances where a therapist is unsure whether the client has received the intended message accurately, he or she may benefit from explaining the need for a mode shift and from seeking feedback from the client that his or her interpersonal message has indeed been interpreted accurately.

An exercise designed to enable continued practice and development of the ability to accomplish mode shifts smoothly is provided in the Activities section of this chapter. Box 7.1 includes a depiction of Michele Shapiro successfully executing a mode shift during her work with an 8-year-old client.

Step 4: Choose a Response Mode or Mode Sequence

For each of the six modes described in Chapter 5, there is a corresponding set of concrete actions or communications that reflect the therapist's use of that mode. These responses are referred to as **response modes**, and they include:

• Advocating responses
• Collaborating responses
• Empathizing responses
• Encouraging responses
• Instructing responses
• Problem-solving responses

For purposes of review, *advocating responses* are communications and actions that respond to a need for physical or interpersonal resources or raise the client's awareness about available resources. Advocating responses may also serve to validate the client's perception of power differentials and injustices and assist the client in taking action to overcome those injustices. *Collaborating responses* are those that encourage and incorporate a

---

Box 7.1 A Mode Shift with Yoni

Yoni is an eight-year-old Israeli boy with cerebral palsy and a severe learning disability (mental retardation). The aim of the treatment with Yoni was to get him to stand for a few minutes. Although this was the reason for referral decided on by the staff during his IEP planning, I felt that without Yoni being highly motivated we would not get though to him. My plan with him was to work with him on standing in the Snoezelen. The treatment would take the following pathway: Go into the Snoezelen with Yoni. Watch his behavior and see what seems to interest him on that particular day. Follow his lead, go to the equipment he seems to prefer. Mirror his behavior—if he bounces up and down I will do the same, if he makes sounds I will do the same. I decided to interpret the bouncing as his way to gain some proprioceptive input into his joints while we both enjoyed the communal interaction. In doing this I was in a situation of completely empathizing with Yoni and mirroring his behavior. I was having a conversation with him by way of our mutual body language, like both of us moving together in some kind of dance.

The natural limitations of therapy prompted a mode shift. Time was up, and I needed to end our session. I prepared Yoni for the end by shifting from the empathizing mode into the instructing mode. First I warned him that we would soon be ending our time together, and I encouraged him to begin our ritual of waving goodbye to the equipment. As I turned off each piece of equipment his face showed definite disappointment, but he had grown accustomed to our ritual and he knew that I would stick to my limits. He also knew that the end of our ritual involved a game, which required me to make yet another shift into the encouraging mode. Yoni knew that when all the equipment had been turned off he would receive a challenge. When he was younger the challenge was to touch the bubble unit. I would then turn it on for a minute before we left the room heading back for the class. Today Yoni knows that more is expected of him. He must make a sound! No sound—no more bubbles. But if he makes a sound he gets the bubbles. Inevitably Yoni makes the desired sounds.

In the first part of our session I was very undemanding and used the empathizing mode. In the next part of the session I was forced to utilize the instructing mode to set a limit because our therapy time was coming to an end. In the final part of the session I present Yoni with a challenge and for this I have to change attitude or shift into the encouraging mode. I think this is right. The same person can "change hats" during treatment without muddling a client.

— **Michele Shapiro**

client's active participation, choice, and decision-making. *Empathizing responses* serve to understand, share, witness, and validate a client's thoughts and emotions. *Encouraging responses* uplift, inspire, complement, and reinforce. *Instructing responses* intend to teach, demonstrate, inform, and provide structure for a client. Finally, *problem-solving responses* engage clients in describing, evaluating, and sometimes questioning a series of options and possibilities. Although the number of possible responses that fall within each mode category is limitless, the responses listed in Table 7.2 are among the most commonly observed in occupational therapy.

Table 7.2   Examples of Therapist Communications and Actions According to Response Mode

Advocating Responses

Interpersonal Focusing
· Encourage the client to be assertive with others about his or her needs
· Validate or point out (if appropriate) an injustice or other power differential that a client is facing
· Openly discuss an injustice or power differential that exists within the treatment setting or within the treatment relationship and its implications for the client

Activity Focusing
· Provide opportunities for and encourage clients to have contact with disabled peer role models who you know will help support his or her pride and identity as a disabled person
· Encourage the client to educate him/herself about his/her entitlements and rights as a disabled individual
· Utilize your professional capacity to advocate/argue on a client's behalf to obtain a needed resource or outcome
· Encourage a client to take action against an injustice, if appropriate
· Assist a client in taking action against an injustice by serving as a witness or becoming involved in a legal or advocacy-type activity

Collaborating Responses

Interpersonal Focusing
· Gather feedback from the client before choosing or recommending any activity
· Encourage a client to make more decisions during the therapy process
· Ask questions to help a client identify life alternatives
· Share with a client how his or her behavior makes me feel
· Ask a critical client about his or her reactions to me as a therapist

Activity Focusing
· Change something about the activity, choice of activity, or environment in response to client feedback that your therapeutic approach is not helpful
· Provide a client with ample choices for occupational engagement
· Ask a client to recommend his or her own goals for therapy

Empathizing Responses

Interpersonal Focusing
· Make summary statements to bear witness to the event and verify your understanding of the client's perspective

· Show emotional resonance or share your personal emotional reactions and thoughts about a client's difficulty
· Strive to understand the nature and source of a client's difficulties through gentle inquiry
· Listen and bear witness silently
· Articulate or describe a client's affect so he or she knows you see and support it
· Admit a mistake you made and apologize for it
· Wonder to yourself if a client's negative behavior is related to something you said or did
· Rely on your emotional reactions to clients to inform clinical reasoning
· Reveal something about yourself or your own life experience to build rapport
· Change my interpersonal style to better match that of a client

Activity Focusing
· Share your emotional reactions with a client (only if appropriate and if they match the client's affect and thought content)
· Mirror a client's breathing, body movements, or facial expressions
· Join a client in an activity (e.g., jumping up and down together on a trampoline)
· Perform the same activity in parallel with a client (e.g., string beads alongside a client)
· Position your body (e.g., sit, stand, or recline) alongside a client
· Use touch to convey empathy (only if appropriate)
· Provide the client with a transitional object, or small token, that he or she can remember you by
· Choose an activity to do with a client that is gratifying, comforting, or conveys an understanding of his or her thoughts or feelings

Encouraging Responses

Interpersonal Focusing
· Use humor
· Encourage or coax a client
· Normalize a concern or event
· Stroke, praise, or label a client's strengths or achievement in therapy
· Reassure the client
· Remind a client of his or her existing strengths or capacities
· Provide a client with hope for improvement
· Tell a client you are confident he or she will be able to complete a task

(table continued on page 144)

Table 7.2 **Examples of Therapist Communications and Actions According to Response Mode (continued)**

Activity Focusing
· Downgrade an activity or select a no-fail activity to be sure the client will have an experience with success
· Choose a pleasurable, comforting, energizing, or mood-enhancing activity
· Engage in entertaining behavior or antics
· Show positive emotion, joy, and enthusiasm through body movements, facial expression, and tone/volume of voice

Instructing Responses

Interpersonal Focusing
· Instruct a client on how to perform a given occupation
· Provide a client with information or advice
· Remind a client of important safety issues
· Remind the client of the likely consequences of a given choice
· Clarify a request or instruction
· Provide a rationale for your request, approach, or behavior
· Label an interpersonal event to raise or heighten the client's awareness of it
· Provide a client with feedback
· Prepare a client for an upcoming discussion, task, or activity
· Share your professional opinion or perspective with a client
· Recommend an alternative way of interpreting the situation

· Question or address a client about his or her lack of follow-through

Activity Focusing
· Model or demonstrate for the client how to perform an occupation
· Introduce a limit or boundary nonverbally
· Choose activities that test or challenge a client's perception of his or her performance capacity

Problem-Solving Responses

Interpersonal Focusing
· Assist the client in evaluating all of the potential consequences of a choice or action
· Assist the client in listing or articulating the pros and cons of a decision
· Assist the client in generating hypotheses (i.e., potential solutions or explanations) to address an unknown or to solve a problem
· Ask questions to help a client correct illogical thinking
· Initiate a process of conflict resolution

Activity Focusing
· Introduce a new technique or technology
· Ignore a client's negativity and focus on intervention strategies
· Redirect an emotional client back to the activity or task

Each response mode is divided into two categories: those that typically involve verbal (or signed) responses of an interpersonal nature (interpersonal focusing) and nonverbal responses, which involve some action or activity (activity focusing). As introduced in Chapter 3, the IRM asserts that it is important to strike a balance between interpersonal focusing and activity focusing—or the amount of time in which interpersonal issues are discussed and processed relative to the amount of time in which the therapist takes some other nonverbal action to address an interpersonal issue. Some clients do not look for or are not able to tolerate much direct dialogue about issues within the relationship, whereas others feel more comfortable if everything pertaining to the relationship is communicated openly and verbally (Fig. 7.3).

When an interpersonal event occurs, it typically serves to intensify any underlying vulnerabilities or challenging aspects of a client's interpersonal style. This increases the need for best-fit matching of a given response mode to a client's interpersonal characteristics. Thus, the same considerations that inform a therapist's decision to shift modes should also guide the category of response mode or sequence of response mode categories selected. These guidelines include consideration of:

• The interpersonal characteristics that underlie the client's preference for one type of response versus another
• The nature and significance of the interpersonal event to the treatment relationship

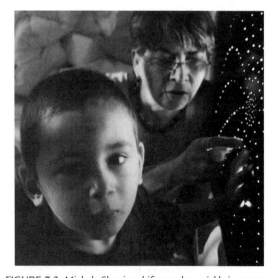

FIGURE 7.3 Michele Shapiro shifts modes quickly in response to a client's changing behavior

• Overarching issues involving the client's safety and other ethical obligations that take precedence and should dictate that the therapist choose a specific response mode (regardless of the client's preference)

A summary of the modes that offer the best chance for a match with various client characteristics was presented in Table 5.1. Although it may be helpful as a rough guide, the summary lacks the context that is otherwise present in live interactions. Thus, it is by no means comprehensive or completely reliable under all circumstances. More complex and challenging constellations of client characteristics make it increasingly difficult to choose the correct response mode consistently. With interpersonally challenging clients, a sequence that includes two or more modes is often what is required to respond to an event in a way that feels satisfying to the client. Conversely, when a client possesses few or no challenging interpersonal characteristics, the therapist has access to a wider range of potential response modes. In these circumstances, the IRM recommends that therapists focus on selecting the response mode that is most appropriate given the interpersonal event that has occurred. If the therapist is successful in his or her selection, one type of response typically is enough to resolve the event. A summary of response modes according to categories of interpersonal events is presented in Table 7.3. As with Table 5.1, Table 7.3 should be considered a rough guide that requires additional judgment that can only occur in a live interpersonal context.

In many clinical interactions, when interpersonal events occur either the therapist's response or the challenging nature of the event itself may precipitate the occurrence of one or more additional interpersonal events. When more than one interpersonal event follows the therapist's initial response to a single interpersonal event, this process is known as an ***interpersonal event cascade***. The example of my interaction with Vera illustrates this phenomenon.

When Vera[2] pushed one of the boundaries of therapy by asking me if she could live with me, her insistence on a yes or no answer forced me to make a statement designed to interrupt the boundary violations. (The first behavior that

---

[2] All client names and geographic information have been changed.

Table 7.3 **Response Modes According to Interpersonal Events**						
Event	**Advocating**	**Collaborating**	**Empathizing**	**Encouraging**	**Instructing**	**Problem-Solving**
Strong Emotion			•	•	•	
Intimate Self-Disclosures	•		•	•		
Power Dilemmas	•	•	•			
Nonverbal Cues			•			
Crisis Points			•		•	•
Resistance and Reluctance		•	•	•	•	•
Boundary Testing			•		•	
Empathic Breaks			•			
Emotionally Charged Tasks and Situations	•	•	•	•	•	•
Limitations of Therapy	•		•		•	•
Contextual Inconsistencies			•		•	•

• indicates that this mode may be most appropriate for the event category.

defined a boundary violation was Vera's asking to live with me, and the second was her demand that I respond in a very specific way by saying "yes" or "no.") Predictably, my use of the instructing mode to explain to Vera why she could not live with me was perceived as hurtful and rejecting. Thus, my response mode, which I perceived necessary, was now considered to represent an empathic break in Vera's mind—the second interpersonal event in the sequence. Vera confirmed that the empathic break took place when she shouted: "I thought you were someone who cared about me." I choose to address the empathic break by empathizing with Vera (e.g., "Vera, I know you took a risk in asking me if you could come live with me, and I can see why you feel hurt that I said no. I want you to know I still care about your happiness here"). At that point, Vera began to sob and stormed away. Thus, a third interpersonal event occurred in the form of Vera's expression of strong emotion.

For complex clinical interactions such as this, it is recommended that the therapist draw upon more than response mode category to address the issue at hand. When a therapist employs more than one category of response mode episodically to address a single or sequence of interpersonal events, it is known as a ***response mode sequence***. In the situation just described, I was first using the empathizing mode when listening to Vera talk about her displeasure about living in the group home. Vera then pushed me to shift to an instructing response that consisted of an explanation of why she could not live with me. When Vera perceived my limit setting as an empathic break, I shifted promptly to provide an empathizing response in which I acknowledged that I had hurt her feelings and conveyed that I still cared. This led Vera to sob and storm away, an expression of strong emotion. At that point I chose to continue functioning within the empathic mode. When Vera returned, I assessed her understanding of what occurred between us, and it appeared as though she no longer wanted to discuss the situation. Responding to her need for less intensity, I suggested we go to the kitchen and prepare Vera's favorite dessert together. Thus, I used a sequence of different response modes to address the cascade of various interpersonal events that occurred.

Another variable that led to the decision to use this particular sequence of responses involved the extent to which Vera was able to tolerate direct conversation about the empathic break that I made. When she returned from her emotional episode, I asked Vera for feedback regarding how she now felt about our conversation. It was clear in her nonverbal behaviors and in her reluctance to provide any feedback that she no longer wished to discuss it. For this

reason, I shifted from utilizing empathic responses that involved interpersonal focusing to an empathic response that consisted of activity focusing—baking Vera's favorite dessert together. Because my verbal response caused Vera to become overwhelmed with emotion, I was prepared to provide a less intense empathizing response that involved engaging in an activity.

Step 5: Draw on Any Relevant Interpersonal Skills Associated With the Mode(s)

Because knowledge of how to respond using a given mode is typically not sufficient when deciding how to preserve the relationship in light of an interpersonal event, step 5 recommends that therapists also draw on their interpersonal knowledge base. Introduced in Chapter 3, this knowledge base is comprised of a continuum of skills that therapists are expected to develop early in their careers and continue to maintain and develop them in more sophisticated and nuanced ways as their careers continue.

Each of the interpersonal skills that the IRM emphasizes is associated with one or more of the six response modes. Thus, the act of drawing on a relevant interpersonal skill should feel natural and consistent with mode use. Ultimately, drawing on the required interpersonal skills that accompany a certain response mode becomes an intuitive process for the more experienced therapist. A summary of the interpersonal skills that are most likely to be associated with each of the modes are presented in Table 7.4. In viewing Table 7.4, it is important to note that the skills that comprise a therapist's interpersonal knowledge base can be applied across the modes. The summary in Table 7.4 is intended to serve as a rough guide that points to the most likely linkages between certain skills and each of the modes.

In the example with Vera, I drew upon the following interpersonal skills.

- Communication skills (i.e., clear verbal communication and therapeutic listening)
- Professional behavior (i.e., setting and maintaining boundaries)
- Conflict resolution including recognizing and resolving empathic breaks
- Self-care in the form of emotional accountability (i.e., I was careful to recognize the possibility that if I did not begin to set limits with Vera I might get irritated with her and respond with less empathy)

- Understanding difficult behavior and recognizing interpersonal hints (i.e., when Vera returned from her emotional episode, it was clear that she did not want to discuss the issue further)

These and other skills are covered in more detail in Chapters 8 to 13.

Step 6: Gather Feedback and, if Necessary, Strive Toward Mutual Understanding of the Response

One of the underlying principles of the IRM is that the client defines what constitutes a successful relationship. Consistent with this principle, the model recommends that therapists check in with clients and gather feedback following their response to an interpersonal event. A therapist's attempts to gather feedback may include:

- Checking in with the client and asking how he or she is feeling about the event and about the way in which the therapist chose to respond to it
- Asking the client if he or she feels comfortable with the therapist's response
- Asking the client if there is anything unresolved that he or she would like to discuss

If an event has been addressed or resolved successfully (i.e., the therapist selected a response mode that was acceptable to the client), clients usually affirm that they are ok, indicate that they have a better understanding of what occurred, or that they now feel somewhat better. In an ideal situation, these feelings of satisfaction are shared by the client and the therapist. However, the client's perception of whether the event has been resolved should always be the priority (Fig. 7.4).

When a client perceives that the event has not been resolved in an acceptable way or remains uncomfortable about the therapist's response, the IRM recommends that the therapist work to strive toward mutual understanding. This process is similar to conflict resolution (discussed in Chapter 13) in that it requires the therapist to initiate a semi-structured conversation with the client. During this conversation, the therapist invites the client to share his or her perspective of the event and then validates the client's perspective (or parts of the client's perspective) to the greatest extent possible. At that point, the therapist is faced with a choice. The therapist may acknowledge that his or her response was not optimal (if it is clear that there could have been a better response), or the therapist may believe that his or her response was optimal and ask for the client's permission to share his or her own perspective or rationale for the response. Therapists should share or reiterate their own perspective only if they remain in disagreement with the client's perspective and if the therapist is convinced that the event necessitated that the therapist stick with one

Table 7.4 **Interpersonal Skills According to Response Mode**						
Skill	**Advocating**	**Collaborating**	**Empathizing**	**Encouraging**	**Instructing**	**Problem-Solving**
Therapeutic Communication	•	•	•	•	•	•
Relating to Clients		•	•	•	•	
Understanding Difficult Behavior			•			
Managing Difficult Behavior and Conflict		•	•		•	•
Professional Behavior	•	•	•		•	•
Therapist Self-Care			•		•	

• indicates that this mode most clearly relates to the corresponding skill set.

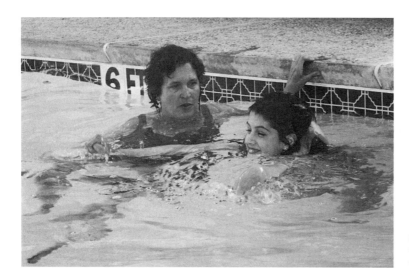

FIGURE 7.4 Kathryn Loukas looks for feedback to determine if a client is satisfied with her response

type of response mode. For example, in the situation involving Vera's request to live with me, her insistence on a yes or no answer compelled me to shift to the instructing mode and be direct about the limits of our professional relationship. If Vera ultimately felt that my telling her the truth about the limits of our professional relationship was not an acceptable response, I would not have been able to validate her need for me to give her the answer she wanted (i.e., allow her to live with me). However, had I not empathized with Vera's feelings of rejection and instead shown my irritation with her for insisting that I answer her, Vera would have been justified in finding my response unacceptable. At that point, I would have had to admit to Vera that I should have shown more understanding of her feelings and that I was wrong in showing my irritation.

Summary

This chapter described the process of therapeutic responding, a process that relies heavily on therapists' use of modes and the extent of development of their interpersonal knowledge base. This process was developed to guide therapists in their decision-making regarding how to react to challenging clients and to the inevitable interpersonal events of therapy. Over time and with sufficient practice, therapists experience the overall process of therapeutic responding as intuitive and automatic. The experience of learning how to

respond therapeutically to clients is no different from the experience of learning any other approach to practice.

To facilitate learning, the Activities section of this chapter contains two examples of reasoning trees that illustrate the response modes and interpersonal skills that might be required to address a given interpersonal event. Interpersonal events have the potential to evoke both therapeutic and nontherapeutic responses. The first reasoning tree (Fig. 7.5) offers a basic example of the reasoning that would be involved if a patient were to express anger during therapy. When clients express strong emotions such as anger, the therapist's selection of modes and use of interpersonal skills is critical to relationship outcomes. For example, if a client is not in control of his or her emotional response and a therapist attempts to encourage or problem-solve with that client, it is likely that the therapist will escalate the client's anger or leave the client feeling misunderstood. The second reasoning tree (Fig. 7.6) depicts the mode choices and skills that I used during my interaction with Vera. These reasoning trees were designed to encourage a process of self-reflection that increases the likelihood that the therapist will select the mode that is optimally therapeutic given the situation. Following these examples, an exercise is provided that encourages you to draw your own reasoning trees to facilitate your own planning and thinking about responding to clients as they face the inevitable interpersonal events of therapy.

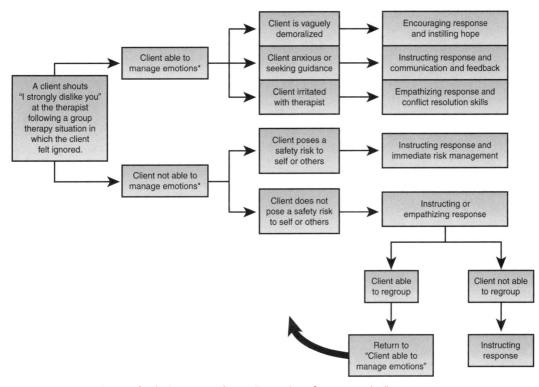

FIGURE 7.5 Reasoning tree for the interpersonal event "expression of strong emotion"

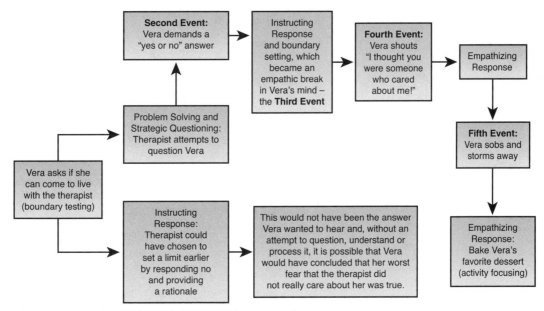

FIGURE 7.6 Reasoning tree for Vera's interpersonal event cascade

ACTIVITIES FOR LEARNING AND REFLECTION

This section contains exercises designed to improve your interpersonal reasoning as well as decision trees to illustrate how the interpersonal reasoning process is utilized in practice. The first exercise is designed to expand your flexibility when using modes during interpersonal reasoning. The second exercise is designed to introduce you to the process of responding to interpersonal events using interpersonal reasoning. These two exercises are appropriate for students and therapists of any level. The third exercise is for therapists with practice experience to develop a new perspective on how reasoning can be used to address interpersonally difficult practice situations.

EXERCISE 7.1

Growing your Capacity to use Modes Flexibly

In the exercises in Chapter 4 you were encouraged to identify whether you have a preferred mode or set of modes and to reflect on other modes you may wish to incorporate into your therapeutic style. In the exercise in Chapter 6, you practiced how to identify the key interpersonal events of therapy that might require you to initiate a mode shift. The objective of this exercise is to allow you to reflect on your ability to change modes in response to social situations in everyday life. The rationale behind this exercise is that the ability to use modes flexibly in everyday life translates into the ability to make smooth transitions when mode shifts are required in practice.

Question 1: Think of a time when you felt very strongly about getting a point across to a close friend, partner, or family member and faced a great deal of difficulty in doing so. Describe the event briefly.

_____

_____

Circle the mode you first used in an attempt to get your point across.

Advocating   Collaborating   Empathizing   Encouraging   Instructing   Problem-solving

Assuming that this did not work, circle the other mode or modes you then attempted to use?

Advocating   Collaborating   Empathizing   Encouraging   Instructing   Problem-solving

Were you ultimately successful in getting your point across? Why or why not?

_____

_____

What modes might you have tried that you didn't think of using at the time?

Advocating   Collaborating   Empathizing   Encouraging   Instructing   Problem-solving

Question 2: Consider a time when a friend approached you with a problem or dilemma, and you wondered whether your response was supportive enough. Describe the event briefly.

_____

_____

Circle the mode you first used in an attempt to support your friend.

Advocating   Collaborating   Empathizing   Encouraging   Instructing   Problem-solving

Assuming that this did not work, circle the other mode or modes you then attempted to use?

Advocating   Collaborating   Empathizing   Encouraging   Instructing   Problem-solving

In your opinion, how effective were you in supporting your friend? Why or why not?

_____

_____

What modes might you have tried that you didn't think of using at the time?

Advocating   Collaborating   Empathizing   Encouraging   Instruction   Problem-solving

Question 3: Remember a time when you tried to demonstrate or teach someone else how to do something and you encountered difficulty. Describe the event briefly.

_____

_____

Circle the mode you first used in your efforts to teach this person.

Advocating   Collaborating   Empathizing   Encouraging   Instructing   Problem-solving

If this did not work, circle the other mode or modes you then attempted to use?

Advocating   Collaborating   Empathizing   Encouraging   Instructing   Problem-solving

Were you ultimately successful in instructing this person? Why or why not?

_____

_____

What modes might have you have tried that you didn't think of using at the time?

Advocating   Collaborating   Empathizing   Encouraging   Instructing   Problem-solving

A client's ability to manage emotion is determined based on the nature and intensity of the emotion being expressed in the moment, the extent to which the intensity of the emotion matches the circumstances, and the therapist's prior knowledge of the client's capacity to express emotion safely, regroup, and reengage in therapy within a reasonable time frame.

In Figure 7.5, the client was irritated with the therapist because he felt that the therapist was paying more attention to other group members. The therapist knew that the client is at no risk for denigrating language or dangerous physical behavior. Because the client was able to manage his emotions and his anger toward the therapist was clear, the therapist chose a response consistent with the empathizing mode. Following an acknowledgement by the therapist that less attention was paid to the client during the group, the therapist then drew upon the foundational skill of conflict resolution in an attempt to achieve complete understanding of the client's concerns and to reach an outcome that would be acceptable to both of them.

EXERCISE 7.2

Using Interpersonal Events to Guide Reasoning

Return to the clinical scenarios in Exercise 6.1 that described various interpersonal events of therapy. For each scenario, draw a reasoning tree similar to those illustrated in Figures 7.5 and 7.6. Try to predict the outcomes of each interpersonal skill and response mode you choose.

EXERCISE 7.3

Recollect and Redefine

Recollect a difficult clinical scenario that you have encountered in practice. Redefine the scenario by labeling the interpersonal events that occurred, the interpersonal skills that were required to manage the event, and the modes you used. Reconstruct the scenario using a reasoning tree. Given the actual outcome of the event, would you have made the same decisions if given a second chance?

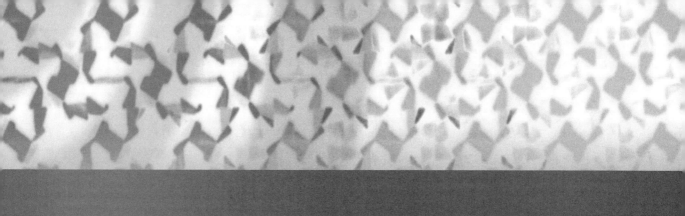

PART II

Building an Interpersonal Skill Base

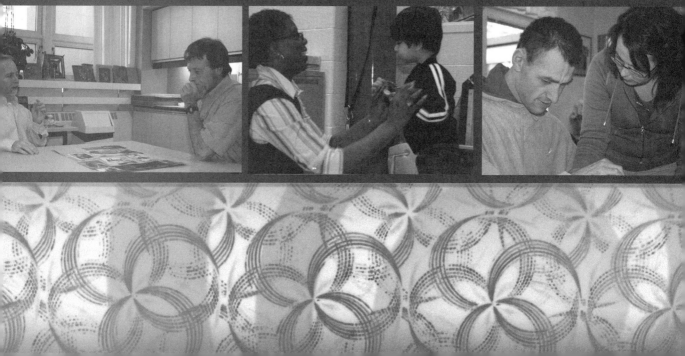

CHAPTER 8

THERAPEUTIC COMMUNICATION

The work of occupational therapy hinges on effective communication, or the exchange of thoughts and feelings between client and therapist. This exchange may occur verbally or nonverbally through the sharing of facial expression, posture, body movements, and other body language, informal gestures, sounds, made-up language, or formalized language such as sign and spoken language. At times communication is limited to the client and therapist, whereas at other times it involves multiple individuals (e.g., group therapy or work with partners, friends, or family members). In some cases communication spans a range of social contexts (e.g., interaction with school systems, places of employment, other health care providers, legal systems, insurance companies). Some forms of communication feel reciprocal and others feel dissatisfying or, in some situations, unbearable.

According to the Intentional Relationship Model (IRM), communication is considered therapeutic when it is characterized by leadership, responsibility taking, empathy, and intentionality on the part of the therapist. This means that the therapist must possess high-level skills in verbal and nonverbal communication. It also means that the therapist must be an expert in listening in ways that are optimally therapeutic. Because so much of what occupational therapists do ultimately involves structuring, educating, and/or guiding clients, therapeutic communication also requires a capacity to act assertively and the ability to provide clients with feedback that is positive as well as feedback that is honest, constructive, or difficult to hear. In turn, therapists should possess enough perspective to receive feedback from clients

gracefully, regardless of whether it is positive or negative. Finally, therapeutic communication requires that the therapist be skilled at asking the right questions at optimal times and in ways that facilitate information-sharing and (when appropriate) client self-refection.

The aim of this chapter is to review the following aspects of communication that comprise the interpersonal skill category that the IRM refers to as *therapeutic communication*.

> Communication is considered therapeutic when it is characterized by leadership, responsibility taking, empathy, and intentionality on the part of the therapist

- Verbal communication
- Nonverbal communication
- Unidirectional versus bidirectional communication
- Therapeutic listening
- Seeking and responding to client feedback
- Providing clients with structure, direction, and feedback

In the Activities section of this chapter, exercises are provided to encourage reflection on these important aspects of therapeutic communication. In addition to being useful for self-evaluation, the scales provided may also be useful in educational settings and for training and live supervision purposes. Because interviewing and strategic questioning are highly specific approaches to communication, these aspects of therapeutic communication are covered in Chapter 10.

Verbal Communication

Regardless of whether our clients possess a capacity for verbal communication, the therapist's verbal communication is an important aspect of the therapeutic relationship. For purposes of this chapter, ***verbal communication*** is defined as the use of a formally recognized spoken or signed language. Verbal communication requires that a therapist's communication be:

- Clear and audible in voice and mouth movements
- Clear, brief, and accurate in terms of the content being transmitted
- Emotionally modulated to match the situation, preference, and comfort level of the client
- Confident in tone of voice about the content of what is being communicated
- Professional, respectful, and tactful in terms of word choice
- Intentional about timing the relation between talking and doing

Being clear and audible in your articulation of words and volume of speech is the first basic criterion for effective communication. The prevalence of hearing impairment in the general U.S. population is approximately 1 in 12 individuals, and rates increase significantly with age and with other impairments that affect hearing and sensory processing. This high prevalence is similar in other developed countries worldwide. Given this high prevalence, the importance of clear, audible articulation during therapy cannot be emphasized enough. Words should be pronounced as slowly, loudly, and clearly as possible given your natural pacing of speech and tone of voice. Many hearing-impaired individuals lip-read. For this reason, it is important that a therapist's mouth movements be obvious and visible when talking. In some cultures, individuals are encouraged not to make obvious mouth movements. Similarly, some individuals develop a habit of covering their mouth with their hand, particularly when they are not entirely confident about what they are saying. This not only muffles the sound, it makes it difficult to read lips and mouth movements. Chewing gum or eating during therapy pose similar challenges and require extra effort to ensure understanding. If a therapist is speaking in a second (or third or fourth) language, has a soft voice, has difficulty hearing the volume of her or his own voice, or has other difficulties with articulation, these skills are even more critical and may warrant extra practice and solicitation of feedback.

Clarity, brevity, and accuracy of the content of your speech or signing similarly constitute important prerequisites for effective therapeutic communication. Clarity and accuracy of content are sometimes difficult to judge

because they are relativistic and can be perceived as such only by the client. This is because the extent to which the content is perceived as clear and accurate largely depends on your cultural background or acquired preferences in terms of your approach to communication.

For example, some cultures favor ***high-context communication***, whereas others favor ***low-context communication*** (Porter & Samovar, 1991). High-context communication places less emphasis on explicit verbal description of events and more emphasis on the context surrounding what is being said, such as the emotional tone, inflection of the voice, or other events in the broader social environment. Thus, there is sometimes a need to make mental leaps or assumptions about what is not being said. For example, wanting to eat an early dinner, I once telephoned a restaurant on a Monday to inquire about what time they planned to begin serving dinner that evening. The voicemail answered and listed the days and hours that the restaurant was open. I listened closely for the Monday hours but they never came. At that point I realized that I had to make an assumption that the restaurant was closed on Monday because the message did not provide hours for Monday. Later I found out that I was correct and concluded that the person who designed the voicemail message must have come from a background in which high-context communication is used (Fig. 8.1).

By contrast, low-context cultures place more emphasis on the literal spoken word and pay less attention to inflection, tone of voice, or the context that frames the communication. People from low-context cultures typically do not hypothesize about what was left unsaid or pay as close attention to subtle changes in inflection or tone. Growing up, I was surrounded by low-context communicators. If my family members, teachers, neighbors, and peers had something to say, they typically described what they meant using spoken language and did not leave much unsaid. Often, but not always, your preferred approach to communication is consistent with the communication that took place during your upbringing. Today, I take the same approach to communicating with others, including my clients. I am always careful to explain what I am saying clearly and with sufficient detail.

However, the IRM would caution me and others from low-context cultures to take extra care when communicating with people from high-context cultures. First, people from high-context cultures may perceive my efforts to be patronizing or as insulting to their intelligence. They may find me too talkative. Likewise, when a client from a high-context culture is attempting to convey something to me,

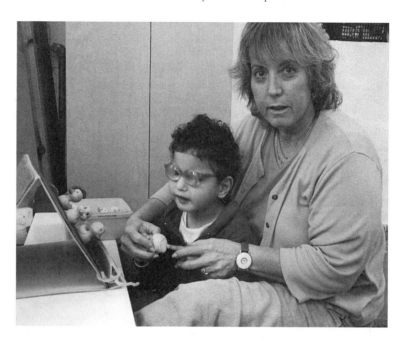

FIGURE 8.1 In her work with nonverbal clients, Vardit Kindler must rely solely on what is implied by the contextual aspects of communication

I always make an extra effort to understand what the client intends to communicate, even if the client is not always as talkative, detailed, or clear as I would be comfortable with. Thus, if I need to ask the client questions to obtain more detail or clarity, I pay particular attention that my emotional tone and inflection do not reflect impatience, condescension, patronization, or judgment. I am careful not to ask questions with a tone that suggests it is the client's fault that I am unable to understand. The important point is that for communication to be perceived as clear and accurate on both ends the therapist must consider whether the client's style matches the therapist's style in terms of emphasis on context. If it does not match, the therapist must make an extra effort to ask questions and accommodate to the client's style to the greatest extent feasible.

The extent to which your verbal communication is marked by emotionality in tone of voice and in choice of words is closely linked to whether your communication is considered to be high-context or low-context. The IRM recommends that therapists be aware of and adjust the level of emotion present in their tone and choice of words to the situation at hand and the client's preference. This process is referred to as ***emotional modulation***. Therapists can make an educated guess about the client's preference and level of tolerance for emotional intensity based on observing these same characteristics in the client. As a

general rule, many clients prefer that a therapist show some emotion in facial expression or voice inflection. Therapists with flat affect are not as easy to understand, and some clients may misperceive the absence of emotion as a lack of caring. Similarly, if the content of what a therapist is saying is inconsistent with his or her affect, it can be confusing to a client. Clients who tend to be more emotional communicators may be more likely to appreciate some evidence of emotion from the therapist. It is important to keep in mind that clients adapt to the therapist's usual level of emotional intensity, and some notice or respond if they notice a change in intensity.

Another aspect of clarity and accuracy of communication involves the extent to which the parties use exaggeration of truth and figurative language to emphasize or embellish what is being said. To some extent, the degree to which an individual is comfortable with exaggeration and figurative speech varies with cultural background and personal preference. However, because the process of occupational therapy relies so heavily on the accurate transmission of information, therapists prone to use exaggeration or figurative language should take extra care to ensure that their clients understand them. Moreover, some clients are unaccustomed to and may doubt the therapist's credibility or misperceive the therapist as unprofessional, rash, arrogant, or overly emotional. Thus, unless a therapist is certain that his or her approach matches or is embraced fully by the client, vague, flowery, overly abstract, or poetic language usually places the therapist at risk for being misperceived. If a client approaches communication in this way, it is important for the therapist to understand that it is likely a communication style to which the client is accustomed. Therefore, the client should be questioned only if it is vital that the communication be absolutely accurate.

Although cultures also vary in terms of the extent to which brevity is favored over loquaciousness, one aspect of communication that almost universally holds, is that people much prefer that people listen to them rather than talk too much. Although norms for what constitutes too much talking vary from culture to culture, a general rule in communicating with clients is to be as efficient and brief as possible. Take care not to provide so much information, detail, and complexity that it is overwhelming for the client.

Similarly, the tone of a therapist's voice should sound professional and confident. Therapists who tend to have young-sounding voices, are soft-spoken and introverted, or are new and lack confidence must make an extra effort to speak to clients in a way that conveys that they are competent and mature enough to be serving them. If a therapist is prone to giggling or nervous laughter, he or she should be made aware of it.

Word choice is another aspect of verbal communication that can be pivotal to the therapeutic relationship. It must be professional, respectful, and tactful. Occupational therapy jargon should be minimized or explained if used. Depending on the norms of the treatment setting and the preferences of the client, therapists should be intentional about their use of colloquial, in contrast to formal, language. Colloquial language, which should not be confused with lay or simplified language, is defined as informal phraseology; and it often is specific to the locale or social context of the setting. Colloquial language always involves a degree of risk in a new or vulnerable relationship because it is less formal and it assumes a level of familiarity with which a client may not be comfortable. Moreover, if a therapist attempts to speak informally with a client or use the local language, he or she must take great care to have social permission to use that language. This level of permission is usually granted with time and with a sufficient level of trust and integration into the setting or community.

Even though a therapist may not have permission to use colloquial or local language, his or her understanding of the language should be consistent with the population being served. For example, therapists working with a group of military personnel or veterans benefit from being familiar with military language so the clients do not have to bear the burden of being questioned or having to explain themselves.

Similarly, therapists benefit from being cognizant and intentional about the use of filler words such as "like," "you know," and other popular phrases that may be used repeatedly and can become habitual. Pet names and nicknames for clients, even children, may also be a sensitive matter. This may be particularly true if the name carries little significance for the relationship or carries a double entendre that might leave a client vulnerable to stereotyping, judgment, or ridicule. Similarly, referring to clients as "you guys," "y'all," "dear," "honey," "sweetie," "hun," or "girl" may also be perceived as condescending, insulting, or unprofessional by some clients. Because a therapist can never predict how a nickname or pet name is going to be received, these names are best avoided in professional situations.

The timing of your speech in relation to the client's performance of a task or activity also plays a role in the way in which your communication is experienced by the client. A therapist must decide how much speech should be initiated and sustained during the client's act of doing. Clients differ in their ability to tolerate informal chatter, formal directives, or questioning during performance. Some may find talking and doing easy to process, whereas others find it confusing or emotionally overwhelming. If unsure, one rule of thumb is to limit the amount of talk that takes place during performance.

Nonverbal Communication

Nonverbal communication is communication that is not based in a formally recognized spoken or signed language. It includes sounds, tone of voice, facial expression, body postures, movements, and gestures. It often provides others with information about an individual's thoughts and feelings that would not otherwise be described or accessed. Thus it has the potential to reveal things that an individual may or may not wish or intend to share but may be critical to understanding and relating. As essential as verbal communication, nonverbal communication influences the way in which communication is experienced in the relationship. It also affects the client's overall impression of the therapist.

People naturally differ in terms of what they focus on when they are observing others. Depending on the extent they prioritize the more emotional and contextual aspects of relating, their abilities to attend to, perceive, and interpret nonverbal communication vary. Some therapists are naturally inclined to notice changes in a client's facial expression, eyes, posture, or tone of voice, whereas others must work more deliberately to learn this skill. However, regardless of a client's abilities, therapists should make a practice of being self-aware and intentional about their own nonverbal communications. There are a number of excellent resources to assist therapists with the nonverbal aspects of relating. One is a book entitled *Body Language* by Susan Quilliam (2004). It is also important to understand what types of nonverbal communication may be interpreted as acceptable or unacceptable to clients from a cultural standpoint. A useful resource for this purpose is a book entitled *Gestures: The Do's and Taboos of Body Language Around the World* by Roger Axtell (1997).

A final element of nonverbal communication that is easy to overlook when multitasking is the importance of orienting your body toward the client and making eye contact when communicating. Turning your back toward the client or looking away while speaking is easy to do when one is focused on enabling a task or activity. However, orienting your body and eyes toward the client demonstrates respect and conveys the feeling of full attention. This is particularly important in situations when there is more than one individual in the treatment room, such as group therapy or therapy with children and families. In these situations, therapists are more vulnerable to having their true feelings

or preferences toward one individual over another revealed through the positioning of their body and eye contact while speaking. This may not be therapeutic if you are attempting to maintain an objective or neutral stance (Fig. 8.2).

Unidirectional Versus Bidirectional Communication

Although it is inevitably shared between the client and the therapist, communication can emerge as predominantly unidirectional or bidirectional in occupational therapy depending on the client's capacities. *Unidirectional communication* is communication that does not feel reciprocal to the therapist because it is initiated and sustained by the therapist without any apparent response from the client. *Bidirectional communication* is communication that feels reciprocal to the therapist because at minimum it involves some indication that the client has received the communication. More typically, bidirectional communication involves an ongoing give-and-take during which both client and therapist may independently initiate and maintain a sharing of body language, thoughts, and/or feelings.

In settings where clients have limited or no apparent capacity for communication, communication may be entirely or predominantly initiated and sustained by the therapist. For example, in a setting that serves children

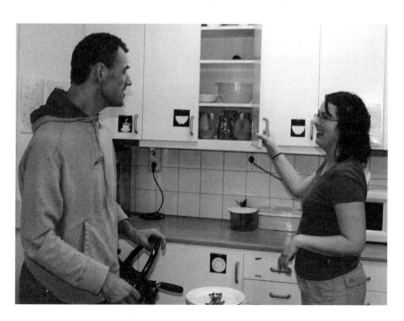

FIGURE 8.2 Kristen Alfredsson Ågren relies on a lot of eye contact to ensure accurate understanding

with severe motor, cognitive, and sensory impairments, therapists often encounter children who lack language and at first appear as though they do not have any interest in communication. With these clients, a therapist may, particularly during the early stages of therapy, communicate in a way that feels unidirectional. This may involve singing to the child, reading or telling stories, or providing sensory or vestibular stimulation using a wide range of modalities, including touch, smell, sound, taste, movement, and visual stimulation. These efforts are clearly rooted in existing practice frameworks (e.g., sensory integration therapy, model of human occupation), but the unique way in which a therapist chooses to deliver them also makes them acts of communication. Their interpersonal impact is inevitably received and felt by the client. Thus, even unidirectional communication must be as intentional as it would be in an exchange that is more clearly reciprocal (bidirectional). This increases the likelihood that the communication will eventually become bidirectional. An example of what was at first unidirectional communication that later became bidirectional is presented by Michele Shapiro in Box 8.1.

Both unidirectional and bidirectional communication can also occur when therapists are working with groups or families. It takes extra effort and a certain level of experience in social systems or group work to achieve bidirectional communication when three or more individuals are present. More information about working with families, groups, and other social systems is provided in Chapter 11 (Fig. 8.3).

Therapeutic Listening

If there is one aspect of therapeutic communication that can be viewed as absolutely fundamental to the initiation, maintenance, and preservation of the client–therapist relationship, it is therapeutic listening. Therapeutic listening involves the therapist's efforts to gather information from a client in such a way that it promotes greater understanding of the client's experience. Its aim is to provide the client with as much validation and support for the client's perspective as possible and appropriate given the goals of treatment. Therapeutic listening involves the following four activities.

- Empathic listening
- Guided listening
- Verbal prompts and sounds
- Enrichment questions

Box 8.1 Witnessing the Transformation from Unidirectional to Bidirectional Communication

I always had a problem because the outcome of the treatment never was the uppermost part of my agenda. The relationship with the client was more important than anything else. When I first started working with her, Eynat's[1] communication (introduced in Chapter 6) felt unidirectional. At first, she would not even look at me. However, I persisted in tracking her eye movements because it was the only reliable means of receiving feedback from her about how she was responding to my attempts at communication.

With Eynat, I couldn't wait for our daily rendezvous because I loved sitting with her and talking to her. I would often tell her how much she meant to me. It was so pleasing to see that through this kind of comforting talk and caring that she became more relaxed. I regarded our eating goal (the reason for referral) as a mere side issue. With time, Eynat reliably smiled and returned my communications with her eyes. At the same time she improved in her eating skills—not so much with a fork (as the teacher had requested) but definitely with her fingers. The most important point to me is that she had learned to relax and had a desire to receive and return communication. I love to think that the quality of her life might have improved through the trust she gained through our gentle relationship. I know that today the class is still having a dilemma regarding her eating habits. Some of the staff members feel she should learn to eat with utensils while others (including me) feel that seeing her prognosis is poor regarding self-help skills, why make her unnecessarily frustrated?

— **Michele Shapiro**

[1]All client names and geographic information have been changed.

Each of these therapeutic efforts is appropriate for specific interactive situations. They must be regulated and timed precisely during the interchange to maximize the likelihood that clients feel heard and understood. These efforts are described in more detail in the following section.

Empathic listening involves the process of recounting, accepting, and affirming any perception or experience a client offers (Gardner, 1991). Its purpose is to allow the therapist to learn about the clients' inner experience and to engage clients more fully in the therapy so their communications are more consistent with their actual emotional experience. To listen empathically, you must first grasp the meaning and purpose of empathy in occupational therapy practice.

According to IRM, empathy is defined as a therapist's ongoing striving to understand a client's thoughts, feel-

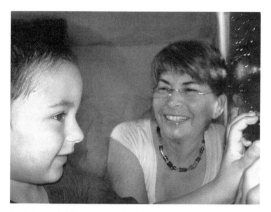

FIGURE 8.3 Through use of a bubble machine, Michele Shapiro achieves bidirectional communication with a client

ings, and behaviors. A number of occupational therapy scholars have written extensively about empathy as a means by which therapists may achieve an understanding of clients' life stories and convey respect for and trust in clients' interpretation of their own lives and experiences (Hagedorn, 1995; Mosey, 1970; Peloquin, 1995, 2005; Punwar & Peloquin, 2000). Suzanne Peloquin has written extensively about the central role of empathy in occupational therapy (Peloquin, 1989, 1990, 1993, 1995, 2002, 2003, 2005). Reviewed in Chapter 1, Peloquin defined empathy as entering into clients' experience, connecting with their feelings, noting similarities and differences, and communicating a sense of fellowship. Although significant contributions have been made in terms of encouraging the development of empathy through literature and the arts (e.g., Peloquin, 1995), how empathy is actually conveyed to the client in occupational therapy has not yet been defined from a skills training perspective.

Although a considerable amount has been written about empathy in occupational therapy, significant contributions have also been made outside the field. Freud (1923) introduced the central prerequisite to empathic listening when he wrote about the importance of "evenly hovering attention." This referred to the desired quality of the therapist's listening. Freud argued that to listen fully the therapist's mind should be free of any conscious judgment, filtering, evaluation, analysis, interpretation, or reflection (Brenner, 2000). According to Freud, a conscious mind that is unencumbered and clear of its own thoughts and formulations is the only means by which a therapist is truly able to listen and come to know the client as a unique individual. When listening in this manner, therapists should not

feel pressured to respond, nor should they attempt to plan their responses. Their conscious minds should be clear and open to the client's input. There are a number of obstacles of which to be aware when attempting to achieve this approach to listening. They are presented in Table 8.1.

Decades after Freud presented his ideas about listening, Carl Rogers (1961) introduced the argument that empathy was both necessary and sufficient for positive psychotherapy outcomes. A prominent psychoanalyst, Heinz Kohut (1984), similarly valued empathy as the most fundamentally healing aspect of the psychotherapeutic process. He defined empathy primarily as an objective mode of observation in which the therapist comes to understand a client's underlying emotions, needs, longings, and motives while at the same time maintaining an impartial viewpoint. Kohut labeled the empathic process of accessing a client's internal world "vicarious introspection," and he consistently emphasized the importance of understanding each client's experiences and behaviors from the client's unique perspective (Gardner, 1991; Kohut, 1984). The world's foremost cognitive therapists (Beck, 1995; Beck, Rush,

Table 8.1   **Common Obstacles to Listening**
· Jumping in to help a client finish a sentence
· Planning your response to such an extent that it distracts you from what a client is saying
· Filtering what the client has said based on what you wish to hear or based on some other prejudiced notion of the client
· Comparing a client to someone else (either in your own mind or aloud)
· Evaluating the accuracy or veracity of the communication
· Judging (either praise or criticism)
· Analyzing, drawing connections, or formulating
· Intrusive thinking (e.g., distracting thoughts that pass through your mind)
· Chronic reliance on nonverbal responding
· Unsolicited advice-giving
· Dropping "hints" at your reaction
· Being "right" or needing to convince the client that you are right
· Introducing a topic that takes the conversation off the original topic
· Reassuring or normalizing (rather than listening—typically motivated by the therapist's anxiety or need rather than by the client's actual preference for reassurance)
· Overutilizing prompts or utilizing them to give a (false) impression that you are listening (e.g., "uh huh")
· Self-disclosing how something would have made you feel or recounting something similar that happened to you
· Asking further probing questions

Shaw, & Emery, 1979) similarly highlighted that clients, rather than therapists, are the experts on the interpretations or meanings they attach to their own experiences.

Taken together, these perspectives form the foundation for the definition of empathic listening according to the IRM. To achieve empathy in occupational therapy, the therapist must consistently maintain a central focus on understanding clients' interpretations of and reactions to the interpersonal events of therapy and any other thoughts, feelings, or circumstances associated with their life experiences in general. Empathy can be used effectively in occupational therapy when:

- A therapist suspects that a client is struggling or upset
- A client openly describes an upsetting circumstance or reveals that she or he is upset
- A client happens upon an obstacle or challenge while participating in therapy
- A client expresses or otherwise demonstrates concern about therapy or the therapist
- A client is angry or frustrated with the therapist
- Some other inevitable interpersonal event occurs (or is anticipated) during therapy
- Anytime a therapist wishes to build rapport or establish more of a relationship with a client
- Anytime a therapist is in doubt about what to say, about what mode to use, or about how to respond to an interpersonal event.

Regardless of how sophisticated an understanding of our clients we achieve, being able to recognize and set aside beliefs, stereotypes, and assumptions about who they are is most fundamental to truly knowing clients' feelings, thoughts, and beliefs about themselves and about their immediate social and physical environments. Only after you separate your own reactions, beliefs, and attributions can you truly understand your clients as unique individuals.

When put into practice, empathy often takes the form of listening in a highly specific and disciplined way. To understand a client's thoughts, a therapist must listen to the client's communications empathically. Empathic listening involves speaking back to the clients' inner reality and reconveying an understanding of what was said after they reveal something about their experience (Gardner, 1991). A central means by which this is done is by making a series of *summary statements*, or brief statements that reflect the main points of what a client has said (Beck, 1995). During this process, a therapist:

- Pays particular attention to the clients' affect and their general opinions and perceptions of experience

- Draws upon his or her own reactions and past experiences in a disciplined way to better understand the client
- Sets his or her own world views and judgments aside
- Refrains from asking questions
- Refrains from summarizing in a way that translates or interprets what was said
- Refrains from summarizing in a way that attempts to structure or guide the client's conversation in any way

Summary statements may at first be challenging to learn. Additional pointers contained in Table 8.2 may be useful as guidelines for what to avoid when making these statements.

A key to understanding empathy within the IRM is that your understanding of the client should never be assumed. Instead, it should be verified and tested for accuracy as appropriate to the clinical situation. Thus, empathy is fully achieved only when sufficient feedback has been provided by the client or by someone acting on the client's behalf. Usually, therapists know that a client feels understood when he or she responds to a summary statement by saying something like "exactly" or "that's correct." Another indication that the therapist has been accurate in making a summary statement is that the client continues to discuss the situation further or in more detail. If a therapist is not 100% accurate in his or her understanding, typically a client corrects the therapist by reexplaining or clarifying what he or she intended to say. The client's corrective feedback is a sign that he or she knows that the therapist is struggling to understand, and this effort by the therapist is usually appreciated by clients and experienced as empathic in itself. Once a client has corrected the therapist, it is the therapist's turn to try again by making a new summary statement or other empathic response that more accurately reflects what the client intended to convey. This cyclical process of feedback and response is central to

---

Table 8.2 What to Limit or Avoid When Making a Summary Statement

- Parroting or repeating every word verbatim
- Extending what the client has said (i.e., putting words into the client's mouth)
- Anticipating what the client might be trying to say or what the client might say next
- Making premature interpretations of what the client has said
- Predicting how something must have made a client feel (when the client has not introduced emotion into the telling of the story or event)

empathic listening. With the IRM, this process is referred to as *striving for understanding*, a term borrowed from the traditions of self-psychology (Kohut, 1984) and humanistic psychotherapy (Rogers, 1961).

In addition to empathizing with a client's thoughts through summary statements, therapists may also choose to listen empathically by simply maintaining what Freud labeled as an "evenly hovering attention" when listening silently to what a client is saying. Other means by which a therapist may empathize with a client is by responding nonverbally. A therapist may respond nonverbally to what a client has said or to something observed in the client's affect or behavior. Empathizing with a client's affect is achieved through a process of emotional resonance in which a therapist strives to understand the client's emotional experience. Emotional resonance may be achieved by observing a client's affect, attempting to feel what the client is feeling, and mirroring it back in your facial expression or tone of voice. Emotional resonance may also be achieved by sharing with the client what you are observing about his or her affect or behavior from what you hypothesize to be the client's perspective.

The decision of whether to approach empathic listening by summarizing, simply listening and responding nonverbally, or commenting on what is observed involves the rhythm and timing of the interaction. By paying close attention to the degree of emotion that accompanies what the client is expressing, the therapist may gauge the intensity with which a summary statement, facial expression, or observational comment is made. For occupational therapy, empathic listening strives to achieve the following outcomes.

- It conveys that the therapist is striving to understand the client.
- It conveys validation and support for the client's point of view.
- It encourages the client to communicate further.
- It decreases the likelihood of presumptions and misunderstandings.
- It helps the therapist maintain attention and remember what the client has said.
- It may help quell a client's anger or frustration toward the therapist.
- Summary statements may prompt feedback that ensures the therapist has understood the client accurately.

Within the IRM, empathic listening assumes that whatever clients choose to say deserves to be heard and reflected back to them in a nonjudgmental way that communicates striving for understanding. Empathic listening also assumes that clients trust and value the therapist enough to be willing to hear their thoughts, feelings, or behaviors summarized or reflected back to them. Thus, unstructured summary statements should be made only when the client has stopped talking and one is confident that the client is expecting a response. In many cases, these statements can be naturally enfolded with other approaches to therapeutic communication, such as the questions, directives, feedback, and suggestions that are also fundamental in occupational therapy. Because they convey validation and support, unstructured summary statements may be the only form of communication that certain clients seeking to vent their thoughts and feelings perceive as therapeutic. In the Activities section of this chapter an exercise and a checklist are provided that encourages evaluation of empathic listening skills. Readers are encouraged to practice empathic listening with a partner and have the partner or a third observer utilize the checklist to rate the extent to which empathic listening is used.

Guided listening is an alternative approach that involves a therapist's attempts to shape what the client is saying by making one or more summary-type statements that serve to clarify or organize what a client has said. Unlike empathic listening, the central aim of guided listening is not to provide the client with empathy by following his or her thoughts in an unstructured and sometimes aimless way. Instead, guided listening is a more strategic approach that may be used to assist a client in limiting, structuring, or organizing what is being said. This is accomplished through the therapist's use of statements that aim to wrap up, limit, or otherwise influence the direction of the conversation. Although some clients find this type of listening somewhat less empathic, others view the structure they provide supportive and empowering if introduced to clients who seek or appreciate guidance and when timed correctly.

Verbal prompts and sounds include expressions such as "Ah," "Uh huh," or "Umm." These utterances may be used to remind a client that you are listening, highlight something a client has just said, or encourage a client to say more. Therapists vary according to the extent to which they are comfortable using this approach. In part, your comfort level may depend on the extent to which you use these expressions in everyday life. There are only two cautions involved in using these expressions. The first is overuse to the point that they sound so redundant that they become irritating to the client. The second is using these expressions as a substitute for more effortful approaches in which the client strives to understand what the client is attempting to communicate at a nuanced level.

Enrichment questions are gentle forms of inquiry designed to encourage a client to continue to communicate and/or to enrich what is being described. They are particularly useful when a therapist needs more information from a client or believes that it would benefit a client to say more about a given topic or life event. The number and nature of questions that an occupational therapist might ask a client to encourage communication or elaboration is unlimited. Some examples of enrichment questions include:

• Would you feel comfortable telling me more about it?
• Would you give me some more details about it?
• When did this happen?
• When did this idea first occur to you?
• Where were you at that time?
• What else do you remember?
• How do you feel about it?
• What stands out in your mind as the most difficult part?
• What is/was passing through your mind?

Each client–therapist interaction is unique in terms of the rhythm of exchange that results from these four styles of listening. More talkative or emotional clients may require more empathic listening coupled with the use of summary statements to help guide and structure the interaction. Less talkative or withdrawn clients may require a therapist to use prompts and ask enrichment questions to convey interest and stimulate the clients' thoughts and feelings.

Clients that interact at a more natural pace likely appreciate a wider mixture of efforts with more frequent shifts between the different approaches to listening (Fig. 8.4).

Seeking and Responding to Client Feedback

Seeking feedback from clients is closely related to therapeutic listening in that it requires therapists to focus on the clients' experience of therapy to such an extent that they remember to ask about it. Like other aspects of therapeutic communication, seeking feedback from clients can be a complex process. When seeking feedback, therapists must strike a balance between projecting a take-charge attitude while at the same time being willing to accept criticism and/or consider the client's viewpoint. When soliciting feedback, an important point to keep in mind is that feedback should be solicited only about aspects of the therapy process that the therapist is willing to alter or correct. One of the most frustrating things for a client is to be asked to provide feedback about aspects of the therapy process (or aspects of his or her personality) that the therapist is not prepared to change. In circumstances where clients and therapists disagree about how therapy is being approached, careful collaboration and conflict resolution strategies are more appropriate. The more specific you are when asking about a given aspect of therapy, the more likely it is that

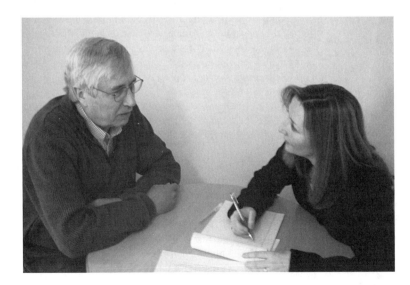

FIGURE 8.4 During an interview, Jane Melton tailors her listening approach according to the needs of a client

the client provides feedback that is realistic, useful, and likely to result in change. Examples of specific ways therapists might solicit feedback from clients while still projecting a take-charge attitude include:

• Asking clients how they felt while performing a task or activity
• Asking clients what difficulties they encountered when following through on a recommendation
• Asking clients if they noticed any problems with an assistive device or environmental modification that was made
• Asking clients if they are finding your style to be supportive enough (Fig. 8.5)

The feedback clients provide may occur in response to your solicitation but it may also arrive unsolicited. Regardless of whether the feedback is solicited or unsolicited, therapists have a

> When therapists do not receive feedback gracefully they put themselves at risk for conflict or other complexities within the relationship.

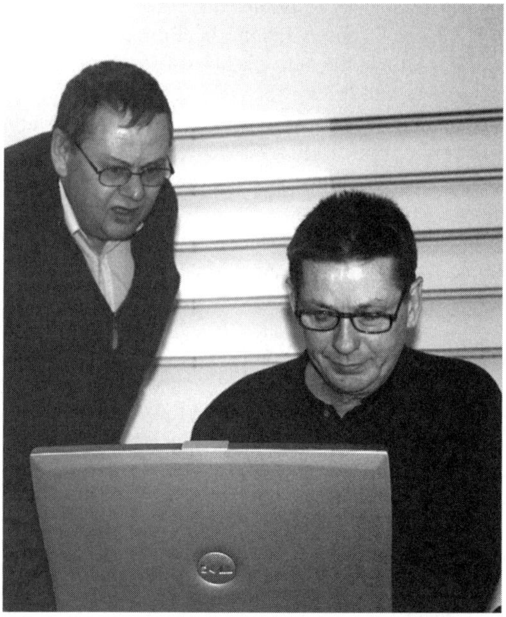

FIGURE 8.5 Roland Meisel incorporates a client's feedback into his search for appropriate job placement

responsibility to receive it gracefully and in a way that encourages the client to continue to feel comfortable providing it in the future. Receiving feedback requires therapists to recognize that they cannot be equally effective with or appreciated by all clients. Moreover, occasionally even the most skilled and experienced therapists make technical mistakes or empathic breaks. All feedback deserves a response. Some examples of graceful ways to receive and respond to feedback include:

• Saying thank you
• Apologizing, if necessary and if appropriate
• Repeating your understanding of the main point of the feedback
• Asking the client what he or she would have preferred
• Offering to alter or correct something if feasible and describing what will be done
• After reflecting on the feedback aloud, and only if appropriate, educating the client about your rationale and then explaining what you will do or what you had been planning to do to address the client's feedback (This one is tricky because you must be careful not to sound defensive or to rely on this strategy because you are uncomfortable with the client's criticism.)

When therapists do not receive feedback gracefully they put themselves at risk for conflict or other complexities within the relationship.

Some examples of behaviors to avoid when receiving feedback include:

• Ignoring or dismissing the feedback without a response
• Questioning the client about the reasons for the feedback
• Rushing to educate your client about your rationale without pausing to make a summary statement and reflect with the client
• Undermining the client for providing the feedback by making jokes or sarcastic comments (e.g., "You never had a problem with this activity in the past")
• Making the client feel guilty about providing the feedback by appearing overwhelmed by it or overly apologetic
• Attempting to overcompensate after receiving the feedback

Providing Clients With Structure, Direction, and Feedback

One of the most critical aspects of occupational therapy involves the ability to provide clients with structure, direction, and feedback in a way that they can understand it, perceive it as constructive, and follow through with it. Guiding clients in these ways serves to relieve any feelings of anxiety they might be having and also communicates that the therapist is being thoughtful about his or her plans for the session. At the most fundamental level, any of the following activities may be required to guide a client sufficiently.

• Setting a basic temporal framework by informing or reminding (if appropriate) the client of expectations for attendance, the regularity of the scheduled appointments, and/or the time allotted for each session.
• Educating the client of the purpose and potential utility of therapy.
• Using goal setting as a means to track progress and assess outcomes.
• Educating the client about your preferred approach to practice or theoretical framework, if indicated.
• Encouraging the client to provide feedback.
• Informing or reminding the client that you are willing to make adjustments in your approach or interpersonal style based on feedback.
• Introducing to the client what is planned for each session at the beginning of the session—even if what is planned simply involves asking the client what he or she would like to work on that day.
• If several activities are planned for the session, the therapist should describe all that is planned and provide the client with a rough estimate of the time frames within which each activity or task is planned.
• Occasionally checking in with the client to monitor his or her experience of therapy.
• Describing your expectations regarding the client's role, responsibilities, and behavior in therapy.
• Projecting an attitude of competence.
• When facing sensitive or vulnerable clients, informing them explicitly about your preferred interpersonal modes and their potential limitations (e.g., "I tend to be the type of therapist who prefers to do more listening than talking. But some people feel lost if I listen too much. Would you give me some feedback so I can be sure I am giving you what you need?")

Many clients naturally conform to the social expectations and cultural norms of the client–therapist relationship within a given setting. For example, in many hospital settings in the United States, clients expect therapists to provide a fair amount of structure, direction, and feedback as part of competent care. However, for clients new to a local culture or for those who are more sensitive and vulnerable, good timing is important when providing instruction and guidance. The therapist must determine when, how often, and to what extent to introduce structure, direction, and feedback into the therapeutic relationship. This is best accomplished by continually monitoring the interaction to assess whether the client is seeking guidance and/or open to receiving guidance. When determining client receptivity or indications that more guidance is needed, points to consider include:

• Is the client asking questions?
• Does the client lack confidence about what he or she is doing?
• Does the client appear uncertain, anxious, or nervous?
• Does the client respond more positively when guidance is provided?

In addition to assessing receptivity and need, there may be some occasions when a client requires guidance for safety reasons or to ensure that a certain standard of care is achieved. Closely monitoring the client enables the therapist to time the introduction of guiding activities appropriately and reduce the chance that these activities will encourage dependence or be perceived as overbearing, controlling, or critical (Fig. 8.6).

An important aspect of providing clients with structure and direction involves providing them with feedback. Regardless of whether the feedback is intended to be positive or negative, the true nature of any type of feedback is that it is a form of judgment. Providing feedback always carries the potential to make the client feel vulnerable, embarrassed, or evaluated. Thus, providing feedback must be approached with care, and it should always be provided in a way that is straightforward and easy to understand. Table 8.3 contains some helpful hints to keep in mind when providing clients with positive and negative (constructive) feedback.

In occupational therapy, the focus of feedback typically involves the client's occupational performance. However, the IRM recommends that feedback of an interpersonal nature is also provided to clients as part of an occasional conversation between the therapist and client about how the client is experiencing the therapeutic rela-

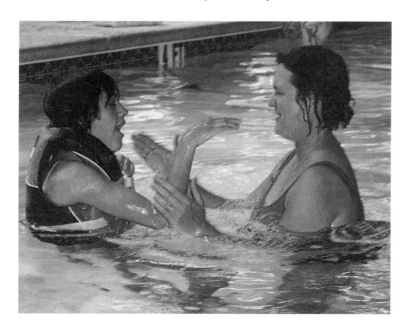

FIGURE 8.6 When conducting therapy in a pool, it is vital that Kathryn Loukas provide adequate instruction and structure to ensure a client's safety

tionship. Thus, occupational therapists should also be prepared to provide clients with feedback about their interpersonal behavior during therapy just as clients are expected to provide therapists with such feedback.

All of these efforts require confidence and assertiveness, which comprise what the IRM labels a *take-charge attitude* on the part of the therapist. A take-charge attitude involves expressing a confident, assertive, and, when appropriate, emotionally self-protective demeanor with clients—particularly clients who test boundaries, are anxious, or prefer structure and direction. The following characteristics may reflect a therapist's take-charge attitude.

• Remaining emotionally centered and managing any anxiety related to your knowledge or performance as a therapist

Table 8.3 **Tips for Providing Clients with Feedback**	
Positive Feedback When praising a client, comment on or describe a specific behavior (e.g., You've gotten that clasp to work") rather than making a more generalized statement, such as "well done" or "great job." This guideline also applies when providing feedback of an interpersonal nature. Rather than stating, "I enjoy working with you," explain why you enjoy working with people or what qualities you appreciate about them. · Use more generalized statements with parsimony. · Never describe a behavior as "perfect" because it encourages clients to strive for an unrealistic level of performance. · Avoid comparisons to other clients or to famous people when providing positive feedback. It robs the client of the chance to experience the accomplishment as an individual.	· Unless the client has put in an unusual amount of effort or accomplished something rare and exceptional relative to his or her abilities, the emotional tone of the feedback should be guarded. · As a general rule, the amount of positive feedback should, at minimum, double the amount of negative feedback provided to a client. · At the same time, be careful not to over-rely on positive feedback as a means of motivating a client or its impact and sincerity may wear off. · If a client does not respond well to positive feedback, stop providing it. Instead, encourage the client to share his or her self-assessment of performance more often during therapy. If the client's self-assessment is unrealistic, work with it using strategic questioning (covered in Chapter 10).

(table continued on page 170)

Table 8.3 **Tips for Providing Clients with Feedback** (continued)

Negative (Constructive) Feedback
· State the feedback in a clear, straightforward manner.
· State the main point of the feedback rather than including other, more peripheral issues.
· When giving constructive feedback, focus on one issue at a time. It decreases the risk of overwhelming clients, so the clients can focus their energy on that single issue.
· Avoid being indirect or vague about the feedback. Overprotecting clients in this way can lead to confusion about the nature of the feedback, a decreased impact of the feedback, or anxious thinking (e.g., "My therapist must think it's really awful because she can't even tell it to me straight").
· Set aside a specific time for feedback in the session (e.g., a wrap-up period at the end of the session). Clients should be prepared for this part of the session in advance (i.e., at the beginning of therapy or at the beginning of each session).
· If a specific time for feedback is established, ask the client for a preference regarding his or her desire to hear constructive versus positive feedback first. This provides a greater sense of control over the vulnerable situation of having to receive feedback.
· You can preface constructive feedback by pointing out strength, but only do this if it is sincere. Avoid prefacing constructive feedback with defensive or protective statements, such as, "You're good at remembering the turn signal, but you need to work on changing lanes" or "I don't mean to criticize your approach, but...." or "I hope this doesn't sound too harsh but,..."
· Avoid comparisons or using others as examples when providing constructive feedback.
· Check in with clients to determine how they experienced receiving the feedback (e.g., ask what they took away from the feedback, how it affected their desire to persist, whether it changed their feelings toward you, whether it provoked any new worries, or whether they found it useful).
· Remain as emotionally neutral as possible when providing constructive feedback. Be particularly careful that facial expressions do not reveal anxiety, disappointment, or irritation.

• Being adequately prepared for the session and rehearsing your plans for therapy before beginning, if necessary
• Using a confident tone of voice and speaking clearly and loudly enough
• Assuming a confident body posture
• Feeling confident about what you are saying
• Making eye contact
• Focusing on making the client feel at ease
• Acting as narrator (describing what will happen next) and emotional buoy (checking in and pausing to assess the client's experience) when necessary
• Not hesitating to maintain the structure, limits, and boundaries of the therapy
• Being adequately self-protective around clients who are behaving in inappropriate or abusive ways.

Regardless of the setting, assuming a take-charge attitude promotes a client's confidence in the therapist and serves to establish the therapist's role as the professional in situations where it is necessary and appropriate to establish such a role.

Summary

One of the most telling indicators that your communication with a client has been therapeutic and successful is the feeling that you are able to communicate with the client in a way that is predictable, straightforward, honest, and comfortable. Feeling that a client is complex or difficult to understand is a sign that additional work on communication is needed within the relationship. This may or may not be possible depending on the client's abilities and tolerance for communication.

This chapter provided a detailed review of six pragmatic aspects of therapeutic communication that are vital to establishing and maintaining an intentional and effective client–therapist relationship. It provided a series of guidelines to ensure that therapists feel knowledgeable and confident about their communication skills. Alone, these guidelines do not ensure that a successful relationship will unfold. As with other guidelines provided in this book, therapists should first consider the client's unique interpersonal characteristics, any interpersonal events that have occurred during therapy, and the overarching social and physical contexts that surround the communication that is taking place. As mentioned at the beginning of this chapter, the Activities section contains an exercise and two self-rating scales designed to facilitate self-evaluation and supervision in the practice of therapeutic communication. Considerations presented in Chapter 9, which includes a focus on cultural competence, should also be incorporated into your thinking about how to achieve effective communication with a client.

GLOSSARY

Bidirectional communication—communication that does feel reciprocal to the therapist because, at minimum, it involves some indication that the client has received the communication. More typically, bidirectional communication involves an ongoing give-and-take during which both client and therapist may independently initiate and maintain sharing of thoughts and feelings.

Emotional modulation—adjusting the extent to which one's verbal communication is marked by emotionality in tone of voice and choice of words according to the situation at hand and one's estimation of the client's preference and level of tolerance for emotional intensity.

Empathic listening—recounting, accepting, and affirming any perception or experience a client offers.

Guided listening—strategic approach in which a client attempts to limit, structure, or organize what the client is saying by making one or more clarifying statements.

High-context communication—places less emphasis on explicit verbal description of events and more emphasis on the context surrounding what is being said, such as the emotional tone or inflection of voice or other events in the broader social environment.

Low-context communication—places more emphasis on the literal spoken word and less emphasis on inflection, tone of voice, or to the context that frames the communication. People from low-context cultures typically do not hypothesize about what was left unsaid or pay as close attention to subtle changes in inflection or tone.

Nonverbal communication—not based in a formally recognized spoken or signed language. It includes sounds, tone of voice, facial expression, body postures, movements, and gestures.

Summary statement—a brief statement that reflects the main points of what a client has said that does not involve asking questions, interpreting, or attempting to structure or guide the client's conversation in any way.

Striving for understanding—a cyclical process that is central to empathic listening. It involves making a summary statement, receiving feedback from the client regarding its accuracy, and, if necessary, making a corrective summary statement that reflects more accurate understanding.

Take-charge attitude—expressing a confident, assertive, and, when appropriate, emotionally self-protective demeanor with clients—particularly clients who test boundaries, are anxious, or prefer structure and direction.

Therapeutic communication—characterized by leadership, responsibility-taking, empathy, and intentionality on the part of the therapist.

Therapeutic listening—therapist's efforts to gather information from a client in such a way that it promotes greater understanding, validation, and support.

Unidirectional communication—communication that does not feel reciprocal to the therapist because it is initiated and sustained by the therapist without any apparent response from the client.

Verbal communication—use of a formally recognized spoken or signed language.

References

Axtell, R. E. (1997). *Gestures: the do's and taboos of body language around the world.* New York: Wiley.

Beck, A. T., Rush, A. J., Shaw, B. F., & Emery, G. (1979). *Cognitive therapy of depression.* New York: Guilford Press.

Beck, J. (1995). *Cognitive therapy: basics and beyond.* New York: Guilford Press.

Brenner, C. (2000). Brief communication: Evenly hovering attention. *Psychoanalytic Quarterly, 89,* 545–549.

Freud, S. (1923). *The ego and the id.* New York: W.W. Norton.

Gardner, J. R. (1991) The application of self psychology to brief psychotherapy. *Psychoanalytic Psychology,* 8, 466–500.

Hagedorn, R. (1995). *Occupational therapy: perspectives and processes* (pp. 259–267). New York: Churchill Livingstone.

Kohut, H. (1984). *How does analysis cure?* Chicago: University of Chicago Press.

Mosey, A. C. (1970). *Three fames of reference for mental health.* Thorofare, NJ: Slack.

Peloquin, S. M. (1989). Sustaining the art of practice in occupational therapy. *American Journal of Occupational Therapy,* 43, 219–226.

Peloquin, S. M. (1990). The patient-therapist relationship in occupational therapy: Understanding visions and images. *American Journal of Occupational Therapy,* 44, 13–21.

Peloquin, S. M. (1993). The depersonalization of patients: A profile gleaned from narratives. *American Journal of Occupational Therapy,* 47, 830–837.

Peloquin, S. M. (1995). The fullness of empathy: Reflections and illustrations. *American Journal of Occupational Therapy,* 49, 24–31.

Peloquin, S. M. (2002). Reclaiming the vision of reaching for heart as well as hands. *American Journal of Occupational Therapy,* 56, 517–526.

Peloquin, S. M. (2003). The therapeutic relationship: Manifestations and challenges in occupational therapy. In E. B. Crepeau, E. S. Cohn, & B. A. Boyt Schell (Eds.), *Willard & Spackman's occupational therapy* (10th ed., pp. 157–170). Philadelphia: Lippincott Williams & Wilkins.

Peloquin, S. M. (2005). The 2005 Eleanor Clarke Slagle lecture: Embracing our ethos, reclaiming our heart. *American Journal of Occupational Therapy,* 59, 611–625.

Porter, R. E., & Samovar, L. A. (1991). Basic principles of intercultural communication. In L. A. Samovar, & R. E. Porter (Eds.), *Intercultural communication: A reader.* Belmont, CA: Wadsworth.

Punwar, J., & Peloquin, M. (2000). *Occupational therapy: principles and practice* (pp. 42–98). Philadelphia: Lippincott.

Quilliam, S. (2004). *Body language.* Dubai, United Arab Emirates: Firefly.

Rogers, C.R. (1961). *On becoming a person: a therapist's view of psychotherapy.* New York: Houghton Mifflin.

ACTIVITIES FOR LEARNING AND REFLECTION

The exercises in this section are designed to improve empathic listening and therapeutic communication skills for both students and practitioners. The first exercise encourages you to select one or two partners and to engage in a series of role-playing exercises. The two checklists may be completed as self-rating tools by a classmate or instructor or by a fieldwork supervisor, employer, or other consultant whose task is to evaluate you in terms of your empathic listening and therapeutic communication skills. For example, the checklist on empathic listening may be utilized in conjunction with the role-plays outlined in Exercise 8.1.

EXERCISE 8.1

Empathic Listening

Empathic listening is vital to the initiation and preservation of an effective therapeutic relationship. It is particularly important when clients are discussing sensitive issues or when facing an interpersonal event in therapy. For some clients, the ability to sustain a relationship depends on it. The purpose of this exercise is to ensure that all therapists develop expertise in this vital area. You are required to role-play each of the following scenarios with a partner. One partner describes an event, and your job is to limit your response to empathic listening only. The role-play scenarios below are designed to evoke a wide range of feelings and impulses in the listener. They become increasingly difficult as the exercise continues. Scenarios 8 through 10 should be attempted only if participants and observers feel comfortable.

You may wish to invite a third individual to observe the process and rate the fidelity with which you adhere to the guidelines of empathic listening. The Empathic Listening Checklist, contained on the following pages, may be used for self-reflection or by your partner or observer to monitor your progress.

- *Scenario 1*: Ask your partner to tell you about his or her favorite occupation and why it is meaningful and enjoyable.
- *Scenario 2*: Ask your partner to teach you about, or explain to you, how his or her favorite occupation is best accomplished.
- *Scenario 3*: Ask your partner to tell you about the neighborhood(s) in which he or she spent childhood years.
- *Scenario 4*: Ask your partner to tell you about someone of whom he or she is fond and to explain why.
- *Scenario 5*: Ask your partner to tell you about someone who is frustrating or upsetting and to explain what about this person makes him or her so.
- *Scenario 6*: Ask your partner to tell you about his or her definition of a community. Ask your partner to tell you about a community to which he or she belongs.
- *Scenario 7*: Ask your partner to tell you about a mentor, teacher, or advisor who influenced his or her life in a positive way.
- *Scenario 8* (for discretionary use only): Ask your partner to tell you about something that is worrisome or that makes him or her nervous.
- *Scenario 9* (for discretionary use only): Ask your partner to describe something that happened that was stressful or irritating.

• *Scenario 10* (for discretionary use only): Ask your partner to tell you about a painful period of his or her life and to explain how he or she managed to cope during that time.

EXERCISE 8.2

Checklist on Empathic Listening

This checklist may be used by practitioners to facilitate self-reflection about empathic listening. It may also be used by educators and fieldwork supervisors to promote learning and gain expertise in this area. It may be used during observation of a live interaction or as a self-rating tool.

Empathic Listening Checklist				
	Strong	**Adequate**	**Needs Improvement**	**Comment/ Reflection**
Clarity of Mind and Attention Span				
Suspended any impulses to interpret, evaluate, judge, formulate, or reflect while listening Maintained concentration and dismissed intrusive thoughts while listening Maintained an impartial viewpoint Sought to understand the client's experience from the unique perspective of the client Did not feel pressured to respond Did not attempt to plan responses while listening Did not attempt to predict what the client might say next				
Summary Statements				
Summary statements reflected the main point of client's comments Summary statements rephrased what the client said rather than parroted Summary statements were accurate on the first try Summary statements did not attempt to extend beyond what the client said Summary statements did not reflect the therapist's interpretation or analysis of what was said				
Striving for Understanding				
Recognized the client's clarification following a summary statement that was not 100% accurate in understanding Understood client's feedback or clarification accurately Responded to client's feedback by making an improved summary statement that was more acceptable to the client Persisted in striving for understanding during the course of the interaction				
Empathizing with Affect and Behavior				
Tone of voice was neutral or mirrored that of the client while making a summary statement Therapist demonstrated emotional resonance Therapist articulated what was observed in the client's affect or behavior No signs of judgment noted in the therapist's facial expression or tone of voice				

Communication Skills Rating Scale

When learning communication skills, it is a good idea to reflect on your interactions with others, including clients. This rating scale is designed to assist practitioners in engaging in this reflective process. It is based on the guidelines associated with each of the aspects of therapeutic communication covered in this chapter. Completing it may be facilitated by referring back to the guidelines. The scale may be completed by the practitioner for purposes of self-reflection or by a supervisor or colleague observing the practitioner's interaction to obtain more objective feedback.

Communication Skills Rating Scale				
	Yes	**No**	**NA**	**Comment/ reflection**
Verbal Communication				
Clear and audible Content of communication clear and accurate Demonstrated brevity/efficiency/parsimony in communication Approach consistent with the client's local norms and/or cultural style Emotionally modulated according to the client's comfort Appropriately confident in tone of voice Word choice professional, respectful, and tactful Intentional about talking while doing				
Nonverbal Communication				
Noticed any changes in the client's facial expression, eyes, posture, tone of 　voice, or other body language Interpreted the client's nonverbal communication accurately Therapist is self-aware and intentional about own nonverbal communication Maintained eye and/or body orientation to client while multitasking				
Unidirectional versus Bidirectional Communication				
Communicated with a client unidirectionally in a way that appeared not to 　upset the client Used unidirectional communication so effectively as to transform unidirectional 　communication into bidirectional communication				
Therapeutic Listening				
Listened empathically Used guided listening to effectively persuade or structure the client Used verbal prompts and sounds intentionally and empathically to promote 　communication Used enrichment questions to facilitate or deepen communication				
Seeking Client Feedback				
Specific and clear in terms of the type of feedback sought from client Maintained a take-charge attitude while seeking feedback				
Responding to Client Feedback				
Thanked client for feedback, even if negative Apologized when necessary and appropriate Repeated understanding of the main point of the feedback Asked the client for input on what she or he would have preferred Offered to alter or correct, if appropriate Educated client about the rationale for the original approach or action, if 　appropriate, and nondefensively				

(table continued on page 176)

Communication Skills Rating Scale (continued)				
	Yes	No	NA	Comment/ reflection
Providing Structure, Direction, and Feedback				
Set a basic temporal framework Educated client about the purpose and potential utility of therapy Used goal-setting to track progress and assess outcomes Educated client about one's preferred approach to practice or theoretical framework, if indicated Encouraged client to provide feedback Informed client about openness to change based on feedback Informed client of plans for the session and timing of activities at the beginning Checked in with client appropriately to monitor his or her experience of therapy Made expectations for client's role in therapy clear Projected an attitude of competence Discussed mode use with client, if appropriate				

NA = not applicable

CHAPTER 9

ESTABLISHING RELATIONSHIPS

Providing information on establishing effective relationships with occupational therapy clients is the central objective of this text. As emphasized thus far, achieving an effective relationship is both challenging and vital to positive therapy outcomes. This chapter covers the most basic criteria for relationship building in occupational therapy. These criteria are critical to emphasize at the beginning of the relationship when a client is still deciding whether and to what degree he or she can trust your personal integrity and professional competence. The criteria convey to the client that you are willing to know the client as a unique individual and that you care about the course and outcome of the relationship. At the most basic level, your ability to relate to clients effectively requires you to have expertise in five interrelated areas.

• Rapport building, impression management, and setting an emotional climate
• Mode matching and versatility
• Managing emotional intensity
• Judicious use of touch
• Cultural competence

Rapport building involves making deliberate efforts to make a client feel comfortable in one's presence and to establish a common ground for communication. *Impression management* consists of intentional statements and behaviors that allow the client to begin to trust in one's personal and professional integrity. The *emotional climate* of an interaction refers to the nature and intensity of affect and the style in which affect is expressed by the client and therapist. *Mode matching and versatility* was emphasized in Chapters 4 and 7. It refers to one's ability to anticipate which interpersonal mode is best suited for a client at any given time and to apply modes flexibly as needed using mode shifts. It conveys to the client that you are willing to orient your interpersonal style to the client's and to respond in ways that facilitate honest communication and

mutual understanding. *Managing emotional intensity* entails knowing how to react when clients exhibit pronounced feelings of sadness, anger, or anxiety. *Judicious use of touch* refers to knowing how to use touch that is intended to have interpersonal effects in a way that respects clients' boundaries and meets their needs for closeness or distance. *Cultural competence* incorporates one's knowledge of, respect for, and ability to incorporate the customs, behaviors, belief systems, world views, and health care practices of individuals with backgrounds other than one's own. Each of these criteria is discussed in more detail in the following sections. In the Activities section of this chapter, a quiz is provided so you can test your knowledge of the concepts reviewed herein.

Rapport Building and Impression Management

Rapport building is an often-used term that varies widely in definition. According to the Intentional Relationship Model (IRM), *rapport building* is defined as one's deliberate overtures to make a client feel at ease, particularly when first meeting and getting to know the client. The aim of rapport building is to establish an initial routine and approach to communication that the client experiences as satisfying and comfortable. Compared with other interpersonal strategies advocated by the IRM, rapport building consists of simple topics of conversation and other basic interpersonal behaviors that allow a client to become familiar with who you are as a professional and as a person. The fact that these efforts may come across to the client as rather simple and superficial should not be confused with the fact that the timing and attitude with which they are delivered are essential to the client's initial impression of you. Because each client gravitates toward different qualities in a therapist, you can gain ground if you are able to anticipate and approximate a match to what the client might prefer in an initial overture. Some examples of rapport building efforts include.

- Making eye contact and greeting the client in an earnest, serious, straightforward professional or friendly manner, depending on the client.
- Asking (rather than assuming) the client how he or she would like to be addressed (e.g., using a formal prefix versus using the client's first name).
- Introducing yourself to a client in a way that you anticipate would be optimal for the therapeutic relationship. Some clients prefer the use of a formal prefix, such as "Ms. [last name]" or "Dr. [last name]." whereas other clients prefer that you use her or his first name. In some circumstances (e.g., working with children, working in a correctional facility), use of a formal prefix is necessary to establish a professional boundary and to communicate that you expect to be respected by the client. With children, some therapists prefer to use a formal prefix along with a first name. This may be motivated by having a complicated last name or by the desire to soften the feeling of formality.
- If uncertain, asking the client how to pronounce his or her name and practicing it until you get it right.
- Orienting the client to the treatment environment (e.g., location of the bathroom) and educating the client about the setting (e.g., types of clients seen or services offered in the setting) and about any routines that occur within the setting (e.g., activities scheduled for the week).
- Making impersonal small-talk with the client (e.g., commenting about the weather, the traffic, noting any interesting facts about the setting, talking about a benign television show, or commenting on any renovations occurring in the treatment environment).
- Asking the client how he or she is feeling today or how his or her day is going.
- Letting the client know that you know a little something about him or her as a person (if appropriate). For example, if a client feels good about his or her referral source, you might inform the client about something positive that the referral source said about him or her. If the client has volunteered, been employed, or has achieved something significant, you might inform the client that you took the time to search the Internet about what he or she does/did to familiarize yourself.
- Sharing some facts about yourself or about the way you approach therapy with a client (e.g., sharing how long

you have been practicing, explaining your approach, or providing other information that qualifies you to be of service to the client).

Each of these efforts is perceived differently by different clients depending on the unique preferences of the particular client. As with other suggestions provided in this book, these guidelines for rapport building should be applied judiciously within the context of the client's particular interpersonal characteristics, the goals for therapy, and any other relevant aspects of the treatment setting or environment (Fig. 9.1).

Impression management is an important aspect of rapport building. It consists of deliberate behaviors and statements that prepare the client to begin to trust in your personal and professional integrity. When clients arrive at a treatment setting, many have a preestablished notion of what they expect to see in the appearance, demeanor, and behavior of a health care professional. Impression management refers to your:

- Physical self-presentation (hygiene, grooming, and clothing, which is impeccable, safe, professional, and nonprovocative)
- Emotional self-presentation (ability to regulate and control your emotions so as to be appropriate for the situation)
- Ability to project a take-charge attitude and to function within the instructing mode, when appropriate
- A sense of pride and energy about your work
- An approachable, nonjudgmental attitude
- Ability to establish and maintain professional boundaries

These aspects of impression management are covered in greater detail in other chapters of this book. A therapist with effective impression management is more likely to have an easier time establishing rapport with a client because her or his appearance and behaviors conform to what the client may be expecting from a health care professional. A therapist with poor impression management may cause clients to feel less comfortable or may cause clients to question some aspect of the therapist's ability to serve them in a professional capacity.

Setting an emotional climate is another important aspect of rapport-building because it frames how the client will experience his or her interaction with you. Moreover, it influences the emotional memory that remains with the client after having interacted with you. For many individuals, the feeling that they come away

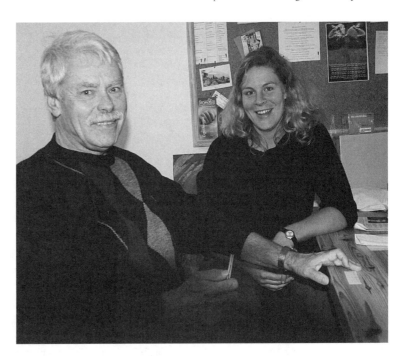

FIGURE 9.1 Anne Reuter understands that with some clients a deliberately formal approach may increase the likelihood of an enduring relationship

with after therapy is the most influential aspect of their entire experience. It affects what content from the session they remember and how accurately they remember it. An emotional climate refers to the nature and intensity of affect and the style in which affect is expressed by both client and therapist.

Generally, the emotional climate of therapy can be thought of as spanning a continuum of intensity. A high-intensity emotional climate is one in which the therapist speaks loudly, shows considerable affective expression, and conveys a lot of energy and animation in gestures and body language. Sometimes the therapist might even cheer, shout, or make other vocalizations to highlight what is being conveyed. High-intensity emotional climates are often evident in therapists functioning within the instructing or encouraging modes. A therapist in the instructing mode might repeat a certain safety reminder with a client. In doing this, the therapist may also use a loud volume or an urgent tone of voice to emphasize its importance. In situations that demand it, a therapist might use a loud, firm voice combined with an upright posture, an athletic-type stance, hands on hips, or other nonverbal gestures to establish his or her role as a leader or authority figure. Alternatively, a

therapist functioning in the encouraging mode might shout out in joy when a client achieves a hard-earned goal (Fig. 9.2).

Conversely, a low-intensity emotional climate is one in which the therapist speaks with moderate to low volume and in a neutral to lower tone of voice. The therapist uses few hand gestures and assumes more control over body language and facial/affective expression. Low-intensity emotional climates typically accompany the advocating, collaborative, and problem-solving modes. Because emotions generally play a secondary role in these modes, they are placed in the background. Instead, the intellectual or cognitive content of the session is emphasized or is used exclusively. The empathic mode is unique in that it is defined by one's complete orientation toward the client's affect, thoughts, and behaviors. Thus, therapists functioning in the empathic mode naturally match their own affective intensity to that of the client, and the emotional climate is defined by the client rather than by the therapist.

Irrespective of the level of intensity, the nature of your affect and the style in which it is conveyed are critical in defining the emotional climate. As a guideline, the nature of your affect should always be consistent with one of the six therapeutic modes. Otherwise, it runs the risk of

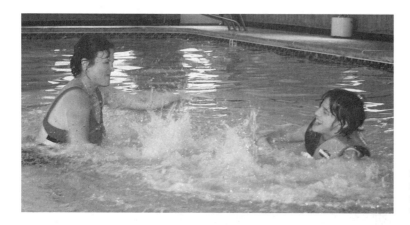

FIGURE 9.2 Kathryn Loukas encourages a high-intensity emotional climate when responding to a client's invitation to have a splashing contest

being nontherapeutic. For example, although a disappointed or even irritated tone of voice may, in certain circumstances, be appropriate within the instructing mode, uncontrolled rage or hostility expressed in the presence of a client is never appropriate. Similarly, an affect that could be interpreted as sexualized is not consistent with any of the modes and is never appropriate in therapy (Fig. 9.3).

Mode Matching and Versatility

In previous chapters, the six interpersonal modes (advocating, collaborating, empathizing, encouraging, instructing, problem-solving) and their application within the

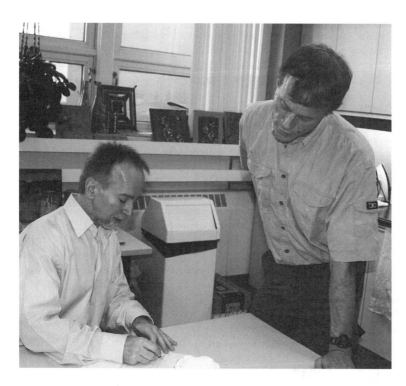

FIGURE 9.3 René Bélanger typically fosters a low-intensity emotional climate, particularly when first getting to know a client

IRM were described. I emphasized the importance of applying them flexibly in response to clients' interpersonal characteristics and in light of the interpersonal event at hand. In this section, the pros and cons of mode matching and mode versatility are elaborated because mode use is so central to establishing effective relationships with clients. *Mode matching* is defined as the therapist's common-sense efforts to select a mode that is most likely to be coherent with the client's interpersonal needs of the day, or preferred way of approaching the therapeutic relationship. Thus, a therapist using mode matching applies general guidelines similar to those presented in Tables 5.1 and 7.3 to select a mode that best fits the client's interpersonal characteristics and/or optimally responds to a given interpersonal event of therapy. In many cases your first intuition that a particular mode is the right one for the client is correct. However, there are exceptions. Some clients are more interpersonally complex than others, and they may respond atypically to your mode choice. Similarly, more than one interpersonal event may occur during a given therapy session, and this may require you to shift modes more frequently than usual. Thus, when mode matching loses its effectiveness, mode versatility is often helpful for managing these more atypical interpersonal circumstances within the therapeutic relationship.

Mode versatility relies on your ability to execute mode shifts, a skill introduced in Chapter 7. *Mode versatility* extends the concept of the mode shift in that it describes the process of trial and error undertaken by a therapist when shifting modes. The aim of this trial-and-error process is ultimately to identify the best-fit mode for the client at that moment in time. To achieve this, you must possess an ability to monitor and read a client's reaction to a particular mode and then utilize the client's reaction as feedback to guide whether to remain in that mode or try a different one.

Mode matching and versatility of mode use both lie at the core of the IRM because they allow you to be maximally in tune with and responsive to a client's interpersonal needs at any given time. These efforts convey to the client that you are willing to orient your interpersonal style so the client is unencumbered by interpersonal concerns and better positioned to get the most out of his or her experience in therapy. According to the IRM, an effective relationship is not a perfect one. Thus, the ideal in mode matching and versatility is not to be able to read the client's mind to predict which mode is the perfect match at any given time. Instead, the goal is to be versatile enough in your efforts and astute enough about gathering client feedback to gradually approximate the best match. Generally, when a mode

matches a client's interpersonal needs (and provided that other elements of occupational therapy have been executed effectively) you may observe any or all of the following in the client's verbal and/or nonverbal communication.

- Relaxation of facial muscles and other body muscles, particularly in the hands, neck, and shoulder region
- Signs of increased interest or engagement in therapy (e.g., more active involvement in therapy, asking pertinent questions, a prompt or effortful response to corrective feedback, greater overall effort)
- Increased ability to attend to and concentrate on the activities and tasks of therapy
- Signs of appreciation, respect, or endearment toward you (e.g., positive feedback about therapy, direct compliments, or attempts to joke in positive and respectful ways with you)

Any of these behaviors indicates that the client feels comfortable and content interacting within a certain mode and can proceed with the tasks and activities of therapy. When your mode choice is not optimal or you do not consistently try to approximate what might be a best-fit mode for the client, clients do not generally exhibit these behaviors.

Managing Emotional Intensity

There are occasions during occupational therapy when clients experience emotions that may be painful, stressful, or upsetting. These difficult emotions may occur in tandem with certain behaviors, some of which, if prolonged or intense, have the potential to interfere with therapy or disrupt the relationship. Three of the most challenging emotions that clients may exhibit include sadness, anger, and anxiety. This section reviews each of these categories of emotion, providing information about how to understand them and offering reminders about how to react and manage them when they emerge during therapy. According to the IRM, there are four central approaches to managing emotional intensity during therapy.

- *Witnessing* the client's expression (without use of language)
- Showing *emotional resonance* (feeling the same type of emotion as the client and allowing your feelings to show it through your affect or in what you say)

• *Labeling* the client's affect or emotional expression
• *Intervening* in the emotional expression

Emotional expression is nuanced in that it can range from being barely noticeable to being frighteningly intense. Each of these approaches to management must be appropriately matched to the unique *emotional dynamic*, or unspoken communication, occurring between the therapist and the client. If observed with empathy and intentionality, this dynamic should guide your next response. Amidst this dynamic, you should be cognizant of and responsive to the type, intensity, duration, and circumstances surrounding each client's emotional expression. Sadness is the first of the three categories of emotion reviewed in terms of its nature and management.

Sadness

Sadness is an emotion that can occur during therapy for a wide range of reasons, most of which link back to some experience of loss. A client's experience of loss may be associated with something that occurred in the present or recent past; it may be linked to one or more cumulative events in the distant past; or it may reflect a combination of all of the major losses the client has experienced in the past and present. During therapy, sadness may show on a client's face as sorrow, despair, or demoralization; or it may be evident in active grieving, crying, or sobbing. A client's eyes may well up with tears; he or she may choke on words or reveal his or her hopelessness or pessimism in what is said or left unsaid.

When it is shared with another supportive person, sadness is more manageable for people because they feel less isolated within their own emotional state. However, people vary in the extent to which they feel comfortable sharing their feelings in your presence. In any case, you must be responsive to the variations in circumstances, intensity, and duration of a client's outwardly expressed sadness.

Sadness is a "given" in some phases of occupational therapy. Many clients demonstrate sadness as a natural reaction to the stress they perceive or to the losses of which they are reminded (either implicitly or explicitly) during therapy. When a client expresses sadness spontaneously and naturally, it is usually an indication that the client trusts you enough to experience emotion freely in your presence. Alternatively, it may be an indication that the client is not self-conscious or ashamed of showing emotion in front of others in general. In either case, when a client freely expresses sadness, you should interpret it as an act of sharing and welcome its expression. If you do not

interrupt or interfere with this natural process, clients usually are able to collect themselves within a reasonable time frame and continue with the work of therapy. Increased trust develops simply as a product of your good timing and efforts to witness the client's sadness in a supportive and nonjudgmental manner. Thus, when a client expresses sadness freely and in a way that makes sense to you, any of the following *witnessing* actions may be initiated to convey respect, support, and empathy.

• Remaining present in the room and showing respect by not talking or by casting your eyes downward (if appropriate)
• If it is not obvious, occasionally looking at the client (rather than staring) to check in to see if the client is inviting you to share or join in the emotion
• Handing a client a tissue

If in the midst of his or her sadness a client looks to you for approval or gives a searching look, it is a likely indication that the client is inviting you to increase your level of involvement in the emotional dynamic. At that point and provided the client is not already escalating his or her emotional reaction, it is appropriate for you to deepen your response by either *labeling* what you observe or by showing *emotional resonance*.

When managing sadness, labeling is most appropriate when you wish to preserve an emotional boundary with the client while at the same time showing support and validation for the client's feelings. An example of labeling would be making a statement such as, "I can see that you are sad about this." You may wish to preserve an emotional boundary through labeling when you suspect that the client is uncomfortable with emotional intimacy or intensity. In this circumstance, labeling may be used to give the client permission to express more emotion while still preserving the client's choice in doing so. For example, you may say something such as, "This is definitely a place where you can cry if you want to" or "Crying can really help sometimes" or "It's okay to cry here" or "People cry here all the time."

Alternatively, you may decide to preserve an emotional boundary out of concern that the client has difficulties regulating or controlling emotions or because of concern that the client may become emotionally dependent. In this circumstance, labeling also helps clients to verbalize what they are feeling, which generally helps them organize their emotions so they can regulate them more effectively. Labeling is also useful when you suspect that the client may have difficulty interpreting nonverbal communication and you want to be clear about what is being conveyed. Thus, additional examples of labeling sadness include comments about what you observe, such as:

• "I can see that you are feeling sad today."
• "You seem sad right now."
• "You are feeling deeply sad right now."
• "It makes sense you would be feeling sad about this."
• "This is a very sad situation."

These are merely examples. When labeling what you observe about a client's sadness, you should use your own words and make statements that are appropriate to the client and the context.

Showing emotional resonance may also be appropriate when a client is sad but restricted in his or her affect, on the verge of tears, or appears to be seeking permission to express emotion. It may be communicated in conjunction with labeling or it may be communicated in the absence of language. When you perceive that nonverbal support would be better than saying anything directly to a client about the sadness, it is best to show emotional resonance rather than attempting any other response.

If a client is receptive to it, emotional resonance typically intensifies what the client is already feeling and may lead to emotional release or to more outward expression. Emotional resonance for sadness may be conveyed by revealing your own reactions of sadness in your facial expression, through allowing your eyes to fill with tears, or even through crying with a client, when appropriate. If you are not comfortable sharing or exhibiting emotion in front of a client, you should not attempt to show emotional resonance for the sheer sake of trying to be therapeutic. Emotional resonance is something that should be experienced as sincere, spontaneous, and natural.

As a general guideline, emotional resonance should be tempered to match the client's level of emotion, and it should be appropriate for the circumstances. When uncertain, you should express less emotion or a level of emotion whose duration and intensity are equivalent to those of the client—never more. Emotional resonance should be shown only if you are confident that the client will perceive it as comforting and will welcome your overture to share in something very personal. Excessive or unregulated use of emotional resonance may have the potential to be misinterpreted by certain clients as disingenuous, as a boundary violation, or as a sign that you are not in control of your emotions. Moreover, for children, too much emotional resonance may startle or distract them, or it may make them feel unsafe. Similarly, some clients react with

worry or by feeling as though they must take care of you. For these reasons, you should express emotion sincerely but intentionally to meet each client's different needs; you should not express emotion without restraint or because you are forcing it as part of an intervention. Most clients, even younger ones, can sense when therapists are not in control or when they are acting a role.

Sadness that is considered adaptive should not be confused with sadness that is considered maladaptive. Although it may be perfectly natural for a client to take an entire session or part of a session to grieve a loss, if a client's expression is uncontrolled or if it does not subside over the course of subsequent sessions, an intervention, and possibly a referral, is necessary. There are some clients for whom witnessing, labeling, and emotional resonance are not sufficient responses to sadness. For these clients, the display of sadness is so prolonged, intense, or chronic that it interferes with therapy goals and/or with the client's occupational engagement. An example of a client who displayed a form of sadness that was maladaptive was provided in Chapter 2 by René Bélanger.

The type of sadness that may interfere with therapy can occur with any client in any setting. It does not occur exclusively in mental health settings. Other signs that a client's sadness requires intervention include:

• Withdrawal from others and/or from the activities of therapy
• Apathy or loss of interest in previous topics or activities
• Ongoing discussion of worries and problems during the therapy session with an absence of commensurate work toward goals
• Sobbing or crying that is prolonged, repetitive, or chronic
• Inconsolability while expressing sadness

Although these behaviors may point to the need for referral, clients likely need to continue in occupational therapy as well. Thus, there are some interventions you should initiate when faced with these behaviors. They include:

• Reassuring the client in a way that does not minimize his or her experience (e.g., "It may be the most difficult thing you have ever faced, but you are going to be okay" or "You have survived this so far, and you will continue to survive" or "It is often most painful in the beginning, but it will get better" or "I can see some improvements already" or "You have been very strong given all you have had to face")

- Assuming a take-charge attitude so the client can rely on someone else to take control (e.g., "I'm here with you now" or "I'm right by your side in this" or "I'm keeping my eye on you to be sure you are okay" or "We will get through this together" or "You are a fighter and I will not allow you to give up on me now")
- Prescribing or suggesting interests or activities in which the client can engage—those that the client has identified as pleasurable, gratifying, or fulfilling (Kielhofner, 2002; Seligman, 2002)
- If the client is unable to initiate these interests or activities independently, you may invite clients to join you in engaging in them jointly

These are only a few suggestions. There are countless specific methods that you may use to support clients who have difficulty with their mood. These and other interventions may be used anytime a client is sad, regardless of whether you consider the sadness adaptive or maladaptive (Fig. 9.4). However, direct interventions are most likely to be effective when clients are in significant need of support. Clients with adaptive (expected) levels of sadness are often able to manage their emotions independently. Many of these clients may be most comfortable with basic efforts at validation (i.e., witnessing, labeling, emotional resonance). Attempts to say or do anything beyond validation may disrupt a client's natural ways of coping. Moreover, saying or doing too much may be perceived as meddling, intrusive, or minimizing. At times, direct interventions in a client's emotional state are perceived by some clients as excessive.

If all efforts at intervention fail, you may ask the client what he or she needs in order to feel more in control (e.g., "What do you think you need right now in order to feel ok?"). If a client is unable to answer, you should make some suggestions and wait for the client's reaction. If (because of symptoms of depression) a client is unable to engage in basic self-care (i.e., eating, drinking, bathing), the assistance of a mental health professional should be recruited immediately by accessing a colleague on staff or phoning the emergency room of a local hospital. In some cases, a client's symptoms and behaviors may point toward an inclination toward self-harm or suicide. If there are any suspicions or concerns about a client's psychological functioning, you should always ask clients if they have any thoughts, plans, or intentions to harm or kill themselves. If a client answers affirmatively, the client should undergo an immediate evaluation by a mental health professional.

Anger

Anger is a challenging emotion for many therapists, particularly those newer to occupational therapy. Despite its challenges, if expressed adaptively it is one of the most useful emotions a client can feel during therapy. This is because anger is powerful in its ability to motivate and activate people to invest and engage in occupation. For most clients, anger is a difficult emotion to access. Many clients feel and express anxiety or sadness before they admit to or even experience any feelings of anger. However, there are other clients for whom anger is their primary means of communicating how they are feeling. Provided it is communicated adaptively, you can learn to use anger to support your clients in accomplishing a wide range of goals in therapy.

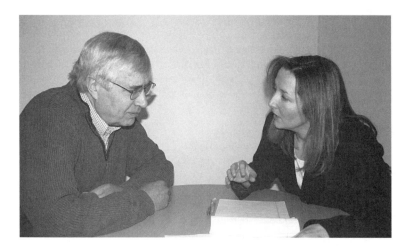

FIGURE 9.4 Jane Melton responds to a client's sadness with emotional resonance

Anger is challenging for many therapists because expression of anger has the potential to evoke fear as it carries an implicit threat of physical or emotional harm. When directed toward the therapist, anger is usually more difficult to manage. Although in most cases anger does not manifest in aggressive behavior, an important point to remember is that aggression is impossible to predict. For this reason, it is important for you to know as much as possible about how to recognize and work with anger in therapy in a way that preserves safety for all involved. During therapy, clients may demonstrate anger in ways that are adaptive or maladaptive. Adaptive expressions of anger may include:

- A client discloses that he or she is feeling angry, frustrated, or irritable and is able to describe or explain those feelings in an appropriate way.
- An angry or tense facial expression or a furrowed brow.
- Irritability or frustration in tone of voice.
- A slightly raised voice (in the absence of shouting, verbal hostility, threats, or aggression toward others).
- Use of strong words or angry vocalizations, provided you are comfortable with the language usage, the language is not directed toward other people, and it is used appropriately given the context. For example, a client grunts in frustration after attempting to string beads only to discover they have fallen to the floor.
- Nonviolent nonverbal behaviors and gestures that convey irritation or frustration (e.g., throwing one's arms up in the air, putting one's head in one's hands, sighing or taking a deep breath, leaving the room to let off steam).

When a client displays adaptive expressions of anger such as these and there is no known risk that the anger will escalate, you should support and validate the client's feelings. In most cases, this does not escalate the anger but, instead, empowers the client and helps quell the intensity of the anger.

By contrast, maladaptive anger should not be tolerated under any circumstance (even if demonstrated by young children). Examples of maladaptive anger include:

- Verbal hostility (e.g., insulting you, calling you or others in the milieu disrespectful names)
- Making verbal threats to act aggressively (e.g., "If I had the chance I would smash that windshield with a hammer") or threats to harm another person (e.g., "That guy better watch his back")
- Subtle insinuations or jokes that are sexually provocative, offensive, disrespectful, or threatening (e.g., "Hello

there little missy" or "You look *very* beautiful in those pants" or "Are *you* supposed to be a therapist?")
- Deriding you in the presence of others (e.g., obviously criticizing, laughing at, or denigrating you during group therapy)
- Nonverbal behaviors or gestures that are menacing or threatening (e.g., raising a hand as if to hit, making an offensive hand sign, performing martial arts moves out of context)
- Physical acts of aggression toward objects (e.g., throwing objects, putting a fist through a wall or window, slamming or breaking down doors, slamming an object onto a table or desk)
- Physical acts of aggression toward people (e.g., hitting, pushing, kicking, biting, or throwing objects at a person)

Any adaptive expression of anger has the potential to become maladaptive. Familiarity with a client's interpersonal characteristics and knowledge of a client's history of managing anger can help you decide how to react. Specifically, historical information about whether a client has ever been verbally or physically aggressive in the past may help to inform whether the anger can be utilized productively to support goal attainment or whether a heightened focus on limit setting is necessary.

Anytime a client chooses to express anger in a maladaptive way it is a cause for concern, and it should be addressed immediately. This cannot be emphasized enough because it has implications for your safety, for the client's safety, and for the safety of others in the treatment setting. In terms of safety, signs of impending physical hostility are the most important to notice. These should be interpreted in context and may include:

- Client rises from a bed or chair and stands
- Client's movements are impulsive, quick, or unpredictable
- Grinding teeth or tensing jaw
- Clenching fists
- Pacing
- Restlessness
- Difficulty articulating feelings reasonably
- Shouting, yelling, or other signs of verbal hostility or rage
- Immediate verbal threats to act
- Approaching you and attempting to break the boundaries of physical space and proximity

To prevent immediate physical aggression, you may attempt any of the following (depending on the context, knowledge of the client's history and characteristics, and the unique interpersonal dynamic at hand).

- Notice the warning signs (listed above) and act to set limits before the behavior escalates.
- Set limits on verbal hostility early (e.g., following the first hostile statement or gesture, warn the client that the next violation will result in a consequence). Consequences might include being asked to leave, ending the session early, being escorted to the emergency room by hospital security, or being expelled from the program, among others.
- Rise when the client rises.
- Urge the client to sit back down to talk (or provide a choice to either talk about it or end the session for the day).
- Instruct the client to describe his or her feelings rather than act on them.
- Remind the client that he or she has a choice in terms of how to communicate anger.
- Remind the client of the consequences for physical aggression and that the behavior is not permitted in this setting.
- Remind clients to leave the room if they feel they may act on their feelings.
- Maintain a safe distance from the client or remove yourself from physical proximity of the client altogether, if necessary.

If timed correctly, delivered in a firm, neutral tone, and if a trusting relationship with the client has already been established, these behaviors are more likely to ensure safety than to provoke or escalate a client's anger. However, with the wrong intervention, the wrong timing, or the wrong client, any of these behaviors has the potential to escalate a client's anger rather than contain it. This is why good timing and careful consideration of context are important variables to consider when deciding how to respond. It is essential that any warning about consequences be followed up when necessary. Warnings about consequences that are not followed up only promote aggressive behavior and weaken your authority in the eyes of the client. The result will be a setting that is less safe for everyone (Fig. 9.5).

When clients' anger escalates, it is often a reaction to a perceived loss. At the most superficial level, clients perceive that they have lost control. This perceived loss of control may be linked to any of the following.

- Loss of control over bodily functioning (e.g., client is no longer able to use the left arm)
- Loss of control over some other aspect of one's life circumstances (e.g., client's spouse asks for a divorce; client is forced to change the nature of his or her employment)
- Loss of a skill the client had been able to achieve in a prior session
- An unfulfilled expectation for performance (e.g., client assumed he or she would have been able to perform a task more effectively following surgery but it did not occur)
- Loss of control over the decisions and activities of therapy (e.g., young client throws a tantrum because the therapist does not allow her to enter the swimming pool in an unsafe way)
- Loss of the therapist's affection, approval, or praise (e.g., a client perceives corrective feedback as disapproval and becomes angry)

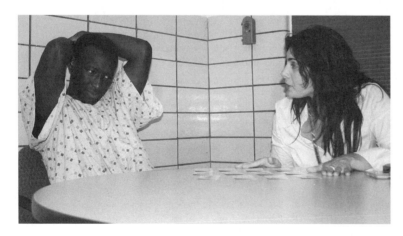

FIGURE 9.5 Stephanie McCammon notices that a client is becoming increasingly frustrated with an assessment

Second to validating the client's feelings, restoring control is an effective means of compensating for feelings of loss and intervening in a client's anger. The most effective way to restore control and de-escalate the anger is to give the client as much choice over decision-making as the client is able to manage safely and responsibly. For example, when a young client begins to throw a tantrum because the therapist sets a limit about entering the swimming pool safely, a therapist might say: "You have a choice—you can enter the pool safely or you can choose an activity other than swimming for our session today." When an older client begins to lose control over angry feelings, one means of providing choice is to say: "What do you need right now in order to feel more in control of this situation?" An unemotional and nonpunitive tone of voice is as essential as the choice of words when offering clients choice.

When providing a client with a choice as a means of de-escalating anger, you must be certain that you are perceived as the authority figure by the client. If you do not have the client's respect, providing choice cannot contain the situation. In some instances, it may only serve to further increase the client's anger or leave an opening for a pre-aggressive client to become aggressive. In addition, when providing clients with choice, you must be careful not to introduce the choice in a way that punishes the client. Otherwise, the offer of a choice is not perceived as genuine. Instead, it may be perceived as an underhanded attempt at manipulation and control. Let us return to the example of the child throwing the tantrum after being instructed to enter the pool safely. If in an angry tone of voice the therapist had said: "You have a choice—you can enter the pool safely or we can leave," the client would have likely continued the tantrum because this second limit would have been perceived as a further threat of loss. In this case, the therapist would have had no other choice but to follow through on the threat and leave the pool with the client.

For certain types of clients, issuing such an abrupt consequence might have been appropriate from a behavioral modification standpoint (even if it did not serve to de-escalate the client's anger). However, attempting to understand the perceived losses that are behind the anger, rather than creating new losses, is often the most effective means of working with such clients. Choice is most effective when you feel that the client is capable of making a choice and that the alternative choice you offer would be equally therapeutic for the client. Understanding choice as it relates to a client's need for control is an essential aspect of learning how to manage anger.

There are additional actions you can take to make a treatment setting more secure even before clients occupy it. This is particularly important in settings where you are likely to encounter clients with affect regulation difficulties or behavioral problems, such as correctional facilities, inpatient psychiatric units, outpatient mental health centers, pediatric clinics, certain educational settings, and treatment settings where clients with certain kinds of neurological disorders are seen. These actions include:

- Using the instructing mode to gain the respect of clients and to establish yourself as a leader or authority figure
- Removing nonstationary objects from the room where potentially aggressive clients will be seen
- Memorizing the phone number of the hospital security officer and keeping a cellular phone close at all times
- Sitting or standing close to the doorway with nothing obstructing it
- Leaving the door to the treatment room open or treating the client in a more public or open setting
- Stationing a security officer inside or just outside of the treatment room, if necessary
- When working with children, learn behavioral modification and safety-restraint procedures, if appropriate
- Learning basic self-defense strategies (with the understanding that you should never attempt to intervene physically with an aggressive client unless you find yourself in the midst of being assaulted and must do so in self-defense)
- Designating a safe room within the treatment setting where clients know they can go to release their aggression in a manner that is safe and acceptable
- Making and posting policies that describe how anger can and cannot be expressed within the setting and ensuring that clients are aware of these policies before they enter the setting
- Emphasizing that clients have choices in how they wish to express anger and reminding them of the consequences for maladaptive choices

If in any setting a client threatens to harm physically or kill another individual, you should have the client evaluated by an emergency room physician or mental health worker immediately. Law enforcement should be contacted, if indicated.

If you are intentional in the way you act to reduce risks associated with the maladaptive expression of anger, your treatment setting will be safer and more comfortable for everyone. Using the strategies reviewed in this section, you can prepare yourself to assist clients in channeling angry feelings constructively to accomplish goals.

Anxiety

Anxiety is the most commonly experienced and the most socially accepted of all of the difficult client emotions (Lepine, 2002). Similar to anger, anxiety is more complex than it appears because it often serves as a mask for a wide range of more painful emotions, many of which revolve around the experience of loss.

For many individuals, anxiety is the most apparent of all of their emotions. Before an individual becomes angry or sad, you may witness a certain degree of nervousness, preoccupation, or worry. In occupational therapy, anxiety is most likely to manifest in any of the following ways.

> Anxiety is more complex than it appears because it often serves as a mask for a wide range of more painful emotions, many of which revolve around the experience of loss.

- Elevated or heightened pitch of voice
- More talkative or talking more rapidly than usual
- Wringing or clenching hands
- Dry mouth while talking
- Scrunching the shoulders
- Raised eyebrows or widened eyes
- Approval-seeking or frequently questioning you about performance
- Hesitating at or resisting an activity or task
- High level of need for reassurance
- Self-doubt about performance
- Medically unexplained increase in fatigue, pain, or other physical or cognitive symptoms
- Slower-than-usual performance or underperformance on an activity or task

Depending on the circumstance, some of these behaviors may not point to anxiety but, instead, represent a manifestation of some other emotion or issue. If you are uncertain whether a client's affect or behavior is linked to feelings of anxiety, you should look to the treatment context and interpersonal circumstances within which the affect or behavior is occurring. In addition, you may utilize emotional resonance or labeling in an attempt to draw out the client's emotion more vividly. Examples of showing emotional resonance for anxiety may include:

- Mirroring a client's affect
- Thinking about what might be worrisome for the client and attempting to feel it yourself
- Admitting to the client that the situation is worrisome (if indeed you feel that it is)

In addition to helping clarify a client's feelings, resonating with a client's anxiety is effective when the client's worries are realistic and you know that reassurance or other suggestions would be insincere or unrealistic. Labeling anxiety is similar to showing emotional resonance in that it may highlight or activate a client's anxiety when the client is just barely aware of it. In addition, it can help clients label and make sense of what they are feeling, and some clients experience this as comforting and orienting. Finally, it may be the only sincere thing you can say to a client if the client's worries are realistic and if there is nothing that can be done about them. Examples of labeling may include:

- Stating what is observed (e.g., "I can see that you are worried about this" or "…seems like you are a bit hesitant about trying this" or "…sounds like you have some concerns about how this will turn out.")
- Validating what is observed (e.g., "It makes sense you would be feeling worried about this" or "This is a big step you are taking")
- Giving the client permission to be anxious (e.g., "You look a little uncertain about this—want to review it again?")
- Normalizing the worry (e.g., "A lot of people are reluctant to try this the first time" or "Many people I have talked to share that concern")

These and similar efforts are likely to help clarify whether a client is anxious. Validation promotes insight and generally serves to increase the intensity of a client's expressed emotion. However, if after these attempts at validation you remain unsure about the nature of a client's affect or behavior, the IRM recommends that you simply ask the client. Examples of questions you might ask clients in order to assess whether they are anxious may include:

- Are you having any questions or concerns today?
- Are you feeling worried or nervous today?
- Does this task/activity worry you?
- Is there something on your mind?
- Is there anything about this that isn't sitting right with you?

Once anxiety is identified correctly, there are some general rules of thumb that may be utilized when intervening to manage the anxiety. The first guideline is to avoid prolonged validation of the client's anxiety. Acts of validation would include silently witnessing the client being anxious without saying anything, showing emotional resonance, or labeling the client's anxiety (as discussed in the preceding paragraphs). Although these are appropriate things to do if the nature of the client's feelings is unclear, once it is established that a client is anxious these efforts serve only to heighten the anxiety.

Instead, the IRM recommends that you make one of the following interventions.

1. Draw more heavily on the instructing mode with the expectation that the client will feel comforted by increased structuring, repetition, guidance, and leadership.
2. Draw upon the encouraging mode to offer incentives, provide reassurance, promote self-confidence, and instill hope.
3. Using the collaborating mode, make deliberate efforts to increase the client's perceived control (e.g., by pointing out the controllable aspects of the situation).
4. Slow the pace of therapy and grade activities more carefully until the client masters and becomes comfortable with less demanding tasks or activities.
5. Reserve a time-out, or break, period in the therapy to discuss the client's worries and problem-solve.
6. Utilize strategic questioning (reviewed in Chapter 10) so the client can begin to examine the validity of his or her worries and analyze the utility of the anxious thinking

If these strategies are insufficient, you may be interested in learning to apply more advanced mental health techniques that are specifically tailored to the treatment of anxiety. They include interventions such as systematic desensitization, cognitive behavioral therapy, and various forms of mindfulness, meditation, and relaxation training. Information on these interventions is beyond the scope of this chapter; some useful references include books by Taylor (2005) and Kabat-Zin (2005).

Judicious Use of Touch

For many occupational therapists, use of touch is a critical aspect of daily work with clients. It is central to physical rehabilitation, hand therapy, sensory integration therapies, training in assistive technologies, and other cognitive rehabilitation interventions. In the literature, touch has also been celebrated as a means of promoting communication and demonstrating sensitivity and caring toward clients (Erhardt, 1997; Erhardt & Deem, 1995). Irrespective of whether your touch is intended to have interpersonal effects or strictly technical outcomes, the IRM contends that the use of touch in occupational therapy always has interpersonal implications. Clients can feel it when your touch is soft, calming, or caringly firm. Conversely, they can also feel it when your touch is rushed, abrupt, tentative, or careless. For some clients, receiving touch can be a powerfully intimate and personal experience. For this reason, the IRM considers it the most risky means of attempting to establish a relationship with a client.

Judicious use of touch refers to knowing how to use touch in a way that respects clients' boundaries and meets their interpersonal needs—whether they be for closeness or for distance (Fig. 9.6). The following guidelines may be useful for using touch judiciously with clients.

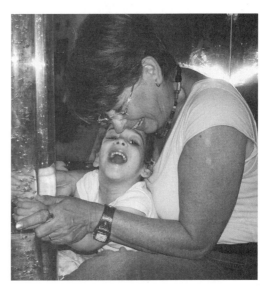

FIGURE 9.6 Michele Shapiro has first-hand understanding that touch is a highly complex form of communication that must be approached thoughtfully

- When first getting to know a client, always ask and explain your rationale before initiating any kind of touch, even if the only purpose of the touch is mechanical or rehabilitative (e.g., "May I touch your wrist to see how the bones move against your joint?" or "I may want to touch you sometimes during our work together in order to correct your position or illustrate how to do something—are you comfortable with that?" or "Sometimes I touch people to convey that I care—are you the type of person who likes that or not?" or "Is it okay if I touch you?").
- If asking the client is not possible or appropriate, announce to the client that you will be touching and explain why (e.g., "I need to lift you up a little to help you into this chair.")
- Be cautious about where you are standing or sitting in proximity to the client when you initiate touch. Avoid touching clients from behind their backs or outside of their visual range, particularly without notifying them first.
- Be careful about where on the body you touch the client. Unless required by your intervention, avoid touching clients on the abdomen, chest, neck, buttocks, pelvic region, inner thighs, or head (avoid the patting or rubbing the head even for young children, as it is perceived as disrespectful by parents in some cultures).
- If touch is being initiated strictly out of an interpersonal intention, then touching a client's hand is the most conservative approach. Touching a client on the arm, back, or shoulder is more intimate.
- Even if you know a client well, avoid initiating a hug or embrace (unless you are confident that it would be therapeutic for the client and that it would be experienced positively). It is always best practice to check with a parent or ask the client first.
- If a client initiates a hug or embrace, do what is most comfortable for you and appropriate for the situation. Keep in mind that you are not required to receive a client's requests or attempts at hugging or embracing. For clients with poor interpersonal boundaries who hug out of context or hug too frequently, it is more appropriate to set gentle limits on the behavior and provide examples of how the client might express these feelings in a way that is more consistent with the nature of your relationship.
- Never accept requests or attempts at sexualized or other inappropriate touch from a client.

These are only a few guidelines for exercising intentionality about touch. As a general rule, you should trust your emotional instincts when initiating and receiving touch with a client. The consequences for not being intentional about use of touch with a client may include:

- Triggering memories of past experiences of physical trauma or abuse
- Increasing the client's anxiety level
- Loss of the client's trust in your personal or professional integrity
- The client feeling less comfortable during therapy
- The client feeling obligated to have a more intimate relationship with you than he or she desires
- Confusion about the nature of the relationship
- The client feeling overstimulated or like a sexual object
- The client experiencing pain (from a tactile perspective)
- The client feeling emotionally or physically violated

When in doubt about a client's level of comfort with and need for touch, the IRM recommends that you limit the frequency of touch or refrain from it entirely (unless it is central to your intervention or the aim of your intervention is to reduce tactile defensiveness, for example). There are many other ways that you may communicate warmth, caring, and reassurance to clients in the absence of touch. They may take the form of verbal statements (e.g., "I like working with you"), facial expressions, tone of voice, and nonverbal gestures (e.g., winking at a child, giving a thumbs up, or clapping).

Cultural Competence

Consider the group of people with whom you are closest. How diverse or similar are they in age, sex, religion, culture, and world view? Do you tend to get along better with others with whom you share things in common? If your answer is yes, you are not alone. When people share world views, religious or spiritual orientations, occupations, cultural or socioeconomic backgrounds, or other important things in common, they may experience this sharing as a powerfully validating and comforting experience. This deep psychological need to connect with others who are perceived as similar has been discussed in the psychoanalytical literature and is referred to as a *twinship need* (Kohut, 1984). It is present in all of us to varying degrees.

The concept of a twinship need has its origins in object relations theory (Kohut, 1998). According to Kohut, the need to feel almost symbiotically attached to another human being is present in everyone at birth. However, as people develop into adults, their twinship needs change and mature to varying degrees. Some individuals continue to have a high level of need for relationships with similar others. They do not tolerate individual differences well. Instead, they prefer relationships that are as symbiotic as possible. Others are able to relate effectively to a more diverse range of people, many of whom may differ from them in fundamental ways. These individuals are considered to have reached a more mature level of development in terms of their need for twinship. For some highly developed individuals, their need for twinship is no more specific than a need for a feeling of connection with others in the human race in general, regardless of the color of their skin, their religious and political viewpoints, or their socioeconomic status.

Applied within the IRM, the extent to which a client and therapist are the same or differ influences the nature and course of their relationship. Consistent with the teachings of Kohut, clients and therapists differ in terms of the extent to which they respect and/or appreciate various aspects of human diversity. *Human diversity* is a term that defines differences between people in any number of characteristics including, but not limited to:

- Age
- Sex
- Race
- Ethnicity
- Language
- Disability status
- Religious or spiritual orientation
- Economic status
- Educational level
- Marital status
- Parental status
- Sexual orientation
- Political viewpoint
- National origin

Our world is becoming increasingly complex in terms of the cultural backgrounds, world views, and other social and demographic characteristics of the people who occupy it. Although diversity may inspire curiosity and facilitate the exchange of new knowledge, customs, or world views, it is equally likely to lie at the source of misunderstandings, conflicts, lost relationships, and, in worst cases, war and violence (Trickett, Watts, & Birman, 1994).

Clients who embrace diversity are likely more resilient when faced with the fact that their therapists differ from them in critical ways. Similarly, therapists who are knowledgeable, curious, and motivated to embrace new behaviors and perspectives are more likely to relate effectively with a wider range of clients. Consistent with the occupational therapy code of ethics (Reitz et al., 2005), the IRM emphasizes that it is not the client's responsibility to manage the complexities introduced by diversity in the therapeutic relationship. Instead, you are responsible for possessing the cultural competence necessary to be able to adjust your practices to better understand and accommodate the ways in which you differ from your clients

> Therapists are responsible for possessing the cultural competence necessary to be able to adjust their practices to better understand and accommodate the ways in which they differ from their clients.

To achieve intentionality, the IRM assumes that we are all more comfortable relating to others like ourselves. Thus, the model asks us to step outside our comfort zones and learn to relate with and be guided by the unique ideologies and behavioral practices of our diverse clients. The extent to which you are able to do so depends, in part, on the specific individual differences that arise between you and your clients.

Because a comprehensive and in-depth review of cultural competence is beyond the scope of this chapter, readers are referred to two excellent occupational therapy texts (Bonder, Martin, & Miracle, 2001; Wells & Black, 2000). The text by Bonder and associates emphasizes self-reflection, assimilation of culturally relevant information, and practice guidelines for work with diverse populations. The text by Wells and Black focuses on explaining the rationale and importance of becoming culturally competent, and it offers information about the health care beliefs and behaviors of specific cultures so readers can begin to expand their knowledge base.

Summary

Establishing functional and trusting relationships with clients is not always easy, particularly when clients are interpersonally challenging, show difficult emotions, have issues related to touch, or differ from you in ways that they perceive are critical to the relationship. In this chapter, I reviewed five critical interpersonal skills that are required for establishing effective relationships with clients. They included rapport building, mode matching and versatility, managing emotional intensity, judicious use of touch, and cultural competence. To test your knowledge of these critical skill areas, a brief quiz is provided in the Activities section of this chapter (see Exercise 9.1).

References

Bonder, B., Martin, L., & Miracle, A.W. (2001). *Culture in clinical care*. New York: Delmar Learning.

Erhardt, R. P. (1997). Case study: Using therapeutic touch. *OT Practice, 2*, 41–43.

Erhardt R. P., & Deem, J. F. (1995). Using touch therapeutically for professional sensitivity and communication. In *Conference abstracts and resources 1995* (pp. 11–12). The American Occupational Therapy Association's 1995 annual conference and exposition, April 1995, Denver. Bethesda, MD: American Occupational Therapy Association; 11–2.

Kabat-Zinn, J. (2005). *Coming to our senses: healing ourselves and the world through mindfulness*. New York: Hyperion.

Kielhofner, G. (2002). *A model of human occupation: theory and application* (3rd ed.). Philadelphia: Lippincott Williams & Wilkins.

Kohut, H. (1984). *How does analysis cure?* Chicago: University of Chicago Press.

Lepine, J. P. (2002). The epidemiology of anxiety disorders: Prevalence and societal costs. *Journal of Clinical Psychiatry, 63S*, 4–8.

Reitz, S. M., Arnold, M., Franck, L. G., Austin D. J., Hill, D., McQuade, L. J., Knox, D. K., Slater, D. Y., Commission of Standards and Ethics (2005). Occupational therapy code of ethics. *American Journal of Occupational Therapy, 59*, 639–642.

Seligman, M. E. P. (2002). *Authentic happiness: using the new positive psychology to realize your potential for lasting fulfillment*. New York: Free Press.

Taylor, R. R. (2005). *Cognitive behavioral therapy for chronic illness and disability*. New York: Springer.

Trickett, E. J., Watts, R. J., & Birman, D. (1994). *Human diversity: perspectives on people in context*. San Francisco: Jossey-Bass.

Wells, S. A., & Black, R. M. (2000). *Cultural competency for health professionals*. Bethesda. MD: American Occupational Therapy Association.

ACTIVITIES FOR LEARNING AND REFLECTION

Test Your Knowledge: Relating to Clients

1. List at least five ways in which you might attempt to build an initial rapport with a client.
   1. _____
   2. _____
   3. _____
   4. _____
   5. _____

2. List the five interpersonal skill sets that are important for establishing relationships with clients.
   1. _____
   2. _____
   3. _____
   4. _____
   5. _____

3. Which of the following is *not* true about impression management?
   a. It includes projecting a sense of pride and energy about your work.
   b. It consists of deliberate behaviors and statements that prepare the client to begin to trust in the therapist's personal and professional integrity.
   c. It is a critical aspect of rapport building.
   d. It involves using one's intuition in order to plan the best interpersonal approach

4. When might labeling serve as an appropriate way of managing anxiety?
   a. When a client tells the therapist that he or she is worried about completing a task
   b. When a client cannot control his or her fears
   c. When a client seems unaware that he or she is anxious
   d. When the therapist knows that the client is anxious

5. Which of the following is *not* part of the emotional climate between client and therapist?
   a. The nature of an individual's affect
   b. The intensity of an individual's affect
   c. The relationship between the client's affect and the environment
   d. The style in which an individual's affect is expressed

6. When would showing emotional resonance not be an appropriate way of managing a client's sadness?
   a. When a client is sad but restricted in his or her affect
   b. When a client is sobbing and completely immersed in grief
   c. When a client is on the verge of tears
   d. When a client appears to be seeking permission to express emotion

7. How do twinship needs affect cultural competence? (choose the *best* response)
   a. If a therapist is emotionally needy it impedes cultural competence.
   b. Therapists are always more effective when they work with clients who are similar to them.
   c. The more developed one's twinship needs are the more likely it is that one is able to work with culturally diverse clients.
   d. Culturally competent therapists do not have a need for twinship.

8. True or False? A therapist should always be receptive to a client's attempts at touch.
   a. True
   b. False

9. When a client's anger is escalating, which of the following behaviors should a therapist avoid doing?
   a. Leave the room.
   b. Remind the client of the potential consequences of expressing anger in maladaptive ways.
   c. Move closer to the client and assume a take-charge attitude.
   d. Provide a client with as much choice as the client is able to manage.

10. Which of the following is an indication that a therapist's mode matches the client's interpersonal needs?
   a. The client appears relaxed.
   b. There are signs of increased interest or engagement in therapy.
   c. The client shows respect, admiration, or appreciation of the therapist.
   d. All of the above

CHAPTER 10

INTERVIEWING SKILLS AND STRATEGIC QUESTIONING

Using interviews and asking questions strategically are highly specific aspects of therapeutic communication designed to elicit the information necessary for treatment planning, progress reporting, outcomes assessment, and making other types of recommendations to employers and insurance companies. When approached skillfully, asking questions is an art that requires good timing and attention to a client's boundaries around disclosure. Interviewing typically involves obtaining information from a client that is accurate and just detailed enough to facilitate appropriate treatment planning. Somewhat distinct from traditional approaches to occupational therapy interviewing, strategic questioning entails using questions to influence a clients' thinking or to facilitate self-reflection. This chapter covers interpersonal strategies involved in administering occupational therapy interviews, and it reviews the essential aspects of strategic questioning (Fig. 10.1).

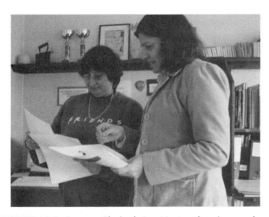

FIGURE 10.1 Carmen-Gloria de Las Heras takes time to clarify a client's response

Occupational Therapy Interviews: Brief Overview

Generally, occupational therapists administer two basic types of interviews. The first type includes semi-structured interviews in which a therapist follows a predetermined protocol and asks a set of questions designed to probe for a specific kind of information. The second type includes open-ended interviews in which questions are formulated more spontaneously and as needed. Semi-structured interviews in occupational therapy are used to gather comprehensive information in a focused way. Although these interviews have a particular structure (i.e., a format designed to gather a specific type of information, a procedure for completing the interview, and a scoring protocol), they are referred to as semi-structured because the actual interview the therapist conducts is adjusted as the interview progresses to allow the interview to feel more like a naturally unfolding conversation. Some excellent examples of semi-structured interviews based on the Model of Human Occupation (Kielhofner, 2002) and commonly used in occupational therapy include:

- Occupational Performance History Interview (Kielhofner et al., 2004)
- Occupational Circumstances Interview and Rating Scale (OCARIS) (Forsyth et al., 2005)
- Worker Role Interview (Braveman et al., 2005)
- Work Environment Impact Scale (Moore-Corner, Kielhofner, & Olson, 1998)

Table 10.1 summarizes the characteristics of these interviews.

Table 10.1 Examples of Semi-Structured Interviews Based on the Model of Human Occupation		
Interview	**Aim or Purpose**	**Average Length of the Interview (mlnutes)**
Occupational Performance History Interview (Second Edition)	To gather a life history of the client and to characterize the client's occupational narrative	45 (can be done in parts)
Occupational Circumstances Interview and Rating Scale	To identify the clients' perceptions of their occupational performance and participation	20
Worker Role Interview	To identify psychosocial factors (volition habituation and perception of the environment) that influence a person's ability to work	30
Work Environment Impact Scale	To determine how the work environment is affecting the productivity and well-being of a given worker	30

Interviewing: Interpersonal Aspects

Some occupational therapy interviews require clients to disclose personal details that are uncomfortable to talk about. When faced with this situation, most clients consciously or unconsciously attempt to influence the interviewer's opinion in a way that serves their own interpersonal needs or some other agenda. Some clients wish to be seen in a positive light, whereas others wish to emphasize their limitations. Interpersonally skilled interviewers are able to make clients feel at ease and at the same time convey the importance of accuracy in reporting and understanding. The more you are able to demonstrate acceptance and evenly hovering attention (Freud, 1923) while listening, the more likely a client is to trust, relax, and respond to questions in an honest and straightforward way.

When conducting an interview with a new client, you must never assume that you are similar to your client in terms of culture, world view, and other aspects of human diversity (e.g., values, religious and spiritual orientation, age, sexual orientation, gender, education, economic status, cognitive ability). By assuming that differences exist (even if they are not visibly apparent at first), it allows you to be more vigilant toward the possibility that certain differences influence the client's approach to the interview, your understanding and inter-

pretation of what the client has said, or both. When there are significant differences between you and the client, the client may:

• Misunderstand the questions because of how they are phrased
• Question your ability to understand his or her life experience
• Detect that you do not fully understand what he or she is saying
• Be more reluctant to disclose information due to fear of judgment
• Feel anxious or uncomfortable responding to questions
• Provide limited responses or request that the interview be discontinued

By contrast, other clients may view the interview process as an opportunity to connect and share things with the interviewer that perhaps he or she has never shared before. In some cases, clients disclose too much intimate information or have a difficult time limiting what they are saying.

Because these and other reactions are common occurrences during interviews, you must be watchful and intentional about how they approach the process of interviewing from an interpersonal perspective. The following section briefly reviews 15 interpersonal guidelines that cut across all types of occupational therapy interviews and increase the likelihood that you will obtain the needed information and the client will experience the interview positively. The guidelines include:

1. Creating a confidential and protective environment
2. Conveying a take-charge attitude
3. Assessing vulnerabilities and sensitivities
4. Orienting the client to the process and requesting consent
5. Rephrasing, reordering, or asking questions creatively (if the interview protocol permits)
6. Detecting and respecting the client's boundaries
7. Listening well
8. Responding (nonverbally or verbally) to a response
9. Responding therapeutically
10. Never apologizing for interview length or the questions
11. Checking in and acting as an emotional buoy
12. Knowing when to stop
13. Redirecting hyperverbal or tangential clients
14. Spotting and clarifying ambiguities, doorknob comments, and contradictions in content
15. Summarizing, seeking feedback, and establishing closure

A checklist is provided in the Activities section of this chapter for use by practitioners, educators, and fieldwork supervisors to assess the learning and use of these important interviewing skills.

Creating a Confidential and Protective Environment

Making clients feel that what they have to say is important and protected is an essential step in obtaining accurate information and maximizing the likelihood that the client will have a positive experience. Thus, the room or area in which the interview takes place should be confidential and contained. Unless otherwise indicated for safety reasons (e.g., a client's behavior may become inappropriate or aggressive during the interview), interviews should take place behind closed doors with no one else present in the room. Otherwise, the environment should be safe for the interviewer and for the respondent (e.g., one-way mirror, door open, security guard or other staff member present, or interviewing in a corridor or other semi-populated area). Provisions for and exceptions (e.g., suicide, homicide, child abuse) to the confidentiality of the client's responses should be reviewed with the client. The interview format and room should be quiet and accessible and accommodating given the client's impairment(s). In addition, the environment should not be excessively visually stimulating (unless indicated as part of the assessment process).

Conveying a Take-Charge Attitude

In addition to providing a protective environment, interviewing is different from regular therapy sessions in that it is more important that you convey a take-charge attitude. This is particularly important in formal semi-structured interviews because you must follow a specific protocol and obtain responses to a highly specific set of questions. In most circumstances, this must be done in a timely manner and, in some cases, within a predefined time frame (e.g., timed assessments). In addition, a take-charge attitude may serve to reduce anxiety for some clients. The prerequisites for a take-charge attitude were reviewed earlier in Chapter 8.

Assessing Vulnerabilities and Sensitivities

It is often helpful for the therapist to try to predict how smoothly the interview process will flow prior to beginning it. This involves determining whether difficulties may be encountered owing to a client's response style, interpersonal behaviors, or attitudes toward the interview. You should make liberal use of small-talk and other casual observations to obtain a best-guess estimate of what a client's response style is before beginning the interview. You should attempt to establish whether a client is likely to be particularly vulnerable or sensitive during the interview. Some behaviors associated with vulnerable and sensitive clients include irritability, nervousness, or reluctance in tone of voice; clenching of fists or jaw; facial expressions that reflect anxiety, mistrust, or doubt; asking an excessive number of questions; requesting special accommodations that are not reasonable or typical; appearing passive or withdrawn; or speaking excessively or in a tangential manner. It is advised that you use your brief first impressions and intuition to guide how you orient the client to the interview and to what extent you need to serve as an emotional buoy during the process. You should not initiate an interview if you suspect that a client has not given consent sincerely or if the client is showing signs of verbal hostility, inappropriate sexual behavior, or a potential toward physical aggression.

Orienting the Client to the Process and Requesting Consent

Once you are ready to begin the interview, the first responsibility you have is to tell the client what is going to happen during the interview and obtain the client's consent to participate. Orienting the client to the interview includes sharing the topic and purpose of the interview with the client and informing the client what will occur at the beginning, middle, and end of the interview. When orienting a client, you should make sure the client knows the difference between an occupational therapy interview and some of the other interviews he or she may have undergone at the hospital. If indicated, you should convey that you are interested in hearing not only about problems, facts, and impairments but, more importantly, the client's perceptions and experiences.

If a client appears anxious, your efforts at orientation may also include informing the client as to how the interview questions are structured and formatted (e.g., "The first part of the interview requires you to give only yes or no answers, and the second part of the interview requires you to provide me with as much detail as you can in response to the questions. That part will feel more as if we are having a conversation."). If it seems indicated, the orientation phase is a ideal time to alert a loquacious or hyperverbal client to time limits and expectations about focused responding and response length (e.g., "Sometimes I may guide the focus of your responses or signal you during your response if I think I have enough information so we can move on to the next question. Is that okay with you?"). Finally, another critical aspect of orienting a client to the process is to ask the client about questions or concerns prior to beginning the interview.

Rephrasing, Reordering, or Asking Questions Creatively

Some more structured interviews, such as those used primarily for research purposes, discourage interviewers from altering the way in which questions are asked or reordering the sequence of questions. However, if the interview protocol permits, you should take liberty to adjust the order or phrasing of questions to promote greater understanding on the part of the client. The sequence in which you ask a series of questions may also be adjusted to better correspond to what a client has just said. This offers interviewers the best chance of showing a client that they are listening and that they care about what is being said in the moment. Alternatively, an interviewer may need to adjust the sequence of questions so material that is more difficult for the client is saved until the end of the interview and material that is easier is presented at the beginning. Similarly, changing the way in which a question is phrased so it sounds more natural to the interviewer or less judgmental is also encouraged. Changing the sequence of questions, rephrasing them, or asking them in more creative ways that match the client's interpersonal needs of the moment is sometimes the determining variable in a client's decision on whether and how to respond to a given series of questions. The Occupational Performance History Interview (Kielhofner et al., 2004) is an example of an interview that allows therapists to rephrase or reorder questions on an as-needed basis (Fig. 10.2).

> Being able to determine where a client's boundaries around self-disclosure and tolerance for revealing strengths or weaknesses lie is essential for maintaining rapport.

Detecting and Respecting the Client's Boundaries

Some clients are more willing to disclose information than others. Being able to determine where a client's boundaries around self-disclosure and tolerance for revealing strengths or weaknesses lie is essential for maintaining rapport.

If you estimate that your client may fall into the sensitive or vulnerable category, you may give the client permission "up front" that he or she does not have to answer any question that makes him or her feel uncomfortable. At the same time, you should not be so protective of clients that you do not ask questions that are a standard part of the interview process. It is important to remember that there is no fault in asking the required questions (provided they are ethical and appropriate for treatment). The only requirement is that you allow a client to refuse to respond or to

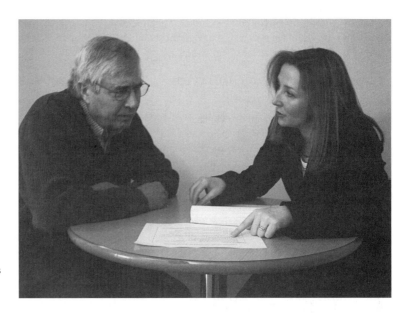

FIGURE 10.2 Carefully, Jane Melton finds a way to ask about content that may be difficult for a client

limit his or her response. If a client sets a limit or boundary around responding, you should never question the client or show disappointment during the interview. This would put the client's trust in you and the interview process at risk. Moreover, it contradicts what was promised to the client at the beginning of the interview. Instead, processing and questions should be reserved for after the interview when the client is providing feedback.

Listening Well

Because of the inherent risks involved in obtaining accurate responses to interview questions, it is imperative that you listen well to clients' responses. Therapeutic listening was reviewed extensively earlier in Chapter 8. As a reminder, key points to keep in mind during an interview include orienting your entire body toward the client, maintaining eye contact, sitting upright and leaning in toward the client, maintaining an evenly hovering attention, which includes not conveying shock, judgment, or other signs of active reflection (Freud, 1923), managing attention and dismissing intrusive thoughts, and responding to a response (covered in the next section).

Responding to a Response

Blank stares or a constricted affect on the part of a therapist is never appreciated by clients because, at best, it conveys that the therapist is absent or not participating fully in the conversation. At worst, it conveys judgment or disapproval. Because interviews increase the likelihood that a client will feel exposed and vulnerable, you should always show some kind of a response when clients answer a question or otherwise disclose key information. Your response can be verbal or nonverbal. Verbal responses may include prompts (e.g., tell me more about that), validating sounds, and summary statements that reiterate what the client has just said and allow for transition into the next question. Nonverbal responses may include a slight nod of the head, a change in facial expression to match the content of the client's disclosure, widening the eyes, or some other validating gesture. When responding to a client's disclosure, it is important to respond in a way that does not interrupt the client's flow of thinking and in a way that encourages the client to say more and stay engaged in the interview.

Responding Therapeutically

Similar to listening well and responding to a response, strategies for responding therapeutically have already been reviewed in Chapter 8. Within the context of an interview, responding therapeutically includes not appearing shocked at a client's disclosure but, instead, matching the client's affect when describing the event. Other already-reviewed strategies include making summary statements to convey empathy, validating what the client has said rather than evaluating it, being judicious about showing emotion when responding, overusing verbal prompts, sounds, and facial expressions as substitutes for making thoughtful summary statements, and listening for the client's strengths.

Never Apologizing for Interview Length or the Questions

Even if a client appears sensitive or vulnerable, you should never apologize for the questions being asked or for the length of the interview. If you have done an adequate job of orienting the client to the process at the beginning of the interview and have the client's full consent, there is no reason to protect the client from the process. Apologizing only undermines your professionalism and the value of the interview. However, if a client is having difficulties getting through the interview, resists responding, or raises a complaint, you should validate those difficulties (if appropriate) and attempt to reach mutual understanding with the client.

Checking in and Acting as an Emotional Buoy

When the content of an interview includes exposing a client's weaknesses or vulnerabilities or if it otherwise contains questions of a personal or sensitive nature, you should continually orient and guide clients through the interview by highlighting shifts in major topic areas by marking how much has been accomplished, how much is left to do, and by describing the questions to come. In addition, you should occasionally check in with sensitive clients regarding their comfort about responding to the questions and their overall emotional well-being. In addition, you might warn a sensitive client before asking a difficult question (e.g., "You may find the next set of questions to be more sensitive in nature"). However, this should be done only if a client has behaved in an emotional, uncomfortable, or mistrustful manner during the interview or if the client's behavior during the interview otherwise indicates that a warning will promote responding rather than inhibit it. If there is no indication that a client is uncomfortable, warning the client beforehand may convey an unintended message that *you* are the one who may be uncomfortable with the questions and potential responses that may arise. Another means of functioning as an ***emotional buoy*** for a client is occasionally to provide positive feedback to the client about his or her behavior during the interview (e.g., "I appreciate what you had to share in that last question" or "You've been able to stay with the questions even though some of them have been difficult for you").

Knowing When to Stop

Inevitably, there are occasions when you have to stop an interview. This can occur when a client requests that it be discontinued or when it is clear that continuing the interview would be physically or emotionally detrimental for the client and/or for you. Some guidelines for knowing when to discontinue an interview entirely include:

- Pausing if a client has become emotional and giving the client permission for self-expression
- Assessing the client's ability to gain composure and continue the interview in the absence of your input or assistance
- Involving the client in the decision as to whether to discontinue the interview
- Discontinuing if the client appears passive, ambivalent, or continues to be highly emotional

You should also discontinue an interview if the client's behavior becomes sexually inappropriate or if the client is verbally hostile or at risk for physical aggression.

Redirecting Hyperverbal or Tangential Clients

Much of this chapter has focused on efforts to establish and maintain enough rapport and trust that a client feels comfortable disclosing the information that you need to complete your job. However, there are many occasions in which you will encounter loquacious clients who are prone to excessive self-disclosure or have difficulty organizing their thinking to respond to questions in a manner that is concise and to the point. When clients communicate to the point that they are unaware of the natural rhythm, shifts, pauses, and boundaries of conversation, they are generally referred to as ***hyperverbal*** in their communication style. When clients digress onto related topics or have difficulty getting to the point of the question, they are described as having a ***tangential*** communication style. In these situations, you must rely on your take-charge attitude and assume a more active role in managing how the client is responding. When encountering this situation, you may interrupt the client by saying, "Pardon me for interrupting...." Following the interruption, a number of strategies may be utilized to limit the client's responses. One may involve simply saying "I have enough information for that question.... Let's move to the next one." Alternatively, you might ask the client if he or she can summarize what is being said. You might also mention that there are several questions remaining in the interview and that it is important that the client try to be as brief as possible when responding. On the first interruption, it may help to reassure the client that you are forced to interrupt everyone on certain occasions and that the limits are necessary so you can get to all of the questions on time.

Sometimes you might make a concrete request, such as, "Would you try to answer in, say, no more than two sentences for each question so we can be sure to finish the interview in time?" or "I am noticing that you are having a hard time staying with the main point of the questions today.... Are you aware of this?... I'm going to interrupt more so we can stay on track." or "If you have more thoughts to share, would you jot them down and we can review them at the end of the interview?" Other strategies may include increasing the firmness and frequency of your limit-setting or providing a rationale that getting to all of the questions provides information that is more comprehensive and relevant to the treatment goals.

Spotting and Clarifying Ambiguities, Doorknob Comments, and Contradictions in Content

Understanding clients is paramount to a successful interview. You should always admit it to a client if you do not follow, cannot hear, or cannot understand what is being communicated. It conveys that you care enough about what the client is saying to ask, and it also demonstrates honesty in communication. If you are listening well and are usually able to hear and understand clients, the fact that you are having difficulty should not be ignored; it may be an important indicator of the client's difficulties in that particular area of communication. When an otherwise articulate client stumbles on words or makes a vague allusion to something that you do not quite understand, it may mean that the client is feeling tentative or insecure about something or is attempting to make an important disclosure. Alternatively, there are times when what a client is saying really does not make any sense, even upon hearing it a second time. Assuming there are no language differences, a client's use of made-up words, statements you find bizarre, or words that are loosely threaded together in a sentence that does not make sense may be symptoms of a neurological or psychiatric disorder.

Some clients, whether intentionally or unconsciously, drop hints or time what they say inappropriately so as to leave you with a choice of whether to pick up on the hint or to ignore it. Sometimes a client might say something vague or emotionally provocative just as the session time is about to end. These are usually referred to as ***doorknob comments***, and they always deserve an attempt on your part to inquire and seek clarification. In addition, when you administer an interview you should always look for contradictions in what a client is communicating and seek clarification when they are recognized.

Summarizing, Seeking Feedback, and Establishing Closure

Clients typically remember the beginning and ending of the interview more than the middle part. The manner in which closure is established at the end of the interview is critical to clients' lasting impressions of their experience as a whole. To ensure a smooth ending, clients should be thanked for their participation and asked if there is anything that was not inquired about that they think might be important for you to know. In addition, you should assess clients' emotional state at the end of the interview (through observation or overtly) and ask for feedback about their experience. If it has been a difficult interview, clients can be informed that it is normal for an interview to stir up residual feelings or memories. If necessary, you should make a support plan for the client before leaving the client alone with his or her thoughts, such as scheduling a follow-up phone call, ensuring that the client will not be alone for the remainder of the day, or ensuring that the client has a plan for activity or self-care (Fig. 10.3).

Taken together, these 15 guidelines form the foundation for a client to feel oriented, clear about expectations, accepted, protected, and appreciated for having undergone an interview. As mentioned earlier, these guidelines are not fixed and should be applied with consideration for a client's cultural background, unique interpersonal characteristics, and circumstances in the immediate social and physical environment. In addition, certain guidelines may be more appropriate in light of any interpersonal events that occur during the interview process. The next section reviews strategic questioning, which typically is not part of any formal interview process in occupational therapy but may be used anytime you wish to encourage a client to reflect upon his or her own thinking and decision-making.

Strategic Questioning

Strategic questioning is an approach to asking clients questions that originated within the tradition of cognitive

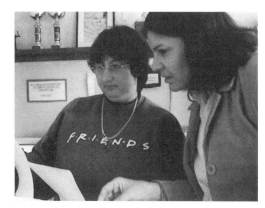

FIGURE 10.3 Interviewing is an art and a critical aspect of occupational therapy practice

therapy (Beck, 1995; Beck, Rush, Shaw, & Emery, 1979). Originally, it was developed to assist clients in transforming various forms of negative and unrealistic thinking into more balanced, neutral, or positive thinking. Applied within the IRM, *strategic questioning* involves asking clients questions in a way that intends to influence their perspective, convey a certain message, or cause them to reflect upon and evaluate their thinking about a given topic. Distinct from enrichment questions (described in Chapter 8), strategic questions are not typically experienced by clients as immediately supportive or empathic. Instead, they subtly challenge clients to question their own thoughts or opinions. In occupational therapy, this kind of questioning may be used in consultation or treatment situations.

- To assist clients in problem-solving about how to approach a situation, activity, or task
- To assist clients in evaluating different treatment options, employment options, goals for therapy, environmental modifications, or assistive technologies
- To address a clients' apprehension about engaging in a novel activity or task
- To raise clients' awareness that their thinking is unnecessarily pessimistic
- To assist clients in achieving a more realistic idea of their own performance capacity—one that neither underestimates nor overestimates their capacity
- To help clients see distinctions between aspects of their lives they can and cannot control
- To help alleviate clients' worries about uncontrollable events

- To help clients plan how to address worrisome aspects of their lives that they can control or influence
- To help a client synthesize information so he or she can develop new ways of thinking or reacting to a given situation or crisis

The potential applications of strategic questioning in occupational therapy are endless. Through this type of questioning, clients examine their thinking from a more objective and logical standpoint, and they are encouraged to test the validity of their ideas by attempting new behaviors.

Strategic questioning relies heavily on the *Socratic approach* (Paul & Elder, 2002). Socratic questioning is an approach originally developed by Socrates to teach students of philosophy how to think critically about information. When applied in occupational therapy, there are five categories of strategic questioning derived from the Socratic approach (Paul & Elder, 2002).

- Origin or source questions
- Questions that probe evidence
- Questions that probe assumptions
- Questions about viewpoint
- Questions about consequences

Some examples of questions that fall into each category are provided in Table 10.2.

Most important to this process is the timing and context in which these questions are presented to clients. Because of their potential to threaten or challenge a clients' existing behaviors and beliefs, strategic questioning should be offered only to clients who are not exceptionally sensitive or vulnerable at the time and then only when it is clear that the client is ready to be questioned in this way. Asking these questions with poor timing (e.g., just before the client is about to undergo surgery) or in an inappropriate context (e.g., in an acute care setting such as an emergency room) may lead to empathic breaks or, more significant, ruptures in the therapeutic relationship.

Summary

When crafted intentionally and delivered thoughtfully, questions asked during interviews and as part of an overall strategy to influence the client can benefit the therapeutic process tremendously. In this chapter, 15 interviewing guidelines were provided for preserving the therapeutic

Table 10.2 **Strategic Questions and Examples of Use in Occupational Therapy**	
Origin or source questions	How did you first get the idea that [you will not be able to work again]? Does your doctor feel otherwise? What has led you to believe that [you won't find accessible housing outside the city]?
Questions that probe evidence	What do you already know that supports your idea that your [friends think that you complain too much]? Do you believe this constitutes enough evidence? Are there any alternative explanations [that you are having more difficulty today]? What evidence do you have that [you are not recovering quickly enough]?
Questions that probe assumptions	Let's assume for the moment that your belief [that your boyfriend no longer finds you physically attractive] is true. What does this say about you? What does that say about your boyfriend? To conclude that [you will never be able to think as clearly as you once did], what must you assume? Do you think someone else would make this same assumption?
Questions about viewpoint	It sounds like you believe that you are being punished for [your affair]. Why have you chosen to explain [your accident] from this perspective? How might someone else that [has had an affair] explain the fact that she also survived [an accident]? How might a friend have interpreted [the physical therapist's behavior]? Would your partner look at this in the same way?
Questions about consequences	If you decide not to [complete your rehabilitation goals], what positive consequences might be involved? What negative consequences might be involved? What are the likely short-term consequences of [not wearing your splint when you go to bed]? What long-term consequences might be involved?

relationship and obtaining information that is accurate and truthful. For those new to conducting interviews and for those seeking to improve their skills, it is often helpful to conduct practice interviews and to reflect on the interview process following the interview. A checklist derived from the interviewing guidelines is provided in the Activities section of this chapter to assist you in engaging in this reflective process. The chapter also reviewed the rationale for and uses of strategic questioning in occupational therapy. Examples of specific applications of strategic questions in occupational therapy were provided. An exercise is provided in the Activities section so that those of you who are newer to the process of strategic questioning may practice with peers or colleagues.

References

Beck, J. (1995). *Cognitive therapy: basics and beyond.* New York: Guilford Press.

Beck, A. T., Rush, A. J., Shaw, B. F., & Emery, G. (1979). *Cognitive therapy of depression.* New York: Guilford Press.

Braveman, B., Robson, M., Velozo, C., Kielhofner, G., Fisher, G., Forsyth, K., & Kerschbaum, J. (2005). *Worker Role Interview (WRI) (version 10.0).* Chicago: Model of Human Occupation Clearinghouse, Department of Occupational Therapy, College of Applied Health Sciences, University of Illinois at Chicago.

Forsyth, K., Deshpande, S., Kielhofner, G., Henriksson, C., Haglund, L., Olson, L., Skinner, S., & Kulkarni, S.

(2004). *User's manual for the Occupational Circumstances Assessment and Interview Rating Scale (OCAIRS) (version 4.0).* Chicago: Model of Human Occupation Clearinghouse, Department of Occupational Therapy, College of Applied Health Sciences, University of Illinois at Chicago.

Freud, S. (1923). *The ego and the id.* New York: W.W. Norton.

Kielhofner, G. (2002). *A model of human occupation: theory and application* (3rd ed.). Philadelphia: Lippincott Williams & Wilkins.

Kielhofner, G., Mallinson, T., Crawford, C., Nowak, M., Rigby, M., Henry, A., & Walens, D. (2004). *Occupational Performance History Interview II (OPHI II)*

(Version 2.1). Chicago: Model of Human Occupation Clearinghouse, Department of Occupational Therapy, College of Applied Health Sciences, University of Illinois at Chicago.

Moore-Corner, R. A., Kielhofner, G., & Olson, L. (1998). *Work Environment Impact Scale* (Version 2.0). Chicago: Model of Human Occupation Clearing-house, Department of Occupational Therapy, College of Applied Health Sciences, University of Illinois at Chicago.

Paul, R., & Elder, L. (2002). *Critical thinking: tools for taking charge of your professional and personal life*. Upper Saddle River, NJ: Financial Times Prentice Hall.

ACTIVITIES FOR LEARNING AND REFLECTION

Interview Review Checklist

When learning to conduct interviews, it is a good idea to reflect on the interview process following the interview. This checklist is designed to assist interviewers in engaging in this reflective process. It is based on the interview guidelines and completing it may be augmented by referring back to the guidelines. It can be completed by the interviewer as a self-reflection or as a means of feedback from a supervisor or colleague who observed the interview process.

Interview Review Checklist	Yes	No	NA	Comment/Reflection
Protective Environment				
Confidential and Contained				
Quiet				
Accessible and Accommodating Any Impairment(s)				
Not Excessively Visually Stimulating				
Safe for the Interviewer and for the Respondent				
Take-Charge Attitude				
Emotionally Centered, Managed Anxiety				
Interview Content/Questions Memorized/ Well Rehearsed				
Professional Attitude/Behavior				
Confident, Clear, Sufficiently Loud Voice				
Confident Body Posture				
Made Client at Ease by Being Navigator, Instructor, Emotional Buoy, and Coach				
Set Limits in Order to Structure				
Orienting Client to the Process				
Shared Topic				
Shared Purpose				
Informed as to Interview Structure and Format				
Informed as to What Will Happen at the Beginning, Middle, and End				
Stated Any Expectations About Focused Responding and Response Length				
Conveyed Intent of OT Interview				
Informed Client of Interest in Client's Perceptions and Experiences, if Appropriate				

(table continued on page 206)

Interview Review Checklist (continued)	Yes	No	NA	Comment/Reflection
Assessed Vulnerabilities and Sensitivities				
Assess/Estimate Client's Response Style				
Identify Vulnerability/Sensitivity				
Used First Impressions to Orient Interviewee/Self				
Respected Boundaries				
Gave Permission up Front to Decline Uncomfortable Questions				
Offered Opportunity to Pause and Receive Support or Go On to Another Topic				
Listened Well, Maintained Attention, Conveyed Interest				
Oriented Body				
Maintained Eye Contact				
Sat Upright or Leaned Toward Client				
Managed Attention/Concentration				
Conveyed Interest				
Always Responded to a Response				
Gave Verbal Responses				
Gave Nonverbal Responses				
Responded Therapeutically				
Without Shock/Judgment				
Validated				
Showed Emotion Judiciously				
Did Not Overuse Verbal Prompts, Sounds, and Facial Expressions				
Heard/Highlighted Strengths				
Used Summary Statements to Convey Empathy				
Never Apologized				
Did Not Apologize for Questions/Interview				
Validated Difficulties/Resistance				
Acted as an Emotional Buoy				
Oriented and Guided Through the Interview				
Highlighted Shifts in Major Topic Area				
Checked in Regarding Comfort				
Warned of Difficult Questions				
Knew When to Stop				
Paused at Emotional Expression				
Gave Permission/Made Room for Emotional Expression				
Assess Ability to Regroup				
Involved Client in Decision to Terminate				
Discontinued Because of Passiveness, Ambivalence, Nonresponsiveness				

	Yes	No	NA	Comment/Reflection
Redirected Hyperverbal or Tangential Interviewee				
Interrupted				
Asked to Summarize Briefly				
Increased Firmness and Frequency of Limit-Setting				
Warned Client of Possible Interruptions/Guidance				
Reassured Client About Limits				
Provided Rationale for Need to Complete All Questions				
Asked Client to Save/Jot Down Thoughts Not Covered for End				
Spotted and Clarified Ambiguous Statements, Doorknob Comments, Contradictions in Content				
Admitted When You Did Not Follow/Understand				
Spotted/Asked About Contradictions				
Picked Up and Followed Through with Doorknob Comments				
Summarized, Sought Feedback, Established Closure				
Thanked				
Asked If Anything Important was Forgotten				
Asked for Feedback				
Assessed Emotional State at End of Interview				
If Difficult, Informed About How It Might Stir Up Feelings/Memories Planned Support				

NA = not applicable

EXERCISE 10.1

Strategic Questioning

Because strategic questioning has the potential to be perceived by clients as unsupportive in certain situations, it is recommended that those newer to strategic questioning practice this process with classmates or colleagues under live supervision before attempting to use it with clients. Ask an instructor, fieldwork supervisor, or consultant with expertise in strategic questioning (or with training in cognitive behavioral therapy) to supervise and observe a role-play interaction with a colleague or classmate. Ask this individual to observe your approach to asking questions and to make suggestions about how you might better use questions as a means of encouraging autonomy in problem-solving and as a means of broadening your clients' thinking about certain issues.

The following exercise is designed to provide just this kind of experience in strategic questioning and to stimulate reflection about its use. You may refer back to Table 10-2 for ideas about how to phrase your questions. When you are finished with the questioning required for each scenario, ask your partner for feedback about how he or she experienced being questioned in this way. If a third observer is present, ask the observer how your questions came across in terms of timing, context, and tone.

Questions that Probe Origin or Source
Ask your partner to think of something he or she is feeling pessimistic or doubtful about. If your partner cannot think of something current, ask him or her to imagine a time when he or she was

feeling pessimistic or doubtful about something that actually turned out well. Once a pessimistic thought has been identified, ask your partner questions that probe the origin or source of his or her thoughts.

Questions that Probe Evidence

Ask your partner to think of something he or she is feeling insecure or worried about. If your partner is not able to provide a current example, ask him or her to think of a time in the past when he or she was feeling insecure or worried about something about which it turned out there was no need to worry. Once a worry has been identified, ask your partner questions that probe the evidence for and against the worry.

Questions that Probe Assumptions

Ask your partner to provide an example of a goal, skill, or activity that might be within his or her reach or capacity but that he or she doubts would ever be possible to do. If your partner cannot provide a current example, ask him or her to think of a time in the past where he or she was faced with a goal, skill, or activity that he or she doubted could be accomplished (but it was eventually accomplished). Once a presumably unreachable goal, skill, or activity has been identified, ask your partner assumption-oriented questions.

Questions that Probe Viewpoint

Ask your partner to state a strong opinion about something important to him or her. Then ask your partner questions that probe viewpoint.

Questions that Probe Consequences

Ask your partner to describe a relatively consequential choice that he or she is facing now or faced at one time in life. Then ask your partner questions that probe the consequences of each side of the choice.

CHAPTER 11

UNDERSTANDING FAMILIES, SOCIAL SYSTEMS, AND GROUP DYNAMICS IN OCCUPATIONAL THERAPY

In many occupational therapy settings, encountering a client in complete isolation is more an exception than a norm. During care, clients and therapists may come into contact with other professionals; other clients; parents, guardians, and caregivers of clients; and partners, spouses, other family members, or friends. When working with children or with adults who require a personal assistant or caregiver, contact with these individuals is likely, even if a particular approach requires that most of the work be conducted with the client alone. Many times, those serving in the role of caregiver occupy dual roles as parents, guardians, spouses, partners, other family members, or friends. At minimum, parents, guardians, or other caregivers interact with therapists when transporting the client to and from therapy, when the therapist provides progress reports or assigns homework, or when the therapist makes other recommendations for resources and equipment. Some parents and guardians prefer to be more involved in a client's care even if a particular intervention does not require it. Still, many occupational therapy approaches require more frequent involvement on the part of the parent or caregiver so the achievements made in therapy will be retained in nontherapy settings. In some circumstances, a therapist might insist on the involvement of others because he or she has identified a dysfunctional dynamic that is interfering with the objectives of therapy. All of these relationships that occur outside the client–therapist dyad represent different types of social systems in which clients and therapists commonly participate during the course of therapy.

Contact with others peripheral to the client–therapist dyad may be initiated by the client, by others close to the client, or by the therapist. Regardless of who initiates the contact, the Intentional Relationship Model (IRM) emphasizes the importance of always making this contact intentional. Intentionality is required because the introduction of another individual or group into the client–therapist relationship inevitably adds complexity to the interaction and increases the likelihood that at least one interpersonal event will occur. Making contact intentional requires knowledge of certain fundamental social systems' principles and knowledge of the structure, process, and dynamics of groups. If contact with others in a client's world is treated with intentionality, it is more likely to support the goals of therapy. If contact with others is not addressed with caution and expertise, maladaptive dynamics may emerge within the social system. These dynamics have the potential to play out in the therapy relationship or otherwise interfere with the goals and outcomes of therapy. In this chapter, I cover the following principles and skill sets that are fundamental to the intentional management of social systems in occupational therapy.

- Preserving confidentiality and boundaries within social systems
- Viewing relationships from a social systems perspective
- Distinguishing between productive and maladaptive dynamics of systems
- Managing maladaptive dynamics of systems

These principles and skill sets derive from a range of family systems theories, group therapy practices, and industrial-organizational approaches that were developed within the field of psychology. Most emphasized are ideas from Murray Bowen's Multigenerational Family Systems

Theory and those from Salvador Minuchin's Structural Family Therapy. Briefly, family systems theories use concepts from the general systems theory to explain the complex interactions that occur in families, couples, and other groups of people. These theories view members of these social systems as emotionally and behaviorally interconnected. Because the members of a system are so connected, any change in the emotional state or interpersonal behaviors of one member is highly likely to affect the thoughts, emotions, and behaviors of other members of the system. Thus, when a problem escalates or when an injury or illness occurs to one member of the system, it is inevitable that other members of the system experience changes in their thoughts, feelings, and behaviors within the system. Similarly, if one member of the system changes his or her perspective or behavior for a reason that is unrelated to an illness or impairment, other members of the system are bound to experience its implications, and they typically strive to resist or counteract that change. More information about these theories can be obtained in Sholevar's (2005) text on family therapy and in the latest book from Minuchin, Colapinto, & Minuchin (1998).

Based on observations of the therapists featured in this book, the particular skill sets highlighted in this chapter were selected because they were determined to be the most relevant to the general day-to-day practice of occupational therapy across different treatment settings. Despite their origins in the field of mental health, they are pragmatically useful when applied to any client population and any treatment setting.

Preserving Confidentiality and Boundaries

Interacting within a social system can create a misperception that it is permissible to share anything about anyone in the system with others in the system. This is particularly likely to occur when you are working with an entire family. However, many social systems (families included) are not open to the uninhibited sharing of information among members. Preserving confidentiality and boundaries within social systems is of high importance. Anytime you interact with someone associated with a client, issues of confidentiality and professional boundaries should always be foremost in your mind. Regardless of how trivial or significant you consider information about a client to be, when information is shared it must be kept confidential

until or unless the client has given you formal permission to share it. For some clients, information to be kept confidential constitutes any type of information, including that related to the impairment or the treatment. Other clients may wish that you keep confidential only personal details that are not directly pertinent to the impairment or treatment. These personal details may range from information that is highly intimate (e.g., information about a client's relationship with a partner) or information that you may consider seemingly banal (e.g., information about what a client did with a friend last week). Even banal personal details may be important to keep confidential because a client may not wish for certain others within the system to know his or her every action.

Similarly, the source with whom you share information about a client is also an important consideration. Regardless of how comfortable a client appears to be with the person to whom information is being disclosed, a client's permission to disclose to a particular individual should always be sought. For example, one client may not mind if certain information is disclosed to a sibling but may mind very much if the same information is disclosed to a parent. Conversely, a different client may mind if information is disclosed to the sibling but may not mind if it is disclosed to a parent. As a general guideline, when talking about a client to any other individual, even a family member, always obtain permission from the client before disclosing any information to anyone. This includes talking to clients about other clients, even if those other clients are unnamed. Not preserving confidentiality is an ethical violation that could lead to distrust, a permanently ruptured relationship, or legal action.

Similar to confidentiality, preserving your own professional boundaries is an important consideration when working inside social systems. It is common for clients to discuss personal details or other sensitive information that has been self-disclosed by a therapist with others. If you do not consider it therapeutic for certain clients, family members, or other individuals associated with the client to know something, you should not disclose the information to any member of the social system. Similarly, if you do not wish for certain information to be shared with coworkers, you should not disclose that information to clients. In many treatment settings, clients interact closely with other professionals and may attempt to engage in casual chitchat or gossip with them. Many clients may be unaware of the implications of sharing personal details about your life with others in the setting. Thus, clients should not be held responsible if they do breach what you assumed was your confidentiality. (This is consistent with the IRM principle of interpersonal self-discipline, introduced in Chapter 3.) Although being able to trust a client's discretion may build feelings of mutuality within the relationship, a client is not obligated to act in a reciprocal manner. As reviewed in Chapter 14, therapist self-disclosures should have a therapeutic purpose and should not be experienced as burdensome by clients. As a general guideline, you should be parsimonious about self-disclosure to protect yourself emotionally and avoid burnout associated with initiating interpersonal risks in the workplace.

Viewing Relationships From a Social Systems Perspective

A social system is defined as any combination of two or more individuals interacting in a defined way. An obvious social system in occupational therapy is one comprised of client and therapist. This social system is dyadic because it involves only two individuals. Multidimensional social systems involve more than two individuals and are generally more difficult to understand for new therapists because they may be comprised of multiple relationships, each of which may have its own unique dynamics. Examples of social systems commonly encountered in occupational therapy may include, but are not limited to:

- Child clients and their parents (or guardians)
- Child clients and their siblings (or friends)
- Adult clients and their parents
- Adult clients and their children
- Adult clients and their siblings (or friends)
- Clients and multiple family members
- Clients and their spouses or partners
- Clients and their nonrelative caregivers
- A formal occupational therapy group or an informal group of clients within a specific milieu or treatment setting
- A formal caregiver group or an informal group of caregivers oriented around a specific diagnosis

Viewing relationships from a social systems perspective requires that you temporarily suspend your focus on the client and instead watch, listen, and reflect upon the nature and emotional tone of the client's interactions with others peripheral to the client–therapist relationship. The client must not be the only member of the system who is viewed as vulnerable or as having a problem or limitation; every other member of the social system must also be evaluated in terms of the vulnerabilities, problems, or limitations they bring into the interaction. This perspective is illustrated in Figures 11.1 and 11.2.

When observing these interactions, you should consider a number of questions that can help you understand the system and decide how to interact with it in a way that serves the client's best interests. Questions to consider include:

- Who are the individuals that comprise the system, and what is their relationship to the client (e.g., parents, friends, extended family members)?
- Who are the most engaged members of the system? Who are the most disengaged?
- Who are the most prominent or influential members? How do they exert their power? How effective are they in influencing the system?
- What topics, general themes, or content of conversations dominate the system?
- What does the client appear to expect or need from others in the system?
- What do others appear to expect or need from the client?
- What is the general emotional tone or mood of the system?
- Is communication within the system shared, open, and direct; or are there certain alliances and indirect routes of communication?
- What productive dynamics exist that support the client's best interests?
- What maladaptive dynamics exist?
- How are disagreements or conflicts of interest managed?

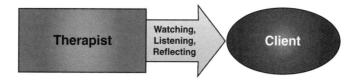

FIGURE 11.1 Viewing relationships from a dyadic perspective

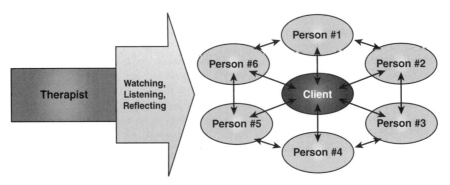

FIGURE 11.2 Viewing relationships from a social systems perspective

One of the most effective ways to begin to understand interactions from a social systems perspective is to observe a group of people interacting. Exercise 11.1, presented in the Activities section, provides an avenue in which you can carry out this observation and reflect upon what you have witnessed. To obtain full benefit, you are encouraged to complete this exercise after you have finished reading the chapter.

Distinguishing Between Productive and Maladaptive Dynamics of Systems

When you attempt to interact with a social system, the entire system becomes a kind of client in itself. As the therapist, you may take on one or more roles within the system and use modes to move into and out of the system in an intentional way to serve a client's best interests. To do this, you must be able to identify and work objectively within any number of dynamics that may occur in a social system.

A dynamic defines the distinctive quality, emotional tone, and specific interpersonal events that comprise an interaction between individuals. Each of the social systems described in the previous section may be further characterized by any number of specific dynamics, many of which may be considered typical of a particular social system. For example, a dynamic involving competition for parental approval may be observed between clients and their siblings. Although it may not always be a productive dynamic, it is observed frequently in practice. If a dynamic

serves a specific purpose in the system (e.g., increased likelihood that at least one of the siblings will receive approval from an otherwise critical parent), a dynamic may become repetitive or even entrenched over time.

Dynamics can be productive or maladaptive. One example of a productive dynamic is a trusting dynamic. A trusting dynamic is characterized by evidence of trust between a client and therapist. For example, if a client feels confident about a therapist's ability to teach and demonstrate a sewing skill, his or her trust in the therapist manifests the client's earnest attempts to learn the skill. When a therapist returns the trust by showing a genuine investment in teaching, it constitutes further evidence of trust that the client has a sincere desire to learn. If a client seeks input to check if the skill is being performed correctly, it constitutes behavioral evidence of this trusting dynamic. Similarly, if a therapist shows pleasure at the client's accomplishment, it is evidence of increased investment and emotional involvement in the trusting dynamic. Other examples of productive dynamics include collaborative dynamics in which client and caregiver work to achieve a desired outcome or problem-solving dynamics in which family members brainstorm solutions and consider potential consequences of various actions. If you are interpersonally self-disciplined and keep personal needs outside of therapeutic relationships, it is likely that most of your relationships with clients are characterized by dynamics that are predominantly productive. This likelihood is increased if you are using one of the six therapeutic modes because each of the modes, if used properly, sets a productive structure and tone for interaction.

However, even when you make all the best efforts to sustain productive dynamics with your clients (and those associated with the clients), you always remain at risk for being invited or drawn into a maladaptive dynamic. This is particularly likely in long-standing social systems in which maladaptive ways of relating can become entrenched over time. For this reason, it is critical that you be able to recognize maladaptive dynamics and differentiate them from dynamics that are productive.

All dynamics serve a specific interpersonal need or purpose. Maladaptive dynamics are similar to productive dynamics in that they serve the needs of at least one individual in the system. Distinct from productive dynamics, however, maladaptive dynamics are usually inefficient and involve negative feelings or outcomes for at least one of the involved individuals. An example of a maladaptive dynamic is one that commonly faces parents

of adolescents that are struggling to differentiate themselves as individuals and take responsibility for the consequences of their actions. In this dynamic, the adolescent continually seeks guidance from the parents only to protest and explain why the guidance offered is unhelpful or would not work. This is commonly referred to as a help-seeking and help-rejecting dynamic. As a result, all individuals in the system end up feeling frustrated and ungratified. Some examples of maladaptive dynamics that have the potential to affect the process or outcomes of therapy are presented in Table 11.1. Although these are systems in which these dynamics are most likely to arise, any of these dynamics may occur in any social system.

(text continued on page 216)

Table 11.1	**Examples of Dynamics That Have the Potential to Interfere with the Process or Desired Outcome of Therapy**
Dynamic	**Description**
Help-Seeking/Help-Rejecting	When an individual establishes a pattern of asking for assistance, guidance, or advice and then explains why it would not work, a help-seeking/help-rejecting dynamic has been established. Potential negative outcomes include frustration or decreased performance in the help seeker. This dynamic is most frequently observed in parent-child relationships or in other relationships involving a power differential. If it is entrenched, it may be replicated within the therapeutic relationship.
Competitive	Individuals often compete to obtain an interpersonal need or a valued resource, particularly if it is perceived to be in short supply. If this competition is sustained, potential negative outcomes include conflict between the competitors or feelings of decreased self-esteem in the loser. Although they may occur in any system, competitive dynamics are often observed between siblings, friends, or client peers within a given milieu.
Enabling Negative Behavior	When individuals permit, facilitate, or support the behavior of another individual even though it is negative or potentially harmful, they further enable the negative behavior. The outcome is a continuation or worsening of the behavior. This behavior is frequently observed in couples relationships or in families where people are not able to show disapproval or take steps to limit the behavior for fear of disappointing the other individual, making the individual angry or losing the relationship altogether.
Dominance/Submission	A nondemocratic system characterized by a clear power differential that involves the consistent oppression of some individual(s) by other(s). Individuals may attempt to dominate others in order to increase their perceived control over their life circumstances or to compensate for feelings of insecurity or inferiority. Individuals may assume a submissive role because they have limited resources or options for independence; they are accustomed to being mistreated; they have low self-esteem; they perceive themselves as less powerful; they perceive themselves as physically, emotionally, or intellectually inferior; or they wish to avoid confrontation. Potential outcomes include passivity, vulnerability, learned helplessness, or feelings of low self-worth in the submissive individual(s). In the worst cases, this dynamic evolves into a pattern of emotional, sexual, and/or physical abuse. These dynamics are most likely to occur in relationships that involve one individual assuming a caregiving role for a more vulnerable individual. Dominant or abusive behaviors suggest that the caregiver is not emotionally capable of functioning in that role and should either seek mental health services immediately or discontinue his or her relationship with the vulnerable individual entirely. More information about how to prevent and intervene with actively abusive or potentially abusive relationships is provided in Chapters 9 and 12.

(table continued on page 214)

Table 11.1	Examples of Dynamics That Have the Potential to Interfere with the Process or Desired Outcome of Therapy (continued)
Dynamic	**Description**
Enmeshment	An enmeshment dynamic is one in which individuals have close ongoing contact. It is expected that individuals share information readily, even if it is highly intimate or personal. There is an expectation that all individuals conform and share similar world views and other behaviors and attitudes. Decision-making is shared, and the concept of individuality is downplayed. Members of enmeshed systems are fiercely loyal to each other despite conflicts or major transgressions. Caregivers in this dynamic often become overinvolved or controlling in reference to a client's treatment. The potential negative outcomes of an enmeshment dynamic include a closed or secretive system that is difficult for health care professionals to enter, psychological dependence between members, a lack of individuality between members, and occasionally feelings of angst or resentment related to the perception that one's efforts are being controlled, stifled, or smothered by the system. Enmeshment dynamics are most often observed in families and couples.
Disengagement	A disengagement dynamic occurs when individuals have little contact and do not share personal information readily. Individuals in the system view themselves as independent of one another in terms of world view, attitudes, behavior, and decision-making. The potential negative outcome is a lack of closeness, loyalty, communication, and connection between members. Caregivers in this dynamic are typically underinvolved in the client's care. Potential negative consequences of this dynamic include feelings of isolation and disappointment in others' lack of presence and investment. In worst cases, disengagement within systems can result in the physical or medical neglect of a client. Although they may occur in any system, disengagement dynamics are most often observed in families and couples.
Approach/Avoidance	When an individual enters a relationship with an expectation that the other will fulfill certain (often unrealistic) needs, there is often a period of intense contact and, in some cases, feelings of closeness. When people are ambivalent about this closeness or when their intentions for the relationships are limited to seeking need fulfillment, they promptly retreat into avoidance. This avoidance may be explained by the fact that they perceived that their needs were not met or by the fact that the relationship became so intense in their minds that it evoked uncomfortable or contradictory feelings (e.g., feeling smothered, fears of abandonment or rejection, feelings of rage, an intense and unfulfilled desire to be admired or unconditionally accepted). When approach-avoidance dynamics occur in couples relationships, they often involve the same partner repeatedly approaching the other partner in order to obtain need fulfillment and the other partner repeatedly finding ways to withdraw. Because the approaching partner's needs are not gratified, the approach behaviors become increasingly intense (and sometimes demanding) over time. In return, the avoiding partner continues to find ways to increase withdrawal (e.g., falls asleep, leaves the environment, becomes emotionally unresponsive, is at a loss for words, remains at work later, spends more time with others, focuses more on the children, or turns to substances or other addictions) to counterbalance the approach behavior. The outcome is a relationship characterized by unpredictability, a lack of trust, feeling smothered or abandoned, and a lack of mutuality. Clients who suddenly appear intensely connected and divulge a tremendous amount of personal details during one session only to appear distant or fail to show up for the next session may be enacting this dynamic in therapy.
Idealizing/Devaluing	Individual(s) can be consistently idealizing of one another, consistently devaluing, or they can change between the two states. An idealizing dynamic is one in which individual(s) filter their perception of other(s) in such a way that the positive characteristics of the other(s) are exaggerated and any negative characteristics are downplayed or denied entirely. A devaluing dynamic is the opposite in which the negative characteristics are exaggerated. Some individuals have a tendency to relate to and know others only in terms of these two categories. Either state is characterized by an unrealistic and superficial knowledge of others. When others unwittingly allow themselves to become a part of this dynamic, they eventually find it uncomfortable, terrifying, or infuriating. At one moment they may be placed unrealistically on a pedestal only to find that they are rejected or even vilified in a subsequent interaction.

Dynamic	Description
	This dynamic is often observed in relationships with health care providers (including occupational therapists), particularly when clients, parents, or partners have unrealistic expectations of the provider and do not want to assume sufficient responsibility for the problem or the solution.
Reluctance/Reassurance	When an individual (couple, family, group) is consistently anxious, skeptical, or self-doubting about engaging in occupation and others reliably attempt to bolster, entice, and reassure them, the dynamic of reluctance and reassurance is occurring. Potentially negative outcomes of this dynamic include psychological dependence, low intrinsic motivation, and limited opportunities for independence and progress.
Demonstrative/Voyeuristic	When individuals become involved in elaborating upon, embellishing, or dramatizing their reactions or hardships, they often have a need for their hardship to be recognized and validated. When others are entertained by this behavior or do nothing but watch or listen, a demonstrative/voyeuristic dynamic is occurring. Negative outcomes include lack of progress and the eventual realization that the voyeuristic party is taking pleasure in the behavior. Although this realization may serve only to increase the demonstrative behavior, it is neither a therapeutic nor a humane way of relating. If committed by the therapist, this kind of voyeuristic behavior is unethical because it does not represent an attempt to provide best practice.
Helpless/Rescuing	A helpless/rescuing dynamic occurs when individuals fall into a pattern of recruiting assistance when it is not necessary. Often the helpless behavior is a maladaptive expression of an entrenched need to be loved, attended to, or cared for. For some individuals this need is strong, and it exists no matter how much love, care, and attention are provided. The other part of the system enables the helpless behavior by rushing in to assist without recognizing that the behavior is maladaptive. The outcomes include increased dependence on the part of the helpless individual and eventual anxiety and/or resentment on the part of the rescuer(s). This dynamic can be culturally contexted and may not always result in maladaptive outcomes for the client. Although it may occur in any system, it is most often observed in parents of disabled children who feel guilty or responsible for the impairment and are unaware of the consequences of enabling the child's helpless behavior.
Chaotic/Organizing	A chaotic/organizing dynamic is one in which one aspect of a system is irresponsible, disorganized, slovenly, undisciplined, and/or lacking in emotional self-control. The other part of the system continually seeks to compensate by replacing lost items, reminding the individual of scheduled appointments or necessary tasks, cleaning up and organizing the person's physical environment, or providing required emotional and logistical support so the person can function. One maladaptive outcome of this dynamic is an ongoing power struggle between the chaotic and organizing aspects of the system. Another consequence is the intensification of the chaotic behavior. Although it may occur in any system, this dynamic is most frequently witnessed in systems in which one member has an impairment that affects cognition, such as attention deficit hyperactivity disorder, bipolar disorder, a psychotic disorder, or another neurological condition.
Manipulating/Conceding	Some individuals are accustomed to getting their needs met through manipulation, particularly when they perceive that there may be an obstacle to getting what they want. This involves a pattern of knowing what the other likes or needs and then giving it out in small doses with the expectation that the other will reciprocate by gratifying the manipulator's needs. When the other party concedes out of feelings of obligation or guilt, the conceding party is fueling the dynamic. Negative outcomes include eventual feelings of resentment and anger in the person enabling the dynamic; it also results in failure to learn to ask for needs to be met in a more direct manner and failure to accept limits imposed by others in the manipulator. In occupational therapy, this dynamic is often observed when working with parents who struggle to feel confident about disciplinary approaches and often feel guilty about setting limits consistently. It may also be witnessed in couples, friendships, or in student–teacher relationships. If it exists, it is also likely to play out in the therapeutic relationship.

(table continued on page 216)

Table 11.1	Examples of Dynamics That Have the Potential to Interfere with the Process or Desired Outcome of Therapy (continued)		
Dynamic	**Description**
Scapegoating	When two or more individuals collude to influence, criticize, reprimand, subjugate, shame, punish, or otherwise control another individual, a scapegoating dynamic has emerged. These dynamics may involve entire families or groups that decide to ally against a single individual. Individuals are most likely to engage in this dynamic when they are allied around a common ideology or when they perceive that the scapegoated individual has threatened the status quo or equilibrium of the system or if they feel that the individual is otherwise problematic. Often triangulation reflects a need to displace anger in the system, and the most vulnerable, powerless, or emotionally safe individual is usually selected as the convenient target. Although this dynamic is most likely to occur within families or groups, it may also occur when a therapist forms an alliance with one of two parents against the other, with one or more clients against another, or with one partner of a couple against the other.

In complex and long-standing relationships, multiple dynamics may emerge, some of which are productive and others maladaptive. At times, it is unclear whether a dynamic is ultimately productive or maladaptive. It is common for families, couples, or other social systems to assume that a maladaptive dynamic is productive because it feels familiar and defines the way people have always interacted in the system. Although uncomfortable or painful at times, members participating in the dynamic may be unaware of any need for change. Also possible is that dynamics that were once thought to be positive become negative over time (and vice versa). The nature

and number of potential dynamics that can occur in a given social system are endless.

If a dynamic is prominent in a system, regardless of whether you are aware of it, it is inevitable that you will be invited or drawn into it when interacting with the system. The difference between being invited to join a maladaptive dynamic or simply drawn into it involves the issue of intentionality. An intentional therapist recognizes the dynamic before becoming involved with it. After identifying the dynamic, the therapist would then use interpersonal reasoning to decide how to interact within the dynamic. An unintentional therapist may not realize that she or he has

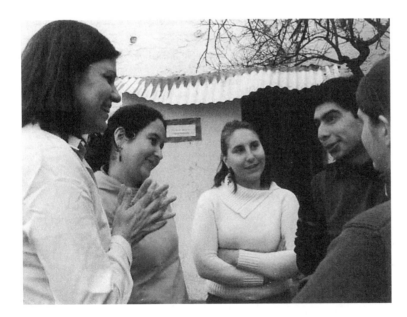

FIGURE 11.3 While leading, Carmen-Gloria de Las Heras observes the supportive dynamics in a group at Reencuentros

become involved in the dynamic until her or his involvement has resulted in interruption or disruption of the client–therapist relationship.

Managing Maladaptive Dynamics of Systems

At one time or another and to varying degrees of intensity, certain maladaptive dynamics are bound to emerge in almost any social system one encounters. The goal of learning about these dynamics is to:

• Understand their implications for the client and for the course of the client's therapy
• Anticipate their effects on the therapeutic relationship
• Remain an objective observer of the dynamic
• Make an intentional decision about whether and how to manage the dynamic

Even though a maladaptive dynamic inevitably involves negative feelings for one or more members of a social system, it is difficult to change. No matter how uncomfortable or unhappy they are, members of the system habitually act together to sustain the dynamic because this is how they are most accustomed to interacting with one another. This is often the case even if members of the system recognize that sustaining the dynamic results in negative outcomes for the client and for all individuals engaged in the client's care. Because systems are, by nature, highly resistant to change, it is important to strive continually toward an empathic understanding of any social system with which you are working. In striving to understand maladaptive dynamics within a social system, you should:

• Look to the system for the problem (e.g., all persons involved in the interaction), rather than to the client alone
• Try to understand why members are invested in sustaining the maladaptive dynamic. What makes sense about the dynamic? What interpersonal needs are served by the members of the system who are enacting the dynamic? How does the dynamic serve the client's needs? What might each of the members lose if he or she were to stop interacting in this way?
• Try to assume a historical or multigenerational understanding of the dynamic. When did it begin? Do members of the system have a history of interacting in this

way? What is known about the childhood family relationships of those most invested in sustaining the maladaptive dynamic? How do their unique histories make them prime candidates to function in their current roles in the system?

After you have achieved an empathic understanding of the system, the next step is to decide whether to remain an objective observer of the maladaptive dynamic or to try to manage or eradicate it. The decision whether to intervene in the dynamic is best made by asking yourself the following questions.

• Is the dynamic interfering with the course of therapy?
• Does the client perceive that this dynamic is negatively affecting his or her quality of life?
• Are certain members of the system attempting to replicate the dynamic in the therapeutic relationship? If so, what are the potential long-term outcomes of this behavior?

If the answer to any of these initial questions is yes, the IRM recommends that you draw upon principles from the family systems theories of Bowen and Minuchin to work actively to manage the maladaptive dynamic. The easiest and most straightforward way to do this is to invite all members of the system to a meeting. During this meeting, you might label the dynamic, encourage shared responsibility for the problem, and educate the system about the negative consequences of the dynamic for the client and for the course of therapy. If the system accepts this explanation, you might encourage members of the system to generate ideas about what each might do differently to create a new dynamic.

Although this sounds straightforward, it typically is not. Even if a social system is otherwise adaptive and characterized by open and direct lines of communication and low levels of conflict, the maladaptive dynamic is likely to reemerge over time. Moreover, many social systems that are deeply entrenched in specific ways of interacting are rarely amenable to recommendations for change. Some members may even feel threatened by any suggestion that the system is not functioning in an adaptive way, and they may turn against a well intended therapist rather than acknowledge that the system needs to be reorganized. If you employ systems principles and attempt to shift the system's attention away from the client's behavior in order to encourage shared responsibility for a negative dynamic, you must first be sure you have established sufficient rapport and trust with all members of the system. Members of a system are most at risk for feeling threatened or offended by a systems perspective on the problem if you have not adequately joined with them through empathy and rapport building during your early interactions. Negative reactions are also likely to occur if you introduce a systems-based intervention too early in your relationship with the members. When asked to take responsibility for their roles in the dynamic at this early point, some members of the system might feel unfairly or inappropriately blamed or tremendously guilty. These understandable reactions would then have to be validated and processed with all members of the system to resolve the empathic break with the system and move forward in therapy.

Thus, an important aspect of managing maladaptive dynamics involves the use of interpersonal reasoning to select and change modes while working to attenuate or eradicate a rigid way of interacting.

If, through the use of modes, you are interpersonally in tune with all of the members of the system, the system is more amenable to any additional systems-focused interventions you might attempt. Table 11.2 provides examples of how each of the six interpersonal modes might be used to address maladaptive dynamics in general. It also designates which modes may be most effective when working to minimize or alter maladaptive dynamics in a system. Explanations are provided for why other modes may not be as desirable for a given dynamic.

As is evident in Table 11.2, the empathizing mode is reliable and effective regardless of the dynamic being addressed. In many cases, it is considered a prerequisite for the use of any other mode because of its powerful ability to allow you to create an alliance with any member of the system who is problematic or otherwise in need of empathy. Maladaptive dynamics create an emotional environment that is often characterized by tension and feelings of vulnerability in various members of the system. The empathizing mode is often effective in reducing tension and bolstering peoples' self-confidence. If you explain in advance the importance of hearing all voices and then take the time and effort to hear and validate the perspectives of

> An important aspect of managing maladaptive dynamics involves the use of interpersonal reasoning to select and change modes while working to attenuate or eradicate a rigid way of interacting.

each member, a precedent for such behavior is set up in the system. The end result of beginning with an empathic approach to the system is that members are ultimately primed to accept other modes and work more receptively toward systems change.

As with all of the guidelines presented in this book, those presented in Table 11.2 may not work with all systems. When selecting the appropriate interpersonal mode you must always consider the client's unique interpersonal characteristics, the timing and nature of your effort to intervene in the maladaptive dynamic, and other contextual issues. For systems that are highly resistant to change, more specific empathically oriented strategies are typically needed to prepare a system to be more receptive to change. One such strategy that is particularly effective is commonly referred to as "joining with the system." This term and its corresponding strategy is derived from Salvador Minuchin's Structural Family Therapy. However, the ideas presented in Minuchin's theory are far more complex and beyond the scope of this book. Ways that you might join with a system include:

- Inviting all members of the system (particularly the most problematic or vulnerable) to participate in one or more therapy sessions.
- Finding a way to build relationships and establish trust with all members of the system (particularly the most problematic or vulnerable) before introducing any other kinds of information.
- Once the problem has been raised for discussion, validate each member's unique perspective on the problem, even if the perspectives differ among members. Let the system know that each member's perspective has some validity because it serves to sustain the dynamic being addressed. During this process you should be functioning primarily in the empathic mode.

Before you attempt this joining process with other members of the system, it is imperative that you first establish a secure and trusting relationship with the client. You should explain the basic premise behind the systems theory to the client (i.e., all members are responsible for con-

(text continued on page 223)

Table 11.2 Modes and Common Maladaptive Dynamics in Social Systems*

	Advocating	Collaborating	Empathizing	Encouraging	Instructing	Problem-solving
General description of modes from a systems perspective	Explicitly support the client's point of view. Raise the client's awareness of any dynamics that are oppressive or subjugating. Encourage members of the system to provide access and resources for the client that support the client's dignity and autonomy.	Shift decision-making power to the client. Assist the client in acting on his or her own behalf to support his or her own best interests within the system. Empower the client to be more assertive/assume more of a leadership role in the system.	Articulate the perspectives of each member of the system. Strive to understand the perspectives of weakest or most problematic members who appear to be in most need of empathy. Validate the utility of the maladaptive dynamic in the system. Assist members in understanding how the dynamic serves the needs of certain members.	Positively reinforce any sign of positive change in the system. Provide members of the system with hope that any difficult or stressful interactions will improve. Assist members in envisioning more positive ways of interacting or what they might be like in the absence of the maladaptive dynamic.	Label the maladaptive dynamic and explain how it functions in the system. Highlight the negative consequences of the dynamic for the system. Teach alternative, more adaptive means of interacting in the system. Provide a rationale that supports the need for change. Support members in experimenting with and practicing more adaptive ways of interacting.	Identify positive implications of the dynamic. Identify negative implications. Compare positive and negative implications.
Help-Seeking/Help-Rejecting	May enable the dynamic because the therapist may be placed in a position of doing too much for the client or being biased toward assuming the client's point of view.	Requires that the client make decisions and take responsibility for therapy. Clients entangled in help-seeking/help-rejecting dynamics are enacting their ambivalence about this very issue.	•	The client or individual enacting the dynamic may perceive encouraging responses as manipulative or naive and may intensify the behavior as a result.	•	Does not directly address the core issue (i.e., that the client feels helpless to function independently and yet is ambivalent about accepting guidance).

(table continued on page 220)

Table 11.2 Modes and Common Maladaptive Dynamics in Social Systems* (continued)

	Advocating	Collaborating	Empathizing	Encouraging	Instructing	Problem-solving
Competitive	Siding with the client may be gratifying but may only intensify the client's competitive behavior with others.	Transferring power to the client does not address the negative consequences of the competitive dynamic. If the client had the capacity to correct the dynamic, he or she would be able to stop it on his or her own.	•	•	•	•
Enabling Negative Behavior	Supporting the client not to enable another member's negative behavior may be effective, but supporting a client in justifying or continuing to act negatively within the system would be counterproductive.	If the client knew how to counteract another member's negative behavior effectively, the negative behavior would not exist. Transferring power to a client who is enacting negative behavior may work in some cases, but in most cases it only empowers the client to continue the negative behavior.	•	The client or individual enacting the dynamic may perceive encouraging responses as manipulative or overly optimistic and may intensify the behavior as a result.	•	•
Dominance/ Submission	•	•	•	•	•	•

	Advocating	Collaborating	Empathizing	Encouraging	Instructing	Problem-solving
Enmeshed	Simply advocating for a client's point of view in an enmeshed system is unlikely to have any effect.	Transferring decision-making power to the client in an enmeshed system is likely to backfire because the system is typically stronger than any single individual. It may help, but it will not be enough.	•	•	Assuming an authoritarian or instructive role in an enmeshed system may backfire because the interests of the system are stronger than those of the therapist. Empathy must be used before instructing.	•
Disengaged		Transferring power to a client in a disengaged system does not influence the system to become more engaged with the client. It may help but will not be enough.	•	Disengaged systems are usually disengaged for a reason (e.g., to avoid conflict or unresolvable differences). Providing encouragement when steps are made toward change can help but will not be enough.	•	•
Approach/ Avoidance	Use of this mode would not address the heart of the problem.	•	•	•	•	•
Idealizing/ Devaluing	Because individuals who at once idealize and devalue others often use this dynamic as a means of displacing responsibility onto another member of the system, a similar explanation as for the help-seeking/help-rejecting dynamic applies.	See explanation for the help-seeking/help-rejecting dynamic.	•	See explanation for the help-seeking/help-rejecting dynamic.	•	See explanation for the help-seeking/help-rejecting dynamic.

(table continued on page 222)

Table 11.2 Modes and Common Maladaptive Dynamics in Social Systems* (continued)

	Advocating	Collaborating	Empathizing	Encouraging	Instructing	Problem-solving
Reluctance/ Reassurance	Advocating on behalf of a reluctant or resistant client may be welcomed by the client if the client is feeling oppressed by the system, but ultimately the client is the one who must become empowered on his or her own.	•	•	•	•	•
Demonstrative/ voyeuristic	•	•	•	•	•	•
Helpless/ Rescuing	An explanation similar to that for the help-seeking/help-rejecting dynamic applies because roles and responsibility taking is not appropriately distributed in the system.	An explanation similar to that for the help-seeking/help-rejecting dynamic applies.	•	An explanation similar to that for the help-seeking/help-rejecting dynamic applies.	•	An explanation similar to that for the help-seeking/help-rejecting dynamic applies.
Chaotic/ Organizing	Use of this mode does not directly address the dynamic.	•	•	•	•	•
Manipulating/ Conceding	Siding with the manipulating member of this dynamic would only intensify it. Moreover, this mode does not directly address the dynamic.	Shifting the right kind of power to the manipulating member of the dynamic may be effective, but if it is the wrong kind of power it only intensifies the dynamic. Moreover, if the conceding member knew how to manage the manipulative behavior it would not be occurring.	•	•	•	
Scapegoating	•	•	•	•	•	•

*A preferred mode for a dynamic is designated by a bullet.

tributing to regression or progress within the group) and prepare the client that there will be a temporary change in the nature of your one-on-one relationship together. By explaining the objectives of the system theory and the need to empathize with all members of the system in order to prime them for change, it reduces the likelihood that the client will feel betrayed by you when you take the time to listen to others' perspectives without judgment or disapproval. Once joined with the system as a whole, you may then apply the interpersonal reasoning process as discussed in the preceding paragraphs.

In some cases, you may be aware of a maladaptive dynamic that is occurring within a system, but key members of the system are physically inaccessible to you. For example, a therapist may be working with a young adult client with a new spinal cord injury who systematically becomes sad and withdrawn following visits from her mother. The client describes an enmeshed dynamic with her mother that is characterized by her mother's constant worry that because of her injury the client will not finish graduate school. In turn, the client has become increasingly guarded with her mother during their visits, which further enrages and worries her mother. The mother has systematically declined the therapist's invitations to join one of her daughter's occupational therapy sessions because she believes these sessions "have no purpose." In this situation, the therapist does not have access to the most influential member of the social system comprised of mother and daughter.

Not all members of the system need to be present to work at changing a maladaptive dynamic in the system. Instead, you can work with the client to effect change in the larger system. This idea stems from Murray Bowen's Multigenerational Family Systems Theory, though the ideas presented in Bowen's theory are more complex and beyond the scope of this book. According to this approach, the therapist focuses on allying with and strengthening the client, who is typically the most vulnerable link in the system. A systems explanation of the maladaptive dynamic is then presented to the client, and the therapist works to bolster and instruct the client to influence other members of the system.

Modes for Parents and Caregivers

In addition to your own use of the six therapeutic modes to identify and work to change maladaptive dynamics in a system, it is important to introduce the six modes and virtues of mode flexibility and shifting to parents and caregivers of clients. This enables them to begin to understand how to sustain systems change on their own. Many times

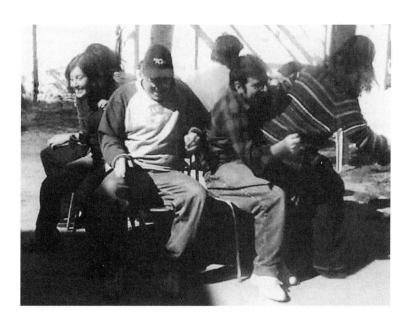

FIGURE 11.4 Carmen-Gloria de Las Heras joins with a group to exert greater influence in the system

maladaptive dynamics develop in systems because the system gets stuck in a fixed way of interacting. Parents and caregivers may grow too comfortable with and dependent on a single mode or set of modes in the same way that therapists may when interacting with a single client for extended periods of time. For example, parents and caregivers who possess a great deal of empathy for a client but lack the necessary ability to empathize enough to know that they must step back and empower the client to think and function more independently may tend to overutilize the empathizing and advocating modes. Parents may use the empathizing mode to validate, witness, and mourn their child's difficulties and the advocating mode to try to create a more facilitative environment for the child at school and in day care. Although overutilization of the empathizing and advocating modes may not overtly harm the client in the short term, over time it undermines the client's capacity and desire for freedom and autonomy. As a result, a dynamic of helplessness and rescuing may develop within the system.

For example, a well intentioned father may be so keenly attuned to his son's needs and vulnerabilities as they relate to his son's learning and attention difficulties that he overlooks the child's needs for natural consequences, structure, self-discipline, and independent thinking. Perhaps the father is locked into the empathizing and advocating modes with his son because he experienced similar limitations during childhood, was punished and misunderstood by adults in his life, or never received appropriate educational accommodations. The father identifies deeply with his son's difficulties. As a consequence of not using other modes, such as the instructing mode to create a structured routine with limits and natural consequences, the collaborating mode to empower his son to set goals and form his own opinions, and the problem-solving mode to encourage thinking about consequences, a child who may already be underdeveloped in these areas may not have the chance to mature in ways in which he would otherwise be capable. As a result, the child may lapse into a helpless role when confronted with a problem or stressor and may expect his father to overfunction in order to resolve the issue. Each time the father jumps in earnest to complete his son's homework for him at the eleventh hour or to confront a teacher for setting what might otherwise be considered an appropriate limit, the father reinforces his son's helpless behavior. Over time, this dynamic not only stifle's the child's development in these critical areas, it may also cause the father to feel emotionally exhausted and manipulated.

When as the therapist you become aware of maladaptive dynamics such as these in a family system, you will be more likely to empower the system and enlist their investment in systems change if you can successfully educate members about the importance of pure and flexible use of modes. With children, adolescents, or adult clients who require ongoing caretaking, parents and caregivers must learn that, as the members with more influence and resources, they are the ones who must take responsibility for sustaining any change that may be necessary in the system to create more functional dynamics. Introducing the importance of mode purity and flexibility may be approached by:

• Defining the six modes using lay terminology and discussing their utility in everyday interpersonal interactions
• Identifying, through observation, the mode or modes that the parent or caregiver seems to be most comfortable using
• Identifying the strengths of the parent's or caregiver's preferred modes
• Discussing the common cautions of those modes and encourage the parent/caregiver to think about the times or situations when these preferred modes do not function as well in the system
• Identifying the mode or modes that may need further development and may lead to improved systems functioning
• Weighing the pros and cons of introducing the new mode or modes into the system with the parent or caregiver
• If collectively you decide that a new mode or modes would be worth a try: identifying the likely short-term consequences (e.g., negative but brief side effects) and long-term consequences (e.g., positive systems change) of introducing the new mode or modes to the system

Exposing parents and caregivers to the concept of modes is a highly challenging task that is not for everyone. It requires a tremendous amount of empathy and trust within the relationship, some preliminary evidence that the parent or caregiver might be capable of learning to use new modes, and making provisions that the parent or caregiver does not feel judged or criticized as a parent when exposed to these ideas. In many cases, it requires a longer-term relationship with the therapist and ample existing experience with successful outcomes in other areas of the therapeutic process.

Summary

In this chapter, the fundamental principles and practices required for successful use of self with social systems and groups were reviewed. If you have not attempted systems interventions with clients or have not had any exposure or training in family systems or group therapies, it is recommended that you receive continuing education and seek supervision in this area from an experienced colleague or a mental health professional before trying these interventions with actual social systems. Working with systems is a highly complex and sensitive endeavor that requires a high level of skill, objectivity, and interpersonal self-discipline when adhering to systems principles. It also requires good judgment as to when systems interventions are appropriate for a client and when they are not. A final recommendation that applies even to experienced occupational therapists is to work together with another professional (mental health professional) to assist in managing the maladaptive dynamic so the issues can be addressed in multiple contexts, with more than one professional, and in a more intense way. A discussion of how you might collaborate with another professional to achieve this end is presented in Chapter 15.

References

Minuchin, P., Colapinto, J., & Minuchin, S. (1998). *Working with families of the poor*. New York: Guilford Press.

Sholevar, G. P. (Ed.) (2005). *Textbook of family and couples therapy: clinical applications*. Washington, DC: American Psychiatric Publishing.

ACTIVITIES FOR LEARNING AND REFLECTION

EXERCISE 11.1

Group Dynamics Observation Exercise

The purpose of this assignment is to provide you with an opportunity to observe a group of individuals interacting and to reflect on the many dynamics and interpersonal events that occur during this complex interaction. The group you observe may be any group of your choice. The only rule is that the group must contain at least three individuals. It may be a formal treatment group, such as an occupational therapy group; it may be a support or self-help group; or it may be an informal group of individuals, such as a group of classmates, a sports team, friends, or family members. When choosing a group, be sure you are able to spend enough time with the group to be able to hear, see, and reflect on the detailed aspects of how members interact with one another. Once you have identified the group, observe them for at least 30 minutes and reflect on the following questions.

1. Who are the members of the group, and what is their relationship to each other (e.g., peers in a support group, teammates, classmates, friends, family members)?

   _____

2. Who are the most engaged members of the system? Who are the most disengaged?

   _____

3. Who are the most prominent or influential members? How do they exert their power? How effective are they in influencing the system?

   _____

4. What topics, general themes, or content of conversation dominated the system?

   _____

5. What do members need or expect from each other?

   _____

6. What is the general emotional tone or mood of the group?

   _____

7. Was communication within the system shared, open, and direct or were there certain alliances and indirect routes of communication?

   _____

8. Did some members emerge as more dominant? Did some participate more than others?

___ No

___ Yes (describe): _____ _____

9. Were there any conflicts between members within the group?

___ No

___ Yes (describe): _____

10. If yes, how were the conflicts resolved?

_____

11. Did you witness members being explicitly supportive of each other?

___ Yes (describe): _____

___ No

12. If no, in your opinion, what prevented support from occurring?

_____

13. What other productive dynamics occurred within the group?

_____

14. Did you witness any of the following maladaptive dynamics occurring within the group? (Check all that apply and provide a brief description. Refer to Table 11-1 for a description of the various dynamics, if necessary.)

___ Help-seeking/help-rejecting _____

___ Competitive _____

___ Enabling negative behavior _____

___ Dominance/submission _____

___ Enmeshment _____

___ Disengagement _____

___ Approach/avoidance _____

___ Idealizing/devaluing _____

___ Reluctance/reassurance _____

___ Demonstrative/voyeuristic _____

___ Helpless/rescuing _____

___ Chaotic/organizing _____

___ Manipulating/conceding _____

___ Scapegoating _____

15. Did you witness any other maladaptive dynamics not listed here?

_____

16. Which, if any, of the following interpersonal events occurred between members (rather than between client and therapist) during the group? (Check all that apply and provide a brief description. Refer to Chapter 6 for descriptions of the various categories, if necessary.)

___ Expression of strong emotion _____

___ Intimate self-disclosures _____

___ Power dilemmas _____

___ Nonverbal cues _____

___ Crisis points _____

___ Resistance and reluctance _____

___ Boundary testing _____

___ Empathic breaks _____

___ Emotionally charged therapy tasks and situations _____

___ Limitations of therapy _____

___ Contextual inconsistencies _____

17. Please write any other thoughts or reactions about the group here:

_____

CHAPTER 12

UNDERSTANDING AND MANAGING DIFFICULT BEHAVIOR

For many therapists, clients' difficult interpersonal behavior is often the source of sleepless nights, concerns about job performance, feelings of burnout, and indecision about how to handle various interpersonal issues that arise during treatment. According to the Intentional Relationship Model (IRM), *difficult interpersonal behavior* is defined as any recurring, enduring, or high-intensity communication or other behavior that prompts one or more negative emotional reactions in another individual. Regardless of whether intended or unintended, these behaviors may cause recipients to feel abandoned, distanced, rejected, insulted, denigrated, unworthy, inadequate, threatened, fearful, worried, victimized, sorrowful, guilty, irritated, angry, or enraged.

As human beings, therapists and clients are equally vulnerable to behaving in a difficult manner toward each other. Your behavior, if negative, has the potential to incite a negative reaction in a client as a client's behavior has the potential to incite a negative reaction in you. The IRM emphasizes the myriad ways in which you must practice a high level of responsibility-taking and interpersonal self-discipline required to ensure that any negative moods, attitudes, or impulses toward clients do not play out in nontherapeutic ways within the relationship. This chapter is more limited to a discussion of how you can recognize, understand, and respond to difficult client behaviors in ways that protect the relationship and are experienced by the client as therapeutic. In learning to protect the client and the relationship as a whole by knowing how to manage difficult behavior effectively, you implicitly learn the skills required to protect yourself from being taken advantage of or from more intense feelings associated with emotional fatigue and burnout (Fig. 12.1).

In a recent survey conducted by our research team (described earlier) (Taylor, Lee, Kielhofner, & Ketkar, 2007), a high frequency of occupational therapists reported that they witness a wide range of difficult behaviors in their clients. For example, 82% of therapists reported feeling not as effective as they could have been because of a client's difficult interpersonal behavior, and 90% acknowledged that a client's difficult interpersonal behavior has sometimes had a negative impact on therapy outcomes. Although difficult behavior may have a negative impact on therapy outcomes, this chapter argues that in some cases the behavior can be managed in such a way that it results in positive therapy outcomes. Details regarding the problematic behaviors most frequently encountered by therapists are reported in Table 12.1.

The number and potential types of difficult behaviors that human beings may exhibit are almost limitless. This chapter addresses a selection of the behaviors that are more frequently encountered within the therapeutic relationship. Because the underlying principles of understanding and management according to the IRM are the same across the difficult behaviors, I selected the most common behaviors observed in occupational therapy practice to illustrate those principles. Therefore, this chapter focuses on understanding and managing the following eight categories of behavior that are reflected in Table 12.1.

- Manipulative behavior
- Excessive dependence
- Symptom focusing
- Resistance
- Emotional disengagement
- Denial
- Difficulty with rapport and trust
- Hostility

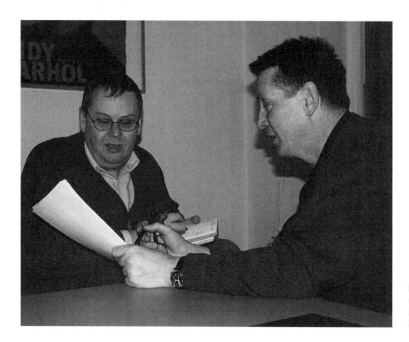

FIGURE 12.1 Being in a position of determining clients' work readiness, Roland Meisel must manage a variety of challenging reactions to the assessment process

An increased understanding of these behaviors and their meanings should lead to greater empathy and more planned therapeutic reactions.

Because they are often part of a larger medical, psychiatric, or interpersonal problem, difficult client behaviors are likely to recur, endure over time, and be acutely

Table 12.1	**Data for Practicing Occupational Therapists Who Encounter Difficult Client Behaviors at Least Some of the Time (n = 568)**

Behavior	%
Attempts to manipulate therapist	85
Excessive dependence on therapist	82
Excessive focus on symptoms	72
Resisting feedback or suggestions	71
Passive or isolative during therapy	70
Fearing judgment from therapist	68
Resistive or oppositional during therapy	68
Emotionally disengaged during therapy	66
Unrealistic expectations of therapy	61
Denial of impairment	59
Difficulty with rapport and trust	55
Hostile toward the therapist	37
Critical of the therapist	35
Questions the therapist's skills	24

intense when they do occur. Moreover, difficult behaviors often cluster together so a number of categories of behavior may be observed in a single client. This chapter focuses on providing information about how you can understand and manage difficult client behavior in your role as a recipient of the behavior. In the Activities section of this chapter, an exercise is provided to encourage you to reflect on and build additional skills in this critical area.

Understanding Difficult Behavior

Understanding difficult behavior is fundamental to being able to address it in a way that preserves and strengthens the therapeutic relationship. Historically, there has been a host of approaches to understanding the mechanisms that underlie difficult behaviors. Most of these approaches have been introduced in the mental health professions. The most frequently cited and widely known contemporary approaches include psychoanalytical/psychodynamic approaches, behavioral approaches, cognitive and cognitive-behavioral approaches, systems approaches, and social cognitive/social constructivist approaches.

At the broadest level, psychoanalytical and psycho-dynamic approaches (Freud, 1923; Kohut, 1984) explain maladaptive behavior as being associated with disruptions in relationships with key figures during childhood and with certain internal subjective beliefs that clients have about their families. Difficult behaviors are deeply rooted in past experiences that were once perceived as hurtful or neglectful by the client. Behavioral approaches (Skinner, 1974) describe dysfunctional behavior as being learned through a process of repetition and reinforcement. For example, if a person learns that the only means of getting her son to visit on the weekends is by making him feel guilty if he does not visit, this strategy is used repeatedly. Cognitive and cognitive-behavioral approaches view mal-adaptive behavior as a consequence of distorted thinking about social events and beliefs about oneself that are ulti-mately rooted in feelings of unlovability and worthlessness (Beck, 1995; Beck, Rush, Shaw, & Emery, 1979). Similar to psychoanalytical and psychodynamic approaches, humanistic approaches (Rogers, 1961) explain difficult behavior as a result of conflicts and other destructive interactions that occur in one's family context during childhood. Systems approaches (Minuchin, Colapinto, & Minuchin, 1998) construe difficult behavior as a symptom or expression of one person's perspective within a broader,

shared dynamic between the person exhibiting the mal-adaptive behavior and the other individuals engaged in the interaction. These five perspectives on difficult behavior and their corresponding recommendations for correcting such behavior are summarized in Table 12.2.

Common among these approaches is that they explain the client's behavior as a product of a social interaction. By implication, then, you can act to trigger, exacerbate, or attenuate these behaviors, depending on how you respond. As is evident in Table 12.2, each of these perspectives has something valuable to offer in the way of understanding and attempting to correct difficult client behavior. Each provides a unique strategy that may serve as an important supplement to the IRM when basic efforts to manage client difficulties fail. If you are interested in learning more about how to incorporate any of these more specialized approaches into your practice, you should seek additional education and supervision from an individual with expert-ise in that particular approach.

Outside of obtaining more advanced training in these specific mental health approaches in an effort to change the behavior, the IRM offers a widely applicable and basic approach to managing (rather than changing) difficult client behavior so the other goals of occupational therapy can be addressed. The approach used in the IRM cuts

Table 12.2 **Common Mental Health Approaches to Understanding and Treating Difficult Behavior**		
Approach	**Explanation**	**Treatment**
Psychoanalytical/psychodynamic	Behavior is a consequence of neurotic conflicts and disrupted relationships early in life.	See client apart from family members and allow for the re-enactment of rearly conflicts. The client can gain insight and experience by reality testing and repair through the therapeutic relationship.
Behavioral	Behavior is learned and reinforced over time through reward or punishment.	Extinguish behavior through active ignoring, discontinued reinforcement, or by replac-ing it with a more adaptive behavior.
Cognitive and cognitive-behavioral	Behavior is a consequence of distorted thinking and maladaptive ways of thinking about events.	Change the way one thinks or interprets events and changes in behavior follow. Behavioral change also reinforces changes in thinking
Humanistic	Behavior is a consequence of a lack of positive regard, affection, and approval from key figures during childhood.	Provide unconditional positive regard and the behavior changes on its own.
Systems	Behavior is a manifestation of a maladaptive dynamic within the larger social system of which the client is a part.	Explain the role the behavior serves in the larger social system and have members share responsibility for correcting the underlying dynamic.

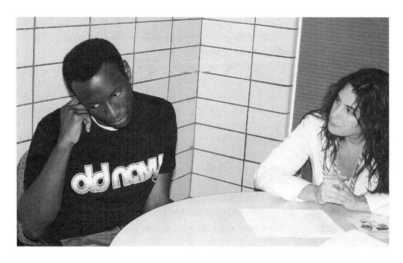

FIGURE 12.2 Stephanie McCammon strives to understand a client's change in behavior

across treatment settings and client populations and can be used in combination with other mental health approaches when necessary. The IRM encourages understanding difficult behavior according to a phenomenological perspective.

A *phenomenological perspective* assumes that whatever the underlying cause of a behavior (be it learned or the result of difficult family relationships) the person who is behaving problematically is doing so on the basis of something he or she is experiencing, thinking, or feeling about the situation at hand. Consistent with a phenomenological approach, the IRM encourages you to do your best to inquire about and use a series of summary statements to approximate an understanding of what a client is thinking or feeling about his or her own experience. It also encourages you to utilize an interpersonal reasoning process to select the appropriate mode (or modes) that respects that person's experience and to help find an alternative behavior that is a more appropriate expression for the client's experience. The latter step is discussed later in the chapter (Fig. 12.2).

A final prerequisite for understanding difficult behavior involves being competent at recognizing the various medical conditions (particularly those affecting the central nervous system) and psychiatric diagnoses that may be contributing to the behavior. Knowing when a behavior may have biological origins or may be mediated by the central nervous system may make it easier to maintain objectivity and emotional balance when attempting to manage it. Although a comprehensive review of all of the possible diagnoses that may, at least in part, explain difficult behavior is beyond the scope of this chapter, information about relevant diagnoses may be obtained by consulting the *Diagnostic and Statistical Manual of Mental Disorders*, Fourth Edition, Text Revision (American Psychiatric Association, 2000) and the *International Classification of Diseases* (World Health Organization, 2006).

Managing Difficult Behavior

Managing difficult behavior, particularly when it manifests within the client–therapist relationship, requires not only understanding but also self-confidence, objectivity, interpersonal self-discipline, and a thorough knowledge of interpersonal reasoning. In this section, general guidelines about how to use interpersonal reasoning to manage difficult behavior are reviewed. Following this review, supplemental information that may aid in understanding and responding to each of the specific categories of difficult behavior described earlier in the chapter is provided.

Many difficult client behaviors are associated with or fall into the same category as inevitable interpersonal events of therapy (introduced in Chapter 6). For example, resistance is both an interpersonal event and a difficult behavior. An empathic break is an interpersonal event that, if not responded to promptly and appropriately, can trigger any number of difficult behaviors. Similarly, difficult behaviors can be triggered by emotionally charged therapy tasks or situations when they are not addressed up front. Difficult behaviors may also result from the natural limitations of therapy, contextual inconsistencies, crisis points, or power dilemmas (when they are not responded to in a way that the client finds gratifying). In some cases, nonverbal cues are harbingers of difficult behavior, or they may represent difficult behaviors in themselves.

Finally, difficult behaviors may be associated with the expression of strong emotion or with boundary testing. Because interpersonal events and difficult behaviors are closely linked, the IRM approaches the management of these behaviors using the same six-step interpersonal reasoning process. However, when managing behavior that is clearly difficult from an interpersonal perspective, each of the six steps of interpersonal reasoning has a much more specific meaning and a more specific set of therapeutic behaviors that accompany it. Interpersonal reasoning as applied to difficult behavior involves the following six steps.

> Managing difficult behavior requires not only understanding but also self-confidence, objectivity, interpersonal self-discipline, and a thorough knowledge of interpersonal reasoning.

1. Anticipate
2. Identify, cope, and strive for understanding
3. Determine if a mode shift is required
4. Choose a response mode
5. Draw on any relevant interpersonal skills associated with that mode
6. Gather feedback

In the following sections, each of these steps is described in greater detail.

Step 1. Anticipate

The first step of anticipating involves preserving a general mindset that difficult client behavior is a natural and inevitable aspect of occupational therapy practice. When people are facing a chronic illness or impairment, they are not always in their best form interpersonally. Carrying a mental expectation that clients may behave in difficult ways prepares you to respond on the basis of understanding (i.e., from a phenomenological perspective) rather than on the basis of your initial emotional reaction to the behavior.

Step 2. Identify, Cope, and Strive for Understanding

The second step involves identifying, coping, and understanding. Identifying difficult behavior involves labeling or categorizing the type of behavior that is occurring. You may do it privately in your own mind if this is what is most appropriate for the situation. The most common categories

of difficult behavior include the eight that are described in this chapter. However, these categories should not limit you from coming up with your own means of identifying and organizing difficult client behaviors. Labeling or categorizing behavior promotes objectivity and allows you to plan an approach that is most likely to be therapeutic for the client.

Once you have identified the difficult behavior, you must cope with the situation at hand. If necessary, you should contain and manage the client's immediate emotional response and ensure that the behavior does not escalate in a way that would be dangerous or inappropriate. Empathizing with the client's perspective is typically the most efficient and effective means of containing a client's emotional response and preventing the negative behavior from escalating. However, when a client is not able to experience empathy as therapeutic, immediate efforts to provide structure and limits may be more appropriate. Additional ideas about how to manage clients' strong emotions can be found in Chapter 9.

Another aspect of coping involves an internal process of thinking through your emotional reaction to the event and putting that reaction into perspective. If you are truly mindful and in touch with your emotional reactions to people, it is natural for you to feel intensely negative feelings when encountering difficult client behavior. By acknowledging those feelings and reminding yourself that they are natural reactions to the behavior, you immerse yourself in the emotional reality of the situation and can begin the process of genuine coping. As discussed in Chapter 7, this occasionally involves actively suppressing any impulses to respond to a client in a way that would be perceived as nontherapeutic and would only escalate the situation. A final aspect of coping involves reminding yourself that, even if an aspect of your behavior served as a trigger, ultimately you are not responsible for the client's negative behavior. There are numerous explanations for a client's choice or impetus to behave in a maladaptive way. In many cases, you are only a convenient conduit for what is most likely a predetermined pattern of behavior or an anomalous acute reaction accompanying a client's current situation or mental status.

If you have coped well with your reaction to the behavior, you are better prepared to make a dedicated effort to understand the negative behavior. As revealed in Table 12.2, there are myriad ways to understand a client's negative behavior. However, the most critical approach to understanding is to determine what a client is thinking and feeling at the moment and potential explanations for those reactions. This informs how you act to manage the behavior in the moment. For example, if a child throws a tantrum during a therapy session, it is the therapist's job to understand what the child was thinking and feeling at that moment so the therapist can select the mode that best responds to it.

Thus, to understand a client's negative behavior, you must embark on a process of instantaneous inquiry and reflection in real time. The objective of this process is to better understand what the client is thinking and feeling just prior to, during, and immediately following the time he or she is engaging in the behavior. A secondary objective is to reflect on what interpersonal need the behavior might fill—or the ultimate purpose of the behavior. Having background information about the nature of interactions in the client's immediate social environment, information about the client's interpersonal history, and knowledge of early dynamics in the client's family of origin may supplement your understanding of the behavior and the needs it may serve. For example, the young client who is throwing a tantrum may be doing so because he was having such a good time playing in therapy and now he is being asked to leave. He may be thinking that the therapist has no right to take the toy away. Because he does not yet understand the concept of limits and boundaries, he may be experiencing the therapist's efforts to take the toy away as a form of interpersonal rejection or as lost affection. As a result, he may be experiencing deeper feelings of loss and rage. The historical context for the behavior may be that the child frequently throws tantrums at home with his father as a means of controlling the father, getting what he wants, and thereby reestablishing a sense of self-worth.

In the interest of inquiry and reflection, you may ask yourself the following questions.

1. What is the origin of this behavior? Is it an isolated reaction to something that occurred during therapy? Or is it part of a pattern of interpersonal behavior? That is, have I witnessed this behavior or similar behavior occurring in the past?
2. What were the circumstances of therapy just before the behavior surfaced?

3. What, if anything, about therapy may have triggered the behavior? Is it associated with an interpersonal event? Is it linked to something I said or did?
4. What was the client thinking before, during, and immediately after the behavior?
5. What did the client hope to accomplish through this behavior?
6. What might the client have wished to be the outcome of this behavior?
7. Does the client engage in this behavior in other settings or with other people?
8. Is the behavior specific to certain settings or certain people? If so, what about these settings or people seem to trigger the behavior?
9. What is the outcome when the client engages in this behavior in other settings or with others?
10. For how long has the client been engaging in this behavior? When did it begin?

This process of inquiry and reflection should involve the client to the greatest extent that it is appropriate for the individual and for the situation at hand. Additionally, the questions you might ask a client are not limited to those contained in this section. Inquiring in an effort to understand a difficult behavior may involve questions that are stated as casually as: "John, what's on your mind right now?" or "What were you thinking just then when you decided not to try using the brush on yourself?" Because questions have the potential to be perceived by some clients as stressful or unsupportive, clients should not be questioned to such an extent that they experience the questioning as an interrogation or as a form of intimidation or mind control. Similarly, questions about a client's immediate social environment, interpersonal history, and dynamics in his or her family of origin should never be asked in a way that the client might perceive as implicating or as disrespectful toward family members.

Step 3. Determine if a Mode Shift is Required

Understanding a client's difficult behavior in real time is likely to help inform whether a mode shift is required to manage the behavior. In determining if a mode shift is required, you must ascertain two things.

1. Whether the client's negative behavior is occurring independently of anything that might be associated with the interpersonal behavior in therapy
2. Whether using a different response mode might be experienced by the client as more comforting, centering, or therapeutic

If the client's negative behavior appears to be unrelated to anything you are saying or doing in therapy, changing your interpersonal style of behavior toward a client may not be what is required to address the negative behavior.

For example, if a client tends to focus more on her symptoms of fatigue and pain when a conflict has occurred between her and her partner and a therapist has been utilizing the instructing mode with the client to address mobility goals, the question of whether switching to a different mode would be more therapeutic is not easily answered. The client may perceive it to be more therapeutic if the therapist remains interpersonally consistent during the behavior and utilizes an alternative intervention that is consistent with the instructing mode. For example, if the therapist decided against a mode shift and, instead, downgraded the mobility task at hand to make it easier to perform, the client might perceive the therapist's action as helpful. In return, the client may even attenuate her physical complaints.

Alternatively, there is the possibility that the client might perceive the therapist's failure to respond to her complaints as dismissive, and in return she might exacerbate her physical complaints or cease attempting the task altogether. If the therapist had decided to switch to the empathic mode in order to notice and better understand why the client focuses more on her symptoms at certain times rather than others, it may make the client feel better, and it may lead her to have some insight into her behavior. However, it may also slow the client's progress toward the ultimate goal of therapy. Thus, as with any guidelines supported by the IRM, feedback from the client (whether behavioral or spoken) and an intentional process of trial and error should ultimately inform the decision making.

If you so much as suspect that something said or done during therapy may have triggered a client's negative behavior, making immediate and deliberate efforts to respond is a necessity. This response may involve switching into the empathic mode to better understand a rift or empathic break that occurred. If you are already functioning within the empathic mode, the situation might call for switching temporarily to an instructing response to guide a process of conflict resolution between yourself and the client.

Because it is sometimes difficult to determine whether a client's negative behavior is linked to something you have said or done during therapy, in some cases it is more important to determine whether using a different response mode might be experienced by the client as more comforting, centering, or therapeutic—regardless of whether the client is reacting to your behavior. Determin-ing whether a different mode might be experienced more positively by a client requires you to make some educated guesses about which mode the client might prefer in a given circumstance. Knowledge of a client's interpersonal characteristics should play a significant role in informing your "guess" about whether a mode shift would benefit the client. Because you never know for sure whether the decision to make a mode shift will result in success, an attitude of trial-and-error that incorporates feedback from the client is important to sustain during this process.

Step 4. Choose a Response Mode

If you have decided that a mode shift is required, you must select an alternative response mode that offers a more desirable approach to addressing the negative behavior. As a general rule, negative interpersonal behaviors are best addressed using the collaborating, empathizing, instructing, and problem-solving modes. The advocating and encouraging modes do not work as well with negative behaviors because they run the risk of reinforcing the behavior and they carry the potential to be perceived by certain clients as ingratiating or insincere. Moreover, some negatively behaving clients may try to take advantage of therapists who use these modes by engaging in more negative behavior that attempts to take advantage of a therapist's time or resources. More information about using modes to address specific categories of negative behavior is provided in Table 12.3 in the following section.

Step 5. Draw on Any Relevant Interpersonal Skills Associated With That Mode

Each of the four modes most likely to be therapeutic in addressing negative client behavior has certain interpersonal skills that are associated with the mode and are likely to be useful when addressing a negative behavior. The two interpersonal skills that are most relevant to addressing negative behavior include resolving an empathic break and conflict resolution (both of which are covered in more detail in Chapter 13). Resolving an empathic break requires that you rely most heavily on the empathizing mode to convey to the client that his or her point of view has been recognized and understood. Conflict resolution is a skill that requires use of all four modes at various time points during the process. You must use the instructing mode to describe the ground rules for conflict resolution and to structure the process. You must rely on the collaborating mode to ensure the client's full and equal participation in the process. The empathizing mode must be used

(text continued on page 240)

Table 12.3 **Modes That May Best Support Efforts to Address Negative Client Behaviors***				
Behavior	**Collaborating**	**Empathizing**	**Instructing**	**Problem-Solving**
	✓ Facilitate the client's active participation in therapy ✓ Encourage the client to make more decisions in therapy ✓ Inform the client that he or she is responsible for the outcomes of therapy ✓ Define the therapeutic relationship as a shared effort to explore and pilot-test new goals or skills ✓ Insist that the client provide direct and honest feedback about his or her experience in therapy	✓ Articulate the client's needs or perspective so the client feels seen and heard ✓ Strive to understand the behavior from the client's perspective ✓ Validate the utility of the negative behavior as perceived by the client	✓ Label and define the negative behavior for the client so he or she is aware of it and aware of the fact that you have identified it. ✓ Set a limit on the behavior, if necessary ✓ Highlight the negative consequences of the behavior for the therapeutic relationship and for the outcomes of therapy ✓ Teach alternative, more adaptive ways that the client may get his or her needs met within the relationship	✓ Ask the client strategic questions that probe the meaning of his or her behavior ✓ Discuss the advantages as well as the negative consequences of the client's behavior ✓ Negotiate with the client to find an alternative way of obtaining gratification of his or her needs
Manipulative	•	•	•	•
Excessive Dependence	•	•	•	•
Symptom Focusing/ Somatization	•	•	This mode rarely works with symptom focusing because clients experience attempts to intervene directly as an empathic rupture (e.g., they feel their experience is being invalidated by the therapist)	This mode may work provided the therapist validates the client's experience and encourages the client to consider ways of accommodating to or working around symptom increases when they occur
Resistance	•	•	Because resistant behavior is often associated with the client's perception of a power imbalance, direct efforts to intervene may be perceived as power plays and may be less effective	•

Behavior	Collaborating	Empathizing	Instructing	Problem-Solving
Emotional Disengagement/ Passivity/Isolative	May be less effective because emotional engagement is a prerequisite for engaging in a collaborative relationship with the therapist	•	Clients typically disengage emotionally, become passive, or isolate themselves when they are emotionally overwhelmed or unable to cope with the demands of therapy or the demands of the relationship. Directly intervening in a client's coping response may cause the client to retreat further	•
Denial	•	•	Clients often use denial to cope with events that are psychologically overwhelming to them. Attempting to break through a client's denial may result in client disbelief or in permanent rupture of the therapeutic relationship	If approached carefully, a therapist may use strategic questioning to help a client identify threats to personal safety and to plan rehabilitation goals
Difficulty With Rapport and Trust	•	•	•	Though it is not counter-indicated, problem-solving is not an efficient approach to improving rapport or building trust
Hostility Toward the Therapist or Critical or Questioning the Therapist's Approach	Provided the client does not pose a safety risk, shifting decision-making power and responsibility for outcomes to the client is often an effective way to manage this behavior	•	•	Negotiating with a client at a time when he or she is hostile, critical, or questioning may only escalate the client's anger

*A preferred mode for a behavior is designated by a bullet.

when listening and striving to understand the client's point of view. Finally, the problem-solving mode is best utilized toward the end of the process when you and the client are attempting to negotiate a satisfactory outcome. There are other skills in the IRM, including limit setting, maintaining professional boundaries (most closely associated with the instructing mode), and strategic questioning (most closely associated with the problem-solving mode) that are also useful when addressing negative behaviors.

Step 6. Gather Feedback

The final step in managing difficult behavior is to gather feedback from the client to determine whether your selection of modes and corresponding interpersonal skills were experienced as positive or therapeutic by the client. When clients exhibit difficult behavior, they rarely are in a mood in which they are capable of providing verbal feedback about their experience of the therapy process. Instead, clients typically provide feedback through their behavioral responses to your actions. The manner in which they provide feedback typically lies at the extreme ends of the continuum. The client's negative behavior either escalates and/or is accompanied by additional negative behaviors, or

the client's negative behavior is attenuated and the client appears more comfortable and relaxed. Thus, when gathering feedback from clients about whether a specific mode choice and/or intervention was effective, you must rely heavily on your observational skills and on the emotions you experience in reaction to the client's behavior (Fig. 12.3).

Summing It Up

The six steps of interpersonal reasoning were developed to facilitate an intentional (rather than an impulsive or emotion-based) response to any difficult behavior a client may exhibit during therapy. This process is somewhat limited in that it does not intend to eradicate difficult behavior permanently or even correct it temporarily. Instead, its purpose is to offer a way of thinking about and adjusting to the behavior that preserves the therapeutic relationship and improves the client's interpersonal experience of therapy. In some cases, it is natural and necessary for you to use this process to prevent nontherapeutic responding and to protect yourself from becoming vulnerable to client behavior that is inappropriate or unsafe. When negative behavior occurs, efforts to think about self-protection as

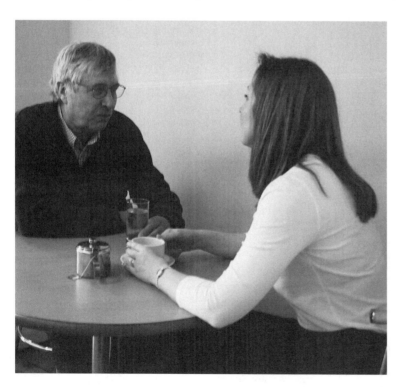

FIGURE 12.3 Jane Melton relies on interpersonal reasoning as she monitors a client's facial expressions

well as the well-being of the client should result in a safe and predictable experience for both you and the client.

Taken together, all of these efforts to use interpersonal reasoning to manage difficult behavior maximize the likelihood that the ultimate goals of occupational therapy are pursued. In the following section, additional information is provided to supplement the understanding and management of the eight categories of difficult behavior most commonly encountered in occupational therapy practice. When reviewing these categories, you may notice that some of the difficult behaviors are consistent with descriptions of some the enduring client characteristics in Chapter 5. This overlap in content is intended to reinforce the idea that difficult client behavior is rarely sporadic and never without meaning. When clients demonstrate difficult interpersonal behavior, it is likely that they have demonstrated the behavior with other people in other contexts. It is also likely that the behavior will not cease on its own.

Specific Categories of Difficult Behavior

As explained in the previous section, identifying and understanding difficult behaviors are the most important prerequisites for intentional management through interpersonal reasoning. In this section, I define each category of behavior and explain the psychological needs or motives that are likely to underlie the behavior. Once a general understanding of the behavior is presented, the interpersonal response modes that may be most effective in managing the behavior are discussed. Table 12.3 provides a summary of the response modes that may be most effective in preserving the therapeutic relationship and managing the behavior so it does not interfere with the ultimate goals of therapy.

As with other guidelines provided in this book, you are encouraged to use your own judgment and to consider the client's interpersonal characteristics and the social and cultural context in which the behavior is embedded.

As mentioned earlier in this chapter, the advocating and encouraging modes are not included. Although these modes can be effective in other contexts (e.g., when responding to certain interpersonal events or when addressing certain maladaptive dynamics within social systems), they are usually ineffective in addressing negative behavior in a one-on-one therapeutic relationship. As an advocate, your role is to serve the client's interests in

some way. As a person providing encouragement, your role is to instill hope and provide vision. The most problematic aspect of using these two modes is that they enable the negative behavior to continue unaddressed, and they place you in a more vulnerable position in the relationship. Using these modes in a one-on-one relationship is likely to encourage the behavior and increase the likelihood that, with time, you may be provoked to respond to the client without intentionality.

Manipulative Behavior

The definition of ***manipulative behavior*** varies widely depending on one's perspective. In general terms, it simply refers to underhanded efforts to maintain control or have one's own way when interacting with others. In mental health settings, the numerous actions that characterize manipulative behavior are defined with greater precision. In the IRM, a more detailed definition of manipulative behavior is utilized so you can become familiar with the myriad ways in which this behavior may manifest during therapy. This definition is, in part, adapted from the work of Messina and Messina (2006). According to the IRM, manipulative behavior may assume any of the following forms.

• Client strives to access a desired social, emotional, or material resource at the therapist's expense or when the therapist is not willing to provide it.
• Client's social presentation is inconsistent such that the client pretends to be cordial, compliant, ingratiating, sincere, or charming toward the therapist to achieve an immediate end when he or she actually harbors underlying feelings toward the therapist that are judgmental, aggressive, or otherwise negative. As a result, the client periodically vacillates between treating the therapist really well and treating the therapist very badly. This behavior keeps the therapist "walking on eggshells" or guessing about what to say or not to say, thereby allowing the client to maintain control.
• A client fabricates stories, distorts reality, or is otherwise dishonest in order to coax the therapist to believe something, do something, or behave in a way he or she might not have behaved spontaneously. For example, a client may convince a therapist to make a special exception or break a professional boundary.
• A client makes a concerted effort to exert a strong influence on the therapist's thinking or to convince the therapist to assume a perspective the client wants him or her to assume.

- A client behaves in a way that causes the therapist to feel responsible or even guilty about the client's thoughts, actions, or overall well-being so the client does not have to bear the burden of taking responsibility for his or her own opinions, decisions, and behaviors in life.
- A client attempts to make the therapist feel pity or sympathy for something that occurred that was actually a result of the client's own actions.
- A client engages in an interpersonally intense or intimate interaction with the therapist so the therapist feels obligated to be present for the client even when the client behaves in an undesirable, hostile, or inappropriate manner. For example, the client engages the therapist by sharing a personal life dilemma to generate a sense of obligation in the therapist to sustain a relationship with the client.
- A client exerts domination or control over the therapist by leading the therapist to believe that the therapist is the one who is dominant or controlling.

This definition of manipulative behavior can be utilized during the first step of interpersonal reasoning when the therapist is attempting to identify and organize the client's negative actions.

In addition to labeling it, making efforts to understand manipulative behavior offers the best chance of selecting a mode that best preserves the therapeutic relationship and allows the client to resume work toward the ultimate goals of therapy. People who behave in manipulative ways are savvy in that they have figured out how to influence people's perception of reality in order to maintain control and achieve a desired outcome of the interaction. They believe that, in most interactions, truth and reality are relative and can be easily distorted to serve their own needs. Because of this, they occasionally have difficulty differentiating between the reality of a given situation and their own perceptions, lies, and distortions. In addition, they approach relationships pragmatically and view others as objects for need fulfillment. If a manipulative strategy is effective, they continue to use it without regard for the potential consequences of the behavior. Individuals who engage in manipulative behavior are attempting to gratify the following psychological needs to:

- Preserve a fantasy that others exist to take care of their every need.
- Have another individual assume responsibility for every decision, behavior, or thought that one might have to free oneself from the burdens of everyday life.

- Gain admiration, control, or other resources from others to improve or preserve feelings of self-worth.
- Prevent others from gaining more resources, looking better, knowing more, or performing better so one can maintain the upper hand in the relationship.
- Keep others locked into intense or dramatic relationships that cause them continually to take care of one's emotional needs. This is a means of ensuring ongoing connection with others and a way of preserving feelings of exclusivity and self-importance. Having others respond to one's emotional crises is a means of meeting needs to be taken care of psychologically and to have alliance and support from others. It is also a means of ensuring that one is the center of attention within the relationship.
- Maintain a false image of flawlessness or omniscience so one does not have to risk being judged as lacking or imperfect by others.

Manipulative behavior can lead therapists to be uncertain about their client's actual goals and preferences during therapy. Over time and once they have been betrayed or hurt by these clients, therapists may come to distrust manipulative clients. If they are not intentional about managing this behavior, they may limit the amount of effort they put into their work with these clients, or they may disengage emotionally in an attempt to protect themselves from the intense interactions that characterize manipulative behavior.

When clients behave in manipulative ways, it is important to respond with intentionality. When using interpersonal reasoning, any of the four modes listed in Table 12.3 may be effective. The collaborating mode may be used to remind power-seeking clients of adaptive ways of retaining and using power within the therapeutic relationship. The empathizing mode is best utilized when a client's manipulative behavior is interfering with the therapy process and you pause to try to understand the reasons behind the client's need to act in this manner. The instructing mode may also be used to inform the client that the manipulative behavior is interfering with therapy or with the therapeutic relationship. It may also be used to remind the client of alternative ways to obtain need fulfillment. If a client accepts the fact that he or she is behaving inappropriately, the problem-solving mode may be used to assist the client in thinking through the pitfalls and alternatives to this behavior on his or her own.

Excessive Dependence

During certain phases of the rehabilitation process, it is natural for clients who are adjusting to an impairment situation to feel dependent on their therapists for various resources, such as emotional support, physical assistance, or advocacy efforts. Experienced occupational therapists come to develop an internal barometer for knowing when, how, and to what degree to empower clients so they may achieve autonomy. However, certain clients are resistant to any attempts by the therapist to promote independent thinking and/or functioning. These clients are considered to be excessively dependent on their therapists. According to the IRM, *excessive dependence* encompasses any of the following behaviors.

- Allowing or encouraging the therapist to do things that one is capable of attempting or doing on his or her own
- Refusing, either passively or actively, to set one's own goals for therapy
- Relying on the therapist to give one's life direction and meaning
- Attempting to become the center of the therapist's life and taking steps to prevent the therapist from interacting with others and carrying out tasks independently of the client
- Lacking independent opinions, world views, preferences, and dislikes—instead, making deliberate efforts to align one's world view and actions with those of the therapist so one can be as close to and similar to the therapist as possible
- Striving to please the therapist and relying on the therapist's approval to determine one's self-worth
- Exacerbating problems and symptoms to gain more of the therapist's attention and time
- Becoming helpless or immobilized in the absence of explicit support, direction, or caring from the therapist
- Downplaying or ignoring one's skills and areas of competence as a means of relinquishing responsibility for one's own life
- Clinging to the therapist or insisting on being in the presence of the therapist as much as possible
- Having a sense of entitlement or an expectation that the therapist will do all of the work required to meet the goals of therapy
- Having unrealistic expectations that therapy will result in more improvement than possible and becoming disappointed with imperfect outcomes

- Using manipulation, intimidation, or threats to ensure connection with or caretaking by the therapist

This definition of excessively dependent behavior may assist you in making sense of clients' behavior during the first step of the interpersonal reasoning process.

After you have identified this behavior in a client, the next step is to strive to understand it. Clients who are excessively dependent on their therapists have very low confidence in themselves and struggle with various fears and feelings of anxiety. Their confidence is so low they often have a need to rely on support and approval from others to feel comfortable with themselves. Some of the fears that individuals who are excessively dependent may harbor include:

- Fear of abandonment, loss of love, or isolation from others
- Fear of facing one's problems and responsibilities alone
- Avoiding success or independence out of a fear of not being able to sustain it over time or a reluctance to take on the additional responsibility required to sustain it
- Fear of the loss of approval that accompanies failing, making an error, or making a decision that is less than optimal
- Performance anxiety or being preoccupied with judgment by others

A natural consequence of clients' overdependence is for therapists to feel smothered or controlled by clients. Once they determine that the client is able to do more than he or she is willing to do, it is common for therapists to become frustrated or angry with clients and to react by confronting them or pushing them to perform. Being intentional in your approach to such clients involves using any of the four modes listed in Table 12.3 to understand and limit the behavior so it does not negatively affect therapy outcomes. The collaborating mode may be used to frame the therapy process as one that requires active involvement, input, and feedback from the client to be effective. The empathizing mode allows the client to discuss openly the meaning of her need to depend on you too much in the absence of judgment or attempts to correct the behavior. However, if not accompanied by one or more of the other modes, it will ultimately be ineffective in facilitating optimal therapy outcomes. The instructing mode may be used to educate the client about his or her dependence issues and provide an alternative perspective. Similarly, the problem-solving mode may be used to allow the client to see both the advantages and the disadvantages of excessive dependence in terms of the ultimate goals and outcomes of therapy. In addition to the modes, other occupational therapy models, such as the model of human occupation (Kielhofner, 2007) and client-centered occupational therapy (Law, 1998), may be used more extensively to promote and support client choice and autonomy.

Symptom Focusing

Symptom focusing is a specific approach to managing an impairment that involves spending a great deal of mental energy, time, and/or physical effort giving in to one's symptoms (or impairment) and spending considerably less time attempting to ignore, implicitly endure, or adjust to symptoms in order to engage in occupations. During therapy, symptom focusing may manifest in any of the following ways.

- The symptoms or impairment become worse during times when a client is facing emotional or interpersonal stressors and the client makes minimal to no effort to manage the stress that he or she is facing.
- A client spends what appears to be an excessive amount of time discussing limitations or symptoms (relative to other clients with similar or more severe conditions).
- A client chronically complains of pain or fatigue but takes little or no initiative to manage these symptoms actively through therapy and/or medication.
- A client utilizes hyperbole or other exaggerated adjectives to describe symptoms (e.g., a client complains that the pain is excruciating but does not consistently behave like someone who is in excruciating pain).
- A client acts helpless or demoralized when challenged to do something.

Symptom focusing is not easily understood because it may serve any number of underlying psychological needs, most of which are not consciously recognized by the person who is engaging in this behavior. At the most general level, symptom focusing may be understood as a coping mechanism that allows clients to avoid occupational engagement for any number of reasons without having to admit it to themselves. Some of the more common ways to understand symptom focusing include conceiving of it as:

- An unspoken communication to the therapist that one is feeling emotionally overwhelmed, vulnerable, anxious, demoralized, or unprepared for something
- A means of expressing an emotional or interpersonal issue that may be present in the therapeutic relationship

- A means of avoiding activity out of fear that it will exacerbate the illness or impairment
- A psychological habit the client has developed because he or she lacks support, stimulation, exposure to more adaptive role models, or alternative resources to cope with the symptoms or impairment

Similar to other difficult behaviors described in this chapter, symptom focusing is a highly stigmatized behavior that often leads health care professionals to make dismissive or minimizing comments, blame the client for having the complaints, attribute the complaints to a psychiatric disorder, push the client harder, overmedicate the client, or ignore the complaints altogether. Occupational therapists have something different to offer in that these kinds of diagnostic and validity issues are less relevant to the main emphasis of therapy, which is occupational engagement. However, a complicating factor is that individuals who engage in symptom focusing often engage in other negative behaviors that are associated with it, such as manipulative, dependent, or resistant behavior. In the end, this common interpersonal profile leaves any professional at risk of reacting without intentionality to clients who focus excessively on their symptoms. For example, an occupational therapist encountering this behavior might risk becoming locked into a dynamic in which they do everything possible to assist the client in pursuing goals that aim to ameliorate the symptoms only to discover that the client remains symptomatic and dissatisfied.

An intentional approach to managing clients who engage in symptom focusing involves choosing a mode sequence that supports the client's experience of his or her symptoms and at the same time attempts to empower the client gradually to take responsibility for participating in occupations of interest. The mode sequence that best reflects these efforts is the empathizing mode followed by the collaborating mode. To work with individuals who experience their symptoms as all-encompassing, you must first honor clients' somatic experience and validate their exaggerated perceptions. Only after a client believes that you are sincerely willing to understand his or her perspective do you have any chance of working collaboratively with the client on issues relevant to occupational therapy.

Resistance

Described in Chapter 6, *resistance* occurs when a client actively refuses to participate in some aspect of therapy. Resistance may also take the form of a client's withdrawal or avoidance of something in therapy. The client may ignore something you have said or fail to follow through with a recommendation for no valid reason. Typically, resistance is directly related to a dynamic that has been established in the therapeutic relationship.

As learned in Chapter 11, it always takes two people to maintain any dynamic. At the same time, dynamics must be initiated by someone. In the case of resistance, the client may initiate a dynamic that is usually related to issues of power and control with little or no influence from the therapist. Most typically, something about a client's recent or distant interpersonal history involving key authority figures causes the client to be exceptionally sensitive to any attempts by others to influence the therapy process in any way that is not consistent with the client's agenda. If the client's agenda is healthy and consistent with activities that are appropriate for therapy, the problem does not surface. However, if the client's agenda is not viewed as being healthy or appropriate by the therapist, the problem of resistance is likely to emerge.

Box 6.6 described a dynamic involving resistance that was faced by Vardit Kindler. The dynamic was triggered by the needs of two recently divorced parents to engage in a sustained conflict over what each thought was best in terms of improving their child's mobility. During her years of work with this family, Vardit had to work hard to resist the unspoken force within the family system that was attempting to draw her into a dynamic that would have created even more resistance in the child's mother.

A well intended therapist acting unintentionally may also serve as a trigger for resistant behavior in a client who is predisposed. This is particularly likely if the therapist chooses an interpersonal mode that is inappropriate for the client, rushes the process, or recommends an activity that is inconsistent with the client's volition (i.e., values, capacities, interests) (Kielhofner, 2007). When this occurs, it is important that the resistant behavior (and the dynamic that accompanies it) are identified promptly and addressed so therapy can progress.

Similar to the other difficult behaviors, interpersonal reasoning may be used to guide the process of mode selection. Modes that are most appropriate for resistant clients include the collaborating, empathizing, and problem-solving modes. When a client is resistant, the empathizing mode is typically a prerequisite for the use of any other modes because it ensures that the client's perspective is heard and understood. If used strategically, the collaborating mode may empower clients to take responsibility for their own rehabilitation goals. Finally, the problem-solving

mode may be used when the therapist and client have achieved enough mutual understanding and trust to be able to begin negotiating a shared plan for therapy.

Box 6.3 described Jane Melton's work with Nickolas,[1] a client exhibiting resistant behavior. Over the course of therapy, Jane discovered that Nickolas was resistant to therapy even before it began because the reason that therapy was recommended was not consistent with his interests. A description of how Jane worked with this client to achieve an eventual positive outcome is provided in Box 12.1.

Jane wisely began her work with Nickolas in the empathizing mode. For a time, she did not try to intervene with Nickolas' way of living but, instead, spent a period of time interacting with him normally in his own environment. Once trust was established, Jane then began to draw upon the collaborating and problem-solving modes.

---

[1] All client names and geographic information have been changed.

Box 12.1 Managing Resistance Using Interpersonal Reasoning

In approaching Nickolas'[2] resistance to work on goals related to hygiene and organization, I was able to form an objective assessment, which allowed me to provide careful feedback to Nickolas, his family, and the other service providers about the nature of his strengths, passions, and difficulties with his occupations. His volition, or motivation for occupation, was a key area for feedback. To reach Nickolas, I knew I would not accomplish his referral goals if I pushed for my own agenda. Instead, I had to join with Nickolas and wear the "no chaos here" spectacles. Overlooking his muddled and frenzied way of living allowed me to unravel his behavior and begin to understand his priorities. By "giving in" to his way of living, I eventually built enough trust to move forward with him in therapy.

It took time and a lot of creativity to foster a situation of negotiation during the sessions. It was essential that some of the "caring for self" tasks were done or facilitated in some way, as hygiene in the home posed a real health risk. We negotiated a system where we would concentrate for part of the session on routine "domestic" tasks and the other part on the leisure tasks. This continued over a long period of time. In parallel to these sessions I was also involved in coaching longer-term care/support workers who eventually took over the routine support that Nickolas needed to use the same patterning with their work.

— Jane Melton

[2] All client names and geographic information have been changed.

Acting within these modes, she communicated to Nickolas that his voice counted in terms of the activities and objectives of therapy. Moreover, she sustained a long-standing negotiation with Nickolas about how to accomplish hygiene and organizational goals.

Given the degree of resistance Nickolas was exhibiting, using interpersonal reasoning to select the appropriate mode sequence was necessary—but insufficient as an intervention in itself. Thus, Jane also incorporated the model of human occupation (Kielhofner, 2007) to discover and work with what motivated Nickolas. More information about how work with motivational issues can be integrated with mode use during the interpersonal reasoning process is provided at the end of this section.

Emotional Disengagement

Emotional disengagement occurs when a client is not experiencing spontaneous and authentic emotional reactions to the interpersonal events of therapy. Emotional disengagement may manifest in any of the following behaviors.

- A client's affect is restricted (e.g., the client appears inhibited in emotional expression or a client's emotional expression is infrequent or barely noticeable).
- A client's affect is completely flat (e.g., client speaks in monotone and/or exhibits a fixed or emotionless facial expression).
- A client has little to say or few ideas to contribute in therapy relative to his or her cognitive capacity.
- A client's actions during therapy or efforts to interact with the therapist appear forced rather than genuine.
- There is an unacknowledged tension between the client and the therapist.
- The client does not seem fully engaged in therapy and lacks adequate effort or enjoyment.

Once it has been identified, emotional disengagement is best understood as a form of psychological self-protection. Some clients learn to make their interactions with the therapist insignificant so they do not have to risk experiencing feelings that would otherwise make them uncomfortable. Some of these feelings may include vulnerability, embarrassment, a desire to have an intense personal relationship with the therapist, or even anger toward the therapist. Instead, the client's emotions "go underground," and he or she interacts with the therapist in a mechanical and regimented way. Accordingly, emotionally disengaged clients are not as open and self-disclosing as other clients.

Like any of the difficult behaviors, emotional disengagement is managed in-the-moment using interpersonal reasoning to select modes. The modes that an emotionally disengaged client is most likely to accept include the empathizing and problem-solving modes. However, unlike some of the other difficult behaviors discussed thus far, the empathizing mode is not necessarily a prerequisite for using the problem-solving mode. Some clients are so emotionally disengaged they do not allow the therapist to get close enough to their inner experience to allow empathic understanding to develop. In these circumstances, you may attempt to utilize strategic questioning to draw out more of the content of the client's thought process. In some circumstances, you may wish to engage in a private mental process of problem-solving about what you might change about the activity or environment to facilitate more engagement and use activity-focusing to engage the client. In some circumstances you may share some of your internal thoughts about how the impasse might be resolved by articulating them aloud or by simply announcing to the client: "Here is what I am thinking…" and asking for feedback. If a client observes that you are trying earnestly and repeatedly to understand and problem-solve about whatever it is that is impeding emotional engagement, he or she may become more open and engaged over time.

Denial

Denial is defined as a way of coping with a painful or uncomfortable event. In many cases, therapists encounter clients who are in denial about some or all aspects of their impairment or illness. However, clients may also be inclined to deny other events or realities that occur during the therapy process. In therapy, denial may take on one of three general forms.

- A client may deny the reality of the event altogether.
- A client may admit that the event has occurred but minimizes its severity or seriousness.*
- A client may acknowledge that the event happens to other people but has a more difficult time admitting that the event has also happened to himself or herself.

When a client denies any or all aspects of the reality of his or her situation, it must be understood as a serious indication that he or she is psychologically overwhelmed. In the moment of denial, the client is not yet ready to endure the pain involved in accepting the fact that the event is a reality. Unlike an addiction—the reality of which must be thrust in a client's face to preserve the health, safety, and well-being of that client—events that are far outside personal choice or control, such as impairments or illnesses, should never be considered reasons to break through a client's denial. Such attempts may result in client disbelief or in a permanent rupture of the therapeutic relationship.

The collaborating and empathizing modes are the only fail-safe modes to use when working with a client in denial. The collaborating mode may be used to shift decision-making and goal setting to clients so they may decide how best to utilize their time in therapy. Even if a client's goals are inconsistent with your agenda, you may decide to allow the client's chosen activity (provided the client is safe) to define the limits of the client's performance capacity, rather than warning or advising the client yourself. Similarly, heavy reliance on the empathizing mode allows an improved opportunity to access the client's understanding of the impairment, regardless of whether or to what extent it is based in reality. In some circumstances (particularly when the client's denial poses a safety risk), you may also draw upon the problem-solving mode and attempt to frame strategic questions for clients that allow them the autonomy to entertain different perspectives on the reality of their situation.

Difficulty With Rapport and Trust

Rapport and trust go hand in hand in the therapeutic relationship. Rapport is necessary for establishing a relationship at the onset of therapy, and trust is necessary to maintain that relationship. **Difficulty with rapport** is evident when a client is unfriendly or unresponsive to any attempts to make casual conversation or to find a common ground for communication. When therapists encounter clients with whom it is difficult to build rapport, they may describe the interaction as:

• Awkward
• Uncomfortable
• Stilted
• Anxiety-provoking
• Intimidating
• Empty
• Infuriating

Difficulty with trust, introduced in Chapter 5, becomes apparent over time as a client expresses various forms of skepticism and uneasiness about the process of therapy. Difficulties with trust may manifest in any of the following client behaviors.

• Questions that reflect concern about the adequacy, ultimate effectiveness, appropriateness, or safety of the therapist's approach or recommendation
• Reluctance to engage in the activities
• Failure to communicate authentically with the therapist (e.g., to provide important feedback about his or her doubts, vulnerabilities, or experience of therapy)
• Engaging in behavior that tests the therapist's dedication or loyalty (e.g., asking personal questions, asking for special exceptions)
• Withholding feedback or other information relevant to the therapy process

When clients have preexisting difficulty trusting others or carry past experiences of being betrayed, abandoned, rejected, or abused by key figures in their lives, issues of trust are more likely to arise in the therapeutic relationship. When behaviors associated with trust issues arise, they can be exacerbated as a result of therapists not being intentional about their approach to the therapeutic relationship.

Within the IRM, a central means of approaching trust issues in the relationship is to acknowledge openly to the client that they exist. You may make statements such as: "I'm wondering if you still need more time to trust this process" or "I'm wondering if you need some time to come to know me and trust that I have your best interests in mind." Making these statements allows the client to reflect on the relationship and provide feedback as to whether you are correct in suspecting trust issues. It also increases chances of dialogue about therapy and minimizes the likelihood that the client will continue to act out trust issues through his or her behavior. Even if you are well intentioned, caring, and kind, if you do not communicate to the client that you have picked up on a behavior that points to trust issues you have no chance of ever establishing genuine trust and rapport with the client.

After the trust-related negative behavior has been identified, you may then draw upon the empathizing mode to work to understand the reasons behind the client's lack of trust. Where trust issues are concerned, the empathizing mode should be a prerequisite for any of the other modes because it forces you to understand what the client wants from therapy and what interpersonal issues are at stake in terms of the client's ability to engage fully in the process. Clients with trust issues are among the most vulnerable. Being an occupational therapist carries a tremendous responsibility that includes not only clients' physical well-being but also their emotional and psychological well-being. If you use empathy respectfully and cautiously, you may discover that particularly vulnerable clients may be willing to begin to trust you—in some circumstances perhaps more than they have ever trusted another human being.

Following use of the empathizing mode, the collaborating mode may feel particularly comfortable for some clients whose capacity for trust depends on their ability to feel a sense of control in the relationship. Alternatively, the instructing mode may be the preference of other clients who want you to reveal your own agenda so they may react to your agenda rather than risk coming up with their own. These clients may find it easier to trust therapists who are more like teachers who work to direct and structure the therapy process and make their thinking about therapy clear and transparent.

Hostility

Hostility is a challenging client behavior for many therapists. *Hostility* is a multifaceted behavioral expression of anger or rage that is not always immediately obvious in the therapeutic relationship. Hostility may manifest in any of the following client behaviors (Messina & Messina, 2006).

- A client makes threats to harm or otherwise make life difficult for the therapist.
- A client emphasizes his or her wealth, status, knowledge, educational level, privilege, connections, talents, or power to intimidate the therapist.
- A client attempts to coerce, force, or blackmail the therapist to get his or her way.
- A client drops verbal and nonverbal hints that lead the therapist to think that he or she better do what the client wants or the client will become upset or enraged.
- A client says or does things that denigrate, belittle, humiliate, harshly criticize, or trap the therapist in a situation where there is no easy escape.
- A client is physically aggressive during therapy.
- A client uses sexually inappropriate language or innuendos or makes actual sexual advances toward the therapist.
- A client finds ways to punish the therapist emotionally for not behaving as desired.
- A client exhibits a quick temper or is easily irritated or enraged by things that do not appear to warrant such a reaction.
- A client is critical or questioning of the therapist's approach or overindulges in providing feedback as a means of controlling and keeping the therapist on guard.

On the most general level, hostile behavior is easy to recognize because it leads to feelings of pain, fear, or both.

Understanding hostility is not always easy, particularly when you are trying to put your own emotional reactions into perspective. For any client, there may be countless possible explanations, some of which were introduced in Chapter 9, and may also include:

- The client utilizes hostility as a means of expressing fear or sadness.
- Hostility is a symptom of the client's illness or impairment or a side effect of a medication the client is taking.
- The client is experiencing physical pain.
- Something negative occurred during the client's interaction with someone else.
- The client was recently made aware of a loss or some other stressful event.
- The client carries a feeling of entitlement that he or she can treat the therapist however he or she feels at the moment.
- The client's self-esteem is fragile, and any perceived threats to that self-esteem are interpreted as a threat to the client's self-perceived power, authority, or status.
- The client carries an unrealistic belief that he or she can control, approve, or disapprove of the behavior of others.
- The client holds a distorted belief that the best way to gain maximal assistance or cooperation from others is through intimidation.
- The client assumes a faulty belief that he or she is superior to others, including the therapist.
- The therapist has made an error that has put the client in danger or has caused emotional or physical harm.
- The client perceives that the therapist has made an empathic break.
- Some other interpersonal quality about the therapist is upsetting to the client.

Once you understand some of the beliefs, circumstances, or events that have caused a client to become hostile, you may attempt to utilize the empathizing and/or instructing modes to stabilize the client emotionally and prevent the behavior from escalating into abuse or violence. If a client is already behaving in an abusive or violent way, you should not attempt to work with the client in that moment and should take measures to ensure self-protection (reviewed in Chapter 9 in the section on anger). However, if the client is amenable to dialogue, you may approach the client using one of two initial modes: the empathizing mode or the instructing mode. The empathizing mode may be used to ensure that the client's perspective is witnessed, acknowledged or validated, and understood, no matter how distorted it may seem. However, not all clients are open to a dialogue that aims to reveal their perspectives. In this circumstance, the instructing mode may be used followed by the collaborating mode to guide the client through a process of conflict resolution. This process is discussed in more detail in the final section of this chapter.

Incorporating a Complementary Occupational Therapy Approach

In addition to using IRM principles and employing interpersonal reasoning to preserve the therapeutic relationship, working on motivational issues with clients may be particularly relevant when addressing difficult client behavior. *Volition* is a term that is used to describe various aspects of motivation as interpreted by the model of human occupation (Kielhofner, 2007). According to the model of human occupation, volition is central to facilitating occupational engagement. Understanding a client's volition involves three central activities (Kielhofner, 2007).

1. Making an effort to discover what interests a client.
2. Determining whether this interest is consistent with a client's values and with the world view reflected by those values.
3. Determining whether a client believes he or she is capable of engaging in that interest.

The model of human occupation offers reliable assessments and empirically validated approaches to working with clients' volition. Like other occupational therapy models, the model of human occupation can be used when interacting in any of the interpersonal modes of IRM. For more information about this approach, it is rec-

ommended that you consult the book, *A Model of Human Occupation: Theory and Application*, Fourth Edition (Kielhofner, 2007).

Summary

In practice, there are occasions when clients exhibit difficult behaviors and when misunderstandings arise between you and your clients. It is essential that you not provoke this behavior or react in ways that exacerbate the situation. This chapter emphasized the importance of accurately identifying and understanding eight categories of difficult client behaviors that occupational therapists encounter most frequently in practice. In addition, I outlined an interpersonal reasoning process that you may use when responding to difficult behavior. Noteworthy is that the empathizing mode may be used effectively with virtually any difficult behavior (provided the client feels contained and is not at risk of harming others). Empathy has a disarming quality that is unmatched by any other response. Imagining why a client might be feeling or behaving negatively is a prerequisite for interpersonal reasoning. To be interpersonally effective, you must not only have a general ability and willingness to try to understand the origins and triggers of a client's behavior, you must also respond to the client, initially, in a way that conveys a willingness to hear and validate the reasons behind the client's statements and actions. Responding to negative behaviors by seeking understanding paves the way for communication and trust between you and the client.

In certain circumstances, there is nothing that you can do to manage a client's negative behavior. For example, when clients are interpersonally hostile, sexually inappropriate, or even subtly abusive and are unresponsive to limit setting and redirection, you should not try to initiate or continue communication. Instead, you should remove yourself from the client and document the nature of the client's behavior in the chart, your specific attempts at intervention, and the reasons it was not possible to treat the client.

References

American Psychiatric Association (2000). *Diagnostic and statistical manual of mental disorders* (4th ed, text revision). Arlington, VA: American Psychiatric Association.

Beck, J. (1995). *Cognitive therapy: basics and beyond.* New York: Guilford Press.

Beck, A. T., Rush, A. J., Shaw, B. F., & Emery, G. (1979). *Cognitive therapy of depression.* New York: Guilford Press.

Freud, S. (1923). *The ego and the id.* New York: W.W. Norton.

Kielhofner, G. (2007). A model of human occupation: theory and application (4th ed.). Philadelphia: Lippincott Williams & Wilkins.

Kohut, H. (1984). *How does analysis cure?* Chicago: University of Chicago Press.

Law, M. (1998). *Client-centered occupational therapy.* Thorofare, NJ: Slack.

Messina, J. J., & Messina, C. M. (2006). *Eliminating manipulation: tools for coping with life's stressors.* Downloaded from the world wide web at www.coping.org on July 27, 2006.

Minuchin, P., Colapinto, J., & Minuchin, S. (1998). *Working with families of the poor.* New York: Guilford Press.

Rogers, C. R. (1961). *On becoming a person: a therapist's view of psychotherapy.* New York: Houghton Mifflin.

Skinner, B. F. (1974). *About behaviorism.* New York: Alfred A. Knopf.

Taylor, R. R., Lee, S. W., Kielhofner, G., & Ketkar, M. (2007). *Therapeutic use of self: a nationwide survey of practitioners.* Manuscript submitted for publication.

World Health Organization (2006). *International statistical classification of diseases and related health problems* (10th revision). Geneva: World Health Organization.

ACTIVITIES FOR LEARNING AND REFLECTION

Reflecting on the Management of Difficult Client Behavior

This exercise is designed to prompt reflection and build skills in managing difficult client behavior. Please complete the following questions and share your answers with your partner, supervisor, or work group.

1. In lay terms, briefly write about a client (or other person you know) who demonstrated behavior that you experienced as difficult.

_____

_____

2. How did this behavior make you feel?

_____

3. How did you react in the presence of the client (or other individual) who demonstrated this behavior?

_____

4. What did you do to try to manage this behavior?

_____

5. Briefly review Table 12.3 and determine what category (or categories) of difficult behavior this client or individual was exhibiting at the time. Write them here.

_____

6. Briefly review Table 12.3 and determine whether any attempts you made at the time to manage the behavior were consistent with any of the modes. If so, list the modes here.

_____

7. In reflecting on the category of behavior, how you reacted, and any modes that you used at the time, are there any alternative or additional modes that you might have used to manage the situation? If so, explain here.

_____

_____

CHAPTER 13

RESOLVING EMPATHIC BREAKS AND CONFLICTS

Empathic breaks and other sources of conflict between clients and therapists are inevitable events of therapy that, depending on how they are managed, can lead to either fortification or deterioration of the therapeutic relationship. Introduced in Chapter 6, an empathic break is defined as a natural consequence of therapy that occurs when a therapist initiates a communication or behavior that is perceived by a client as hurtful or insensitive. On some occasions, this does not involve any direct action on the part of the therapist but, instead, consists of failure to notice, understand, or validate some communication that a client perceives as important.

When a client perceives that a therapist has made an empathic break, it can trigger uncomfortable thoughts and feelings that ultimately result in difficult interpersonal behavior. For example, if a therapist suggests that a client consult a nutritionist because of a weight issue and a client is offended by the suggestion, it may trigger a pattern of negative behavior in a vulnerable client. The client may become emotionally disengaged from therapy or hostile and critical of the therapist's approach. Because empathic breaks may lead to undesirable behavior that negatively affects the therapeutic relationship and detracts from the process and outcomes of therapy, this chapter focuses how to resolve them as promptly and completely as possible before they escalate. Even when you are vigilant about recognizing and resolving empathic breaks, there are occasions when differences in opinion remain or other issues arise that are not easily resolved. These differences may occur between therapist and client or between a client and another person, such as a peer, family member, or other treatment provider. On some occasions, conflicts occur between therapists and coworkers. For this reason, information about how you can approach conflict resolution

with others and mediate conflict between others is provided in this chapter (Fig. 13.1).

Resolving Empathic Breaks

The Intentional Relationship Model (IRM) contends that it is inevitable that some of clients' difficult behavior during therapy is the direct result of an empathic break that clients perceive was made by the therapist. Being able to resolve an empathic break promptly once it has occurred can prevent a host of difficult behaviors from developing or enduring over time. It can also strengthen the relationship and increase levels of trust and communication. Resolving an empathic break requires that you accomplish six critical actions.

1. Recognize that the empathic break has occurred.
2. Avoid behaviors or comments that deflect/minimize the break.
3. Avoid behaviors or comments that inflame the break.
4. Raise it with the client.
5. Repeat your understanding of the injury.
6. Say something that soothes or reassures the client.

If you expect to have any chance of resolving an empathic break, the first step, recognition, is the most difficult and the most critical to accomplish. Recognizing that a break has occurred involves drawing on your working knowledge of the many potential causes of empathic breaks. If you are vigilant to the types of therapist behaviors that may represent an empathic break, you are more likely to avoid the behaviors and recognize them when they have occurred. Examples of therapist behaviors that may constitute an empathic break in the minds of some clients are included in Chapter 6.

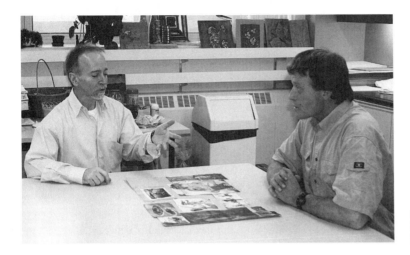

FIGURE 13.1 A client listens while René Bélanger attempts to resolve an empathic break

The second responsibility in resolving an empathic break is to avoid behaviors that deflect or minimize the break. It is common for therapists to attempt to protect themselves and their clients from the discomfort, pain, or embarrassment that accompanies situations that involve an empathic break. Examples of typical ways in which therapists act to downplay emotional intensity include:

- Apologizing prematurely before fully acknowledging one's actions and having the patience to hear the client's reactions
- Apologizing excessively in an effort to shield oneself from the client's emotions
- Excessive self-effacement (e.g., "typical me, I always seem to put my foot in my mouth!")
- Changing the subject or saying or doing something that distracts the client's attention away from the situation
- Saying something that minimizes the seriousness of the injury or allowing the client to say something dismissive, such as "It's not that big of a deal" or "It's ok, it happens to me all the time"
- Using humor or joking about the situation with the client

Although these behaviors may provide some short-term emotional relief, they prevent the empathic break from being resolved as fully as possible in the minds of both client and therapist.

A third effort required to resolve an empathic break involves avoiding behaviors or comments that have the potential to be inflammatory. When a client reacts negatively to something you have said or done, it is natural to react in a defensive way. Some examples of behaviors that may exacerbate the situation rather than resolve it include:

- Denying or distorting what one has done or said
- Saying something that makes the client feel guilty or blamed for his or her reaction (e.g., "You really took this the wrong way" or "C'mon, not this again")
- Using adjectives or other language that exaggerates the situation in an attempt to be sarcastic or to shame the client for having reacted negatively

If you have successfully avoided comments and behaviors that would minimize or provoke the situation, it is likely that you can raise the issue with the client in an intentional and therapeutic way. When you suspect that an empathic break has occurred, you should immediately raise it with the client. Examples of comments that introduce the possibility that a break has occurred include:

- "I think I may have said something insensitive."
- "I think I may have missed something important."
- "I can't put my finger on it, but I have a hunch I have said or done something hurtful."
- "I'm wondering if that comment I made about your sister's behavior toward you was out of bounds as an outsider to your family."
- "Your face tells me I may have said something wrong."

There are countless ways you can introduce the possibility that you have caused a client to experience an empathic break. With nonverbal clients, a mode shift may be enough to let a client know that you recognize that a change in your approach is needed. Most important is that

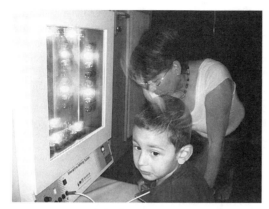

FIGURE 13.2 Michele Shapiro pauses to reflect on a client's worried look

the issue is raised so the client knows it has been acknowledged (Fig. 13.2).

Once you have an approximate idea of what was said or done to cause the client to react negatively, the next step involves repeating your understanding of the injury. Even if a client reluctantly acknowledges disappointment or attempts to minimize his or her reaction, it is still vital that you not take the situation lightly. This is because, in addition to recognizing that a break has occurred, the next most vital step in fully resolving that break is to admit what you have done or said to cause the break and to validate the client's reaction to it.

Thus, the fifth step of resolving an empathic break involves repeating and summarizing your understanding of what you said or did to cause the injury while being careful not to apologize prematurely. For example, if a therapist has said something about the behavior of a client's sister that offended the client, he or she might say: "When I said that your sister does not seem willing to accept the fact that you need additional support right now, it was hurtful to you." Similarly, if a therapist is forced to miss an appointment with a client because of a traffic jam and senses that the client may be upset about it, the therapist may say something like: "I missed your appointment entirely and you waited here for an hour when you could have been doing something else."

After you have summarized the injury, you should look for feedback from the client that the injury has been adequately summarized and understood. Sometimes a client simply nods the head or otherwise indicates that you are correct. Other times, your summary and acknowledgement prompts the client to elaborate more on feelings of

disappointment, hurt, or anger. Regardless of whether the client continues to elaborate on his or her feelings, it is vital that you validate the client's negative reaction (again without apologizing prematurely). Examples of ways to validate a client's reaction include:

- "When I didn't show up, you were wondering if maybe I forgot about you."
- "When I didn't show up, you began to wonder if you weren't as important to me as other clients are."
- "When I didn't show up, it made you wonder whether I really care about working with you."
- "When I said that about your sister, it made you think that I was unfairly judging her."
- "When I said that about your sister, it reminded you of other times when she has let you down in the past."
- "When I said that about your sister, it made you worry that she might not be there for you when you most need her."

Once you are certain that the client has said everything possible that he or she needs to say about the incident, the final step in resolving the break involves showing some acceptance of responsibility for the oversight and providing reassurance to the client. At this point, it may be appropriate for you to apologize. Other examples of means of apologizing, accepting some responsibility, or providing reassurance may include statements such as:

- "I'm sorry that what I said (or did) caused you to feel that way."
- "You are correct. I could have left earlier so as to plan ahead for the traffic, but my lack of planning does not mean that I do not care about our work together."
- "When I hear these types of stories, I tend to share too many of my opinions about clients' family members. I am sorry for overstepping my bounds."

Within the IRM, the interpersonal mode that is most useful to draw upon when resolving an empathic break is the empathizing mode. This mode allows you to focus on understanding the client's perspective of the situation rather than attempting to clarify, fix, distract, or provide a rationale for why the situation occurred. When you make sincere efforts to recognize and resolve empathic breaks with clients, you not only prevent negative interpersonal behaviors from escalating into conflict but you also maximize the likelihood that an open and trusting relationship will develop.

Although the IRM emphasizes the importance of being able to recognize and respond therapeutically to an empathic break, it is important for you to remain emotionally balanced and objective while doing so. There must be a balance between recognizing an empathic break and assuming too much responsibility for it. This is not an easy balance to strike. Some clients are so prone to perceiving empathic injury that a pattern may develop in which you allow yourself to feel at fault for behaviors that are ethical, well intended, necessary, and/or interpersonally benign, such as setting limits and establishing professional boundaries. Similar to other stepwise guidelines presented in this book, these steps should not be implemented rigidly. You should use your own judgment about the timing, inclusion, and sequence of steps utilized to resolve an empathic break. An exercise for practicing how to resolve an empathic break with a partner is provided in the Activities section of this chapter.

Conflict Resolution

Conflict resolution represents the final means of addressing negative client behavior that is covered in this chapter. In certain circumstances, there is nothing that you can do or say to avoid engaging in conflict with a client. Within the IRM, there are two major categories of conflict.

1. Conflict that begins with a minor misunderstanding or small difference in opinion and progressively escalates into a more emotionally intense and personalized exchange
2. Conflict that begins as an emotionally intense and personalized exchange because of the magnitude of the particular issue that is at stake

With reference to the first category, conflict does not always have to be emotionally charged. In therapy, conflict may take the form of unspoken tension, or it may represent a minor misunderstanding or difference in opinions between you and the client. Because this more nascent category of conflict is likely to grow if left unaddressed, the IRM recommends that you regard any complex dialectical situation that involves distinctive viewpoints as a conflict, even if both perspectives are warranted and there is no apparent emotional intensity within the exchange.

Within the IRM, conflict may be addressed in one of two ways. It may be minimized, or it may be contained. Minimizing conflict involves recognizing situations in which opposing viewpoints are present and acting early to implement conflict resolution strategies. Containing conflict involves setting limits to preserve the emotional and physical well-being of participants and then returning to implement conflict resolution strategies once strong emotions are quelled and participants' physical safety is ensured.

When managing conflict, some general guidelines to keep in mind include the following.

• Cope in order to retain perspective and emotional control.
• Avoid any need to be right or to win the argument; focus more on understanding the other person's perspective.
• As a rule, do more listening than talking.
• Use "I" statements that take responsibility for your perspective (e.g., "I acknowledge that I could have been easier on you" or "I prefer that the rules be established collectively"). Simply stating an opinion (e.g., "I think you were wrong") is not considered an "I" statement because there is no evidence of responsibility-taking in the statement.
• Use "why" statements that explain why you feel the way you do rather than "you" statements that blame or describe what the other individual did wrong (e.g., "You always forget to clean the microwave" or "You seem to use that as your excuse a lot these days").
• Avoid using absolute adjectives and statements such as "always" or "never" to characterize the situation (e.g., "You never show up to appointments on time" or "I'm always the one who ends up cleaning up the toys afterward").

These general guidelines may help reduce the chances that the conflict will escalate. Similar to resolving an empathic break, the formal approach to conflict resolution is a stepwise process that involves the following actions.

• *Step 1*: Exercise emotional restraint and invite the client to join you in attempting to resolve the issue. Be willing to initiate and guide the resolution of the conflict.
• *Step 2*: Explain the structure and the ground rules for discussing the issue at hand. Explaining the process may involve saying something like: "We are each going to have a chance to talk about what is on our minds, and then there will be a chance to problem-solve about how to resolve this situation." Establishing ground rules for communication with the client may involve explaining the importance of rules such as a *no cross-talk rule* or a *no retribution rule*. A no cross-talk rule means that the other individual must listen fully and never interrupt

the person who is explaining his or her point of view. A no retribution rule means that each participant must not blame the other for having raised an issue or disclosed a perspective.

- *Step 3*: Invite the client to share his or her perspective on the issue and work hard to just listen to the client's perspective no matter how distorted or irrational it may appear.
- *Step 4*: Summarize your understanding of the client's perspective and ask for feedback about accuracy.
- *Step 5*: Ask the client if he or she is willing to listen to your perspective. Tell the client that you will be asking him or her to summarize your perspective once you are finished. If the client tries to argue with you before you are finished explaining your perspective, remind the client of the no cross-talk rule.
- *Step 6*: Ask the client to summarize your perspective. Reinforce the client for attempting to see the situation from your point of view. If necessary, correct any misperceptions or major details the client may have left out.
- *Step 7*: Problem-solve about solutions. This involves identifying issues that you and the client agree on by making a mental list or by writing them down on a piece of paper. It also involves identifying the major points on which you disagree. Once you and the client are clear about the issues on which you agree and disagree, you have three options. The first is to agree to disagree and offer no concessions. You do not always have to "give in" if you believe that your perspective is what is most ethical, safe, or best for the situation. The

second option is to offer your "deal-makers" or points on which you are willing to compromise. The third option involves informing the client of any "deal-breakers" or points on which you are not willing to compromise. You should invite your client to do the same.

In terms of mode use, the modes that are most consistent with engaging in conflict resolution include the instructing, collaborating, and empathizing modes. The instructing mode allows you to take the lead in structuring and guiding the process. The collaborating mode encourages clients to take responsibility for their perspectives and reactions and to participate as equal partners in the conflict resolution process. The empathizing mode ensures that your first priority is listening to and striving to understand the client's perspective.

When you are intentional about your communication with clients, conflicts are less likely to occur, and the need for a formal process of conflict resolution may not be as great. It is more likely that conflicts will arise between clients and their peers or between members of a client's family.

Occasionally, you may find that a conflict with a coworker arises that requires resolution. The same steps for resolving conflicts with clients may be applied with others. You may find that it is actually easier to guide others through the steps of conflict resolution as a third party than as an involved participant. An exercise for practicing the process of conflict resolution as a third-party mediator is provided in the Activities section of this chapter (Fig. 13.3).

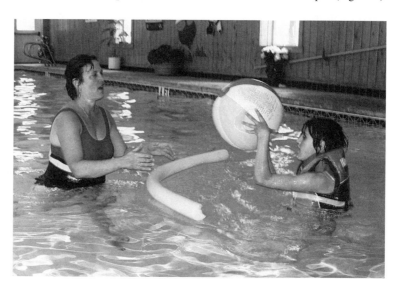

FIGURE 13.3 Kathryn Loukas and a client reach an agreement about ground rules for playing volleyball

Summary

In this chapter, two approaches are described that can help prevent difficult behavior from escalating or becoming chronic. When you suspect that something you have said or done has caused a client to perceive an empathic break, you may look to the guidelines provided in this chapter to resolve the break as promptly and completely as possible. When differences in opinion surface, you may rely on your conflict resolution skills to contain or minimize the disagreement. All of these efforts are intended to preserve and fortify the therapeutic relationship so the original objectives for therapy can be pursued.

ACTIVITIES FOR LEARNING AND REFLECTION

EXERCISE 13.1

Resolving Empathic Breaks

This exercise is designed to allow role-play practice in resolving empathic breaks. The two scenarios described below are situations in which it is clear that some kind of an empathic break has occurred. Find a partner and practice taking the roles of therapist and client in each of these scenarios. As the therapist, your only job is to employ the guidelines you learned in this chapter in an attempt to resolve the rift. As the client, your job is to embellish the complaint and not let the therapist off the hook too easily.

At the end of the exercise, more space is provided for you to describe any actual empathic breaks that you have experienced or witnessed and to role-play optimal scenarios for resolving them.

Scenario 1: Subject to Criticism

Your supervisor phones you to tell you that a parent has made a vague complaint about you and has requested to work with another OT. The supervisor reports that the parent believes her son is not making enough progress in therapy with you. Because the supervisor was not able to get any more details about what it was that you said or did to upset the parent, the supervisor is asking you to go back to the parent and try to resolve the issue.

Scenario 2: Angry about Lack of Progress

You have been working with a client with a spinal cord injury who has been reluctant at times to participate in the steps of the rehabilitation program. The only means by which you have been successful in getting him engaged in therapy has been to remind him that he will get more movement and function back if he works hard enough. Right before discharge, he expresses disappointment in you and accuses you of lying to him regarding the benefits of therapy. He complains that he has not gotten the movement and function back that you told him he would.

Actual Empathic Breaks

In the space provided write a brief description of any empathic breaks you have witnessed or experienced in your own life or practice. Once fully described, role-play an optimal scenario for resolution with your partner.

_____

_____

_____

_____

EXERCISE 13.2

Conflict Resolution

This exercise is designed to allow for role-play practice in resolving conflict as a third-party partic-ipant. The two scenarios described below are situations in which a conflict is taking place or about to take place between your client and another individual. Please find two partners and practice tak-ing the roles of the client, the individual involved in conflict with the client, and the therapist. As the therapist, your only job is to employ the guidelines you learned in this chapter in an attempt to minimize or contain the conflict. As the participants in conflict, your job is to embellish the details surrounding the conflict and not to let the therapist off the hook too easily.

At the end of the exercise, more space is provided for you to describe any actual conflicts that you have experienced or witnessed and to role-play optimal scenarios for resolving them.

Scenario 1: Failure to Follow Through

By the request of your adolescent client's mother (the teenager agreed), you have worked for weeks to assist the family in planning for and implementing home renovations that will allow improved mobility within her home environment (grab bars, hardwood flooring, ramps, widened doorways, bathroom renovations). You have also obtained a scooter for her and have trained her to use it. The goal is to improve energy conservation and mobility with the hope that the client will become more involved in extracurricular activities and social contact with friends. You return to assess changes in her mobility following these efforts only to find that she is uncomfortable using the scooter, insists on walking, and continues to retreat to the couch absolutely exhausted after school and on weekends. At this point you are disappointed and upset, but the client's mother is even more disappointed in the client. She begins to scold the client in front of you.

Scenario 2: A Client and her Physician

A client comes to you very disappointed in her physician's recent behavior and treatment plan. She raises the following issues with you about her physician: (1) "He prescribes medications for me without regard for their side effects." (2) "He doesn't listen well enough." (3) He doesn't seem to have a comprehensive treatment plan for me." Just then, her physician enters the room, and the client begins to argue with him about why he prescribed a medication for her to which she con-tends she is allergic.

Actual Conflicts

In the space provided, write a brief description of any conflicts that you have witnessed or experi-enced in your own life or practice. Once fully described, with your partners role-play an optimal scenario for resolution.

_____

_____

_____

_____

CHAPTER 14

PROFESSIONAL BEHAVIOR, VALUES, AND ETHICS

In occupational therapy, professional behavior, values, and ethics encompass a broad spectrum of attitudes and behaviors that are fundamental to practice. As individuals, our training and exposure to various value systems throughout our development influence the occupations we choose and the ways in which we interact with other people. In turn, the professional behavior, values, and ethics that we embrace as occupational therapy professionals reflect our personal values and ethics as individuals. This chapter covers the values, ethics, and professional behaviors that are most relevant to therapeutic use of self according to the Intentional Relationship Model (IRM). In addition to summarizing the major aspects of the core values and attitudes of occupational therapy practice (American Occupational Therapy Association, 1993) and the American occupational therapy code of ethics (American Occupational Therapy Association, 2005), which remain in use within the field today, the following topics are emphasized.

• Core values and therapist interpersonal modes
• Behavioral self-awareness
• Reliability
• Confidentiality
• Professional boundaries

In 1993, Elizabeth Kanny, together with Ruth Hansen and the Standards and Ethics Commission of the American Occupational Therapy Association (AOTA), produced a statement of the core values and attitudes of occupational therapy practice (AOTA, 1993). Based on a task inventory of what practitioners actually do in practice, this statement describes the attitudes and values that form the foundation for the profession. In this document, values are defined as beliefs or ideals to which an individual is committed. Attitudes are defined as the disposition to respond positively or negatively to a given person, idea, object, or situation. These seven basic concepts around which the core values and attitudes are organized are presented in Table 14.1.

The value system of occupational therapists is also reflected in the most recent revision of the AOTA Code of Ethics (AOTA, 2005). The AOTA ethics code strives to promote and maintain high standards of conduct for the profession by educating professionals and the public about established principles of accountability, socializing novice occupational therapists to the expected standards of conduct, and assisting all occupational therapists in recognizing and resolving ethical dilemmas that occur in practice, research, and educational settings. The seven principles upheld by the AOTA (2005) ethics code are summarized in Table 14.2.

One of the most effective ways to become familiar with the ethics of occupational therapy practice is to read about common ethical dilemmas that practitioners face and to think about viable solutions. Exercise 14.1 in the Activities section of this chapter describes a series of ethical dilemmas faced by therapists and calls for planning and discussion about how to resolve those dilemmas (Fig. 14.1).

Together, our personal and professional values and ethics contribute to our interpersonal styles, or preferred modes of interacting during therapy. Occasionally, competing values clash, and it becomes difficult to determine which more ethical value should be upheld in a given clinical situation. Inevitably, you will be forced to choose which values and ethics you see as being of greatest benefit and least harm to the client in the situation at hand. The core values statement (AOTA, 1993) acknowledges that it is impossible to apply all the values simultaneously and

Table 14.1	Summary of the Seven Core Values and Attitudes of Occupational Therapy Practice
Altruism:	Oriented toward others rather than oneself. Actions and attitudes reflect commitment, dedication, caring, responsiveness, and understanding.
Equality:	Embraces equal rights and opportunities for all humans regardless of diversity in culture, values, beliefs, or lifestyles. Actions and attitudes reflect a deep respect for human diversity, fairness, and impartiality.
Freedom:	Encourages clients to exercise choice and demonstrate independence, initiative, and self-direction.
Justice:	Upholds fairness, equity, truthfulness, and objectivity. Relationships tend to be goal-directed and objective. Respects and is knowledgeable about clients' legal rights and the laws that govern practice.
Dignity:	Views each individual as unique and as having inherent worth. Upholds attitudes of empathy and respect for self and others. Supports the promotion of feelings of competence and self-worth through participation in relevant and valued occupations.
Truth:	Demonstrates accountability, forthrightness, and honesty. Accurate and authentic in all actions and attitudes.
Prudence:	Exercises self-governance and self-discipline through the use of reason. Demonstrates judiciousness, discretion, vigilance, moderation, care, and circumspection in relationships.

Source: American Occupational Therapy Association (1993)

that you must choose the values you see as most relevant to a given practice situation. Although in some cases these choices are situation-specific, in other cases the values favored by occupational therapists may, in part, reflect their own personal priorities and world view. The following section describes some potential linkages between your core values and the interpersonal modes you may utilize in various practice situations. A summary of this information is provided Table 14.3.

Core Values and the Therapist's Interpersonal Modes

Introduced in Chapter 4, each of the six therapeutic modes defines a unique style of relating to clients. To varying degrees, each of these styles is associated with certain core values of the profession. In the section below, the values most closely associated with each of the modes are elaborated. While reviewing this section, you are encouraged to reflect on your preferred interpersonal modes and to determine the extent to which those modes are consistent with the professional values you tend to emphasize in practice.

Advocating Mode

Therapists who prefer the advocating mode place a high value on social justice, equality, empowerment, participation, and access to opportunities and resources in a client's broader community. Because they are keenly sensitive to

the roles of power and injustice in the lives of individuals with disabilities, therapists who favor the advocating mode are quick to recognize and assist their clients to respond to the physical, social, economic, and occupational barriers they encounter. They are careful not to undermine their clients' autonomy, dignity, sense of personal power, and judgment by functioning as an expert or as someone interested in repairing them. Instead, those who favor the advocating mode serve in the modes of facilitator and consultant to clients. Some may engage in consciousness-raising with their clients about their legal rights and about the barriers to access and independence they may face as individuals with disabilities. Therefore, the occupational therapy core values that are most closely associated with the advocating mode include equality, freedom, justice, and dignity (Fig. 14.2).

Collaborating Mode

Therapists who emphasize use of the collaborating mode tend to value client empowerment, independence, and personal choice. They believe that clients are more likely to achieve positive outcomes during therapy if they function as equal participants in the process and assume a significant amount of responsibility for the therapy outcome. Therapists who favor collaboration view clients as capable of determining what they need from therapy and, with appropriate education and guidance, selecting occupational therapy goals and tasks that address those needs. In concrete terms, they prefer that clients set their own goals for therapy, monitor their own progress toward those goals, and, in general, choose their preferred occupations.

Table 14.2 **Summary of the Seven Ethical Principles of Occupational Therapy Practice**	
Principle	**Description**
Beneficence	Concern for the safety and well-being of clients · Provide services in a fair and equitable manner · Embrace all aspects of human diversity · Ensure that fees are fair and commensurate with services; consider context and ability to pay · Advocate for recipients to obtain services through available means · Promote the public health, safety, and well-being of individuals and groups
Nonmaleficence	Ensure safety and avoid imposing harm · Relationships must not exploit clients sexually, physically, emotionally, psychologically, financially, socially, or otherwise · Avoid dual relationships or activities that conflict or interfere with professional judgment and objectivity · Refrain from undue influences that may compromise provision of service · Exercise professional judgment and critically analyze directives that could result in potential harm before implementation · Practice self-care and identify and address personal problems that may adversely affect professional judgment and duties · Bring concerns regarding impaired professional skills of a colleague to the attention of the appropriate authority when or if attempts to address those concerns independently are unsuccessful
Autonomy and confidentiality	Respect recipients of service and ensure their rights · Collaborate with recipients in setting goals and priorities for intervention. Fully disclose the nature, risk, and potential outcome of any intervention · Obtain informed consent when involving recipients in research or educational activities · Respect an individual's right to refuse services or involvement in research or educational activities · Protect all privileged confidential forms of written, verbal, and electronic communication unless otherwise mandated
Duty	Should achieve and continually maintain high standards of competence. · Hold appropriate national, state, or other credentials · Conform to AOTA standards of practice and official documents · Be responsible for maintaining and documenting competence in practice, education, and research through continuing education and professional development activities · Be competent in all topic areas in which one provides instruction to consumers, peers, or students · Critically examine available evidence to perform duties on the basis of current information · Protect service recipients by ensuring that duties assigned to other therapists match their credentials and qualifications · Provide appropriate supervision to OT personnel and students for whom you are responsible in accordance with AOTA and laws · Refer to or consult with other service providers in collaboration with the recipient when it could be helpful to the recipient
Procedural justice	Comply with laws and association policies guiding the profession · Understand and abide by institutional rules, association policies, local, state, national, and international laws · Be familiar with revisions to those laws and inform employers, employees, and colleagues · Encourage those one supervises to adhere to the code of ethics · Take reasonable steps to ensure that one's employers are aware of the ethics code and the implications for OT practice, education, and research · Record and report in a timely manner all information related to professional activities
Veracity	Occupational therapists should provide accurate information when representing the profession · Represent one's credentials, qualifications, education, experience, training, and competence accurately, particularly with recipients and during professional interactions · Disclose any professional, personal, financial, business, or volunteer affiliations that may pose a conflict of interest to those with whom one may establish a professional, contractual, or other working relationship

(table continued on page 264)

Principle	Description
	Table 14.2 **Summary of the Seven Ethical Principles of Occupational Therapy Practice** (continued)

Principle	Description
	· Refrain from using or participating in the use of any form of communication that contains false, fraudulent, deceptive, or unfair statements or claims · Identify and fully disclose to all appropriate persons errors that compromise recipients' safety · Accept responsibility for professional actions that reduce the public's trust in OT services
Fidelity	Should treat colleagues and other professionals with respect, fairness, discretion, and integrity · Preserve, respect, and safeguard confidential information about colleagues and staff unless otherwise mandated by national, state, or local laws · Accurately represent the qualifications, views, contributions, and findings of colleagues · Take adequate measures to discourage, prevent, expose, and correct any breaches of the Code and report to the appropriate authority · Avoid conflicts of interest and conflicts of commitment in employment and volunteer roles · Use conflict resolution and/or alternative dispute resolution resources to resolve organizational and interpersonal conflicts · Familiarize oneself with established policies and procedures for handling concerns about this Code

Source: American Occupational Therapy Association (2005)

Thus, the occupational therapy core values that are most closely associated with the collaborating mode include equality and freedom (Fig. 14.3).

Empathizing Mode

Therapists who embrace the empathizing mode value the act of bearing witness to clients' experience of therapy over all other aspects. They may focus particularly closely on striving to understand the clients'

• Emotional experience (e.g., clients' outward affect and the internal feelings that drive affective expression)
• Psychological experience (e.g., clients' thoughts about themselves as participants in therapy and their interpretations of their impairment situations)

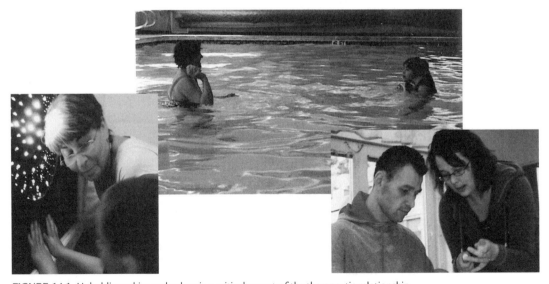

FIGURE 14.1 Upholding ethics and values is a critical aspect of the therapeutic relationship

Interpersonal Mode	OT Core Values
Collaborating	Equality—equal rights and opportunities for all humans, deep respect for human diversity, fairness, and impartiality Freedom—choice, independence, initiative, and self-direction
Empathizing	Altruism—oriented to the other rather than to the self Dignity—emphasizes the uniqueness and self-worth of each client, upholds attitudes of empathy Truth—accurate and authentic
Encouraging	Dignity—emphasizes the inherent worth of clients
Instructing	Justice—goal-directed and objective Truth—accountable and forthright Prudence—judiciousness, discretion, vigilance, moderation, care and circumspection
Problem-solving	Justice—goal-directed and objective Prudence—judiciousness, discretion, vigilance, moderation, care, and circumspection

Table 14.3 **Therapist Interpersonal Modes and Occupational Therapy Core Values**

- Physical embodiment of the impairment (e.g., clients' bodily experience and their interpretations of that experience)
- Interpersonal experience (e.g., their thoughts and feelings toward the therapist and/or others in the treatment milieu at any given time)

Therapists in the empathizing mode value clients' experience to such an extent that they do not try to speed the pace of therapy or work to modify a client's perceptions, even if those perceptions are negative. Rather than hypothesizing about or assuming what a client might be thinking or feeling, therapists who emphasize the empathizing mode take the extra time required to under-stand thoroughly these experiences from the client's perspective. They actively and continually seek input and feedback from the client. They value patience and empathic listening as necessary requirements not only for understanding clients' experience accurately but also for communicating with clients in a truthful and authentic way. Although they maintain the focus on the clients rather than themselves, these therapists also know how to reference their own physical and emotional reactions to clients as a guide for moving as close as possible to their clients' experience during therapy. Accordingly, therapists in the empathizing mode tend to value the process of therapy over the outcomes; they view positive outcomes as a natural consequence of their careful attention to the process.

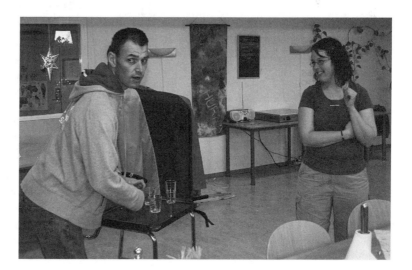

FIGURE 14.2 Clients deserve advocacy efforts on the part of the therapist

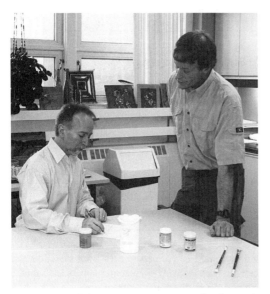

FIGURE 14.3 Collaboration conveys an attitude of mutual respect and belief in clients' capacities

Therefore, the occupational therapy core values that are most closely associated with the empathizing mode include altruism, dignity, and truth (Fig. 14.4).

Encouraging Mode

Therapists who emphasize the encouraging mode place a high value on hope and view it as a priority for occupational therapy practice. They tend to be optimistic and are

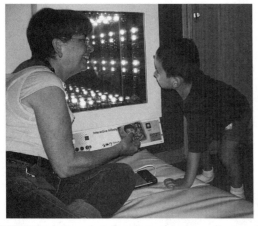

FIGURE 14.4 Empathy is foundational to any application of core values

comfortable imaging clients' futures in the most positive light possible. These therapists also tend to emphasize clients' potential rather than focusing on the problems or obstacles in their current life situations. They view all clients as having inherent worth and as being capable of achieving positive outcomes in therapy. They may work tremendously hard in an attempt to make this belief a reality for their clients. They put a lot of effort into instilling and preserving hope in the minds of their clients. They may utilize a lot of positive language and spend a great deal of time discussing future possibilities with clients. In addition, therapists who emphasize the encouraging mode tend to value humor and good cheer in their interactions with clients. They want clients to enjoy the experience of therapy as much as possible. Because these therapists believe in hope and in promoting experiences of self-efficacy in clients, the occupational therapy core value that is most closely associated with the encouraging mode is dignity (Fig. 14.5).

Instructing Mode

Therapists who focus on the instructing mode value the importance of structure, leadership, education, and the transfer of knowledge as powerful avenues for participation and change. These therapists believe that the empowerment of clients occurs primarily through skills-based learning and other teaching approaches aimed at facilitating adaptation to impairment and occupational engagement. They perceive all clients as being capable of learning and growth at some level and hold a general expectation that clients will experience successful outcomes if they strive to learn and adhere to the therapist's recommendations. These therapists are of the opinion that therapy is best accomplished when the therapist functions as a leader who guides the client through the therapy process. They may value a social-learning approach to occupational therapy in which they view themselves as role-models for their clients. In addition, some instructor-coaches may believe that therapy occurs best in a highly structured and contained setting, even in a community context. Because they tend to be goal-oriented, they tend to value performance and outcomes. Instructor-coaches view therapy as being most successful when clients show improvement over time and when they are able to accomplish the objectives and goals of therapy. Being competent, having a particular expertise, and keeping current with the latest technical developments may be particularly important to these therapists' professional identity as occupa-

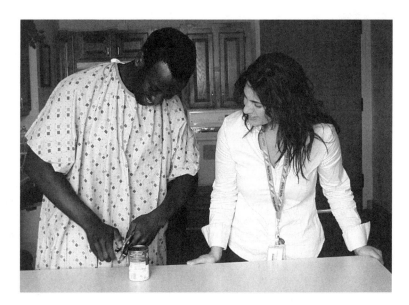

FIGURE 14.5 It is an obligation to provide our clients with hope

tional therapists. Therefore, the occupational therapy core values that are most closely associated with the instructing mode include justice, truth, and prudence (Fig. 14.6).

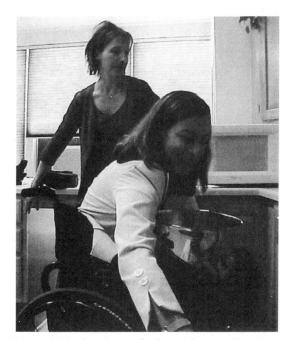

FIGURE 14.6 Education is a fundamental aspect of occupational therapy

Problem-Solving

Therapists who prefer the problem-solving mode are true believers in solutions and techniques, using the correct and most contemporary procedures and technologies as means of ensuring therapeutic effectiveness. When problems arise, they value a reasoned and analytical approach that involves weighing options in an attempt to reach a solution. Therapists who emphasize the problem-solving mode tend to value evidence-based practice and scientific approaches to care that include hypothesis generation, hypothesis testing, deductive reasoning, and evaluation of outcomes. When interacting with clients, these therapists may come across as highly disciplined, logical, and circumspect. Thus, the occupational therapy core values that are most consistent with this mode include justice and prudence (Table 14.3).

Overview

When reflecting on the values that are most closely associated with a preferred interpersonal mode, it is important to bear in mind that there is no reason why other values not linked to a particular mode in this section may also be utilized with that mode. Moreover, the fact that one mode may be associated with a greater number of values than another says nothing about whether a therapist who emphasizes the mode with the highest number of values is a more value-driven therapist. These guidelines were established not to promote competition between the modes but, instead, to generate thinking about the ways in which your use of self at any given time may reflect your professional values.

Behavioral Self-Awareness

Behavioral self-awareness refers to therapists' ability to observe and restrict their nonverbal communications with their clients so they convey a *professional presence*, or a feeling of centeredness and professionalism. Introduced in Chapter 8, nonverbal communications consist of vocal utterances and tone of voice; body postures, movements, gestures, and stance; physical appearance; and facial expressions. Nonverbal communication provides clients with information about your thoughts and feelings that may not be directly articulated.

Thus, it has the potential to reveal things that you are thinking or feeling but may not wish or intend to share with the client. For example, most of us have idiosyncratic habits or quirks that occur when we are not conscious of them. Examples of such behaviors include:

> Nonverbal communication provides clients with information about your thoughts and feelings that may not be directly articulated.

- Playing or fidgeting with writing utensils or office supplies
- Rocking, wiggling, or swinging your body, legs or feet
- Nodding your head excessively when interacting
- Excessive use of verbal prompts (e.g., "uh hmm" or "that's good")
- Stereotypically rubbing or stroking an object or a part of your body in an attempt to soothe yourself
- Arranging, twirling, or otherwise playing with your hair
- Eye contact that is prolonged or intense
- Lack of eye contact or darting eyes
- Excessive blinking of eyes
- Cracking your knuckles or biting your nails or cuticles
- Scratching, picking, or other grooming habits that should occur in private
- Exhibiting a facial tick, wince, or slight snarl in reaction to something
- Showing fatigue or exhaustion in your facial expression

- Obvious referencing of the clock or your wristwatch at poorly timed moments during the session
- Clenching your fists or grasping tightly to furniture or other objects
- Clenching your jaw, grinding your teeth
- Chewing on gum or candy
- Shifting body weight or posture too frequently or in ways that are unrelated to the occupation at hand while sitting and listening to or observing the client
- Exhibiting a posture or stance that appears judgmental, disappointed, or closed during times when communication of these messages would not be therapeutic
- Using a high, tense, shrill, or overly loud tone of voice
- Nervous giggling or excessive laughter

If allowed to occur in the presence of clients, some of these habits or quirks may communicate that a therapist is preoccupied or feeling geared-up and not completely centered and attentive during the interaction. Clients may interpret any of these behaviors as the therapist being impatient, restless, full of too much energy, bored, uneasy, nervous, or uncomfortable (even when a therapist is not conscious of such feelings or is thinking about and reacting to something that has nothing to do with the client). When practicing according to the IRM, it is important to exhibit behavioral self-awareness so your nonverbal communications convey a feeling of professionalism and centeredness. Closely associated with a take-charge attitude, you may develop a professional presence through self-observation and by practicing the following behaviors.

- Sitting or standing solidly and quietly in the presence of a client and feeling your weight within your center of gravity
- Allowing your arms to drop at your sides or to rest in your lap slightly in front of your body without feeling compelled to do something with them
- Allowing your palms to face slightly forward when standing or slightly turned upward when sitting and allowing your fingers to cup the air naturally and gently in order to communicate an attitude of openness and tranquility

• When you want to convey an attitude of attentiveness, sitting upright with the back as straight as possible and shoulders as far back as possible

• Leaning forward slightly if you need to convey a heightened level of interest

• Allowing yourself to sit back or recline in a chair if you wish to convey an attitude of relaxation

• Folding your hands in classroom fashion to demonstrate self-restraint and patience

• While sitting, cupping one hand around the fist of the other hand to convey strength, confidence, or a take-charge attitude

• Maintaining a deliberately lower, more soothing tone of voice

• Keeping your forehead, eyebrows, cheeks, mouth, and jaw relaxed at rest and in fluid and natural movement while speaking (Fig. 14.7)

If you are having difficultly relaxing before therapy sessions or when seeing particularly challenging clients, you may consider receiving training in meditation or relaxation techniques and engaging in these exercises in a quiet room just before interacting with the client. If you have received feedback that you are not naturally self-aware, you may wish to ask a supervisor or peer to observe your nonverbal behaviors during a session, or you may choose to videotape a therapy session. If this is not possible, you may wish to role-play a clinical interaction and videotape it or have someone present who is assigned to observe and point out your nonverbal behaviors.

In addition to your behaviors, your physical appearance represents another form of important nonverbal com-

munication that is readily seen and interpretable by clients. It is not only essential that your appearance is clean and safe for clients, it is also important that it is not offensive or provocative in any way.[1] Ways in which you may maintain a desirable physical appearance in the presence of clients include:

• Brushing teeth and bathing or showering daily to promote good hygiene and reduce odors that may be interpreted as offensive by some clients

• Hygiene and care of fingernails

• Good hair care

• Clothing that is flexible and easy to move in, with no sharp or protruding objects

• Clothing that has minimal to no chance of being interpreted as sexually provocative by clients (e.g., neckline not too low, shirt buttoned up to second button, skirts, if worn, should be knee-length or longer)

• Jewelry should be simple or absent when having close physical contact with clients to prevent ripping, breaking, or choking hazards

• Footwear should allow for easy movement and should not have open or exposed toes, protruding objects, or heel types that could be dangerous to clients

Although students sometimes tell me that such a list is unnecessary because they already know how to maintain good hygiene, I consistently hear of stories about students

[1]Requirements for physical appearance are culture-specific and vary according to where you might be practicing in the world. The guidelines presented here represent practices that are generally supported in institutions in the United States.

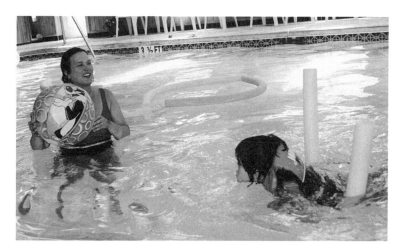

FIGURE 14.7 Regardless of setting or activity, it is important to convey a strong professional presence during therapy

from various programs whose physical presentation has caused some type of difficulty for them during training. So, although it may seem obvious to some, my hope is that this list helps prevent more students from facing what could be an embarrassing situation for them.

In addition to basic safety and hygiene considerations, you should have a general awareness of the interpersonal image you wish to project to clients. Your clothing, hairstyle, eyewear, footwear, jewelry, tattoos and body adornments, facial hair choices for men, and makeup choices for women project a unique social image that is plainly visible to clients. When considering your physical appearance during therapy, it is important to think about how you would like to be perceived. Examples of images therapists may project to clients simply by virtue of their physical appearance include:

• Authoritative or professional
• Relaxed or approachable
• Simple or neutral
• Youthful
• Mature
• Sophisticated
• Successful or status-oriented
• Particularly feminine, particularly masculine, or neither
• Conservative
• Artistic or creative
• Fashionable or trendy
• Alternative or outwardly different
• Identified with a certain religious or social group

There are countless images therapists can project through their physical appearances. In turn, there are numerous ways clients may interpret these images. In mental health settings, some professionals espouse the value of consistency and neutrality in dress and appearance (i.e., dressing as plainly and conservatively as possible, keeping makeup simple, keeping long hair under control or away from the face, and wearing few to no adornments). The ideal is to dress in a way that has no potential to be overstimulating or to detract attention away from clients. The rationale behind this value is that neutrality and consistency allow clients to focus on themselves and on the activities of therapy rather than on how you look or on what you are wearing on any given day.

Although neutrality and consistency decrease the likelihood that clients will pay attention to your physical appearance, the reality is that even if you attempt to be neutral in your physical appearance it is inevitable that some clients will focus on or interpret this neutrality in some way. Natural aspects of our appearance as basic as our height, weight, skin color, and facial features are bound to generate reactions in our clients, especially if they are distinctive or unusual in some way. Therefore, you are encouraged to choose an image that does not intentionally offend, upset, or otherwise detract attention away from the therapy process but at the same time feels natural and true to you. If you happen to naturally possess a certain distinctive physical characteristic or if you deliberately choose a nonneutral image that may generate more of a reaction, it is important that you take responsibility for and actively address any interpersonal consequences that may accompany a client's reaction.

Reliability

Reliability is defined as being utterly consistent and predictable with clients. It includes being present and on time to all therapy sessions without deviation. In addition, it involves following through on whatever you say you will do no matter how much effort it takes. It is an essential professional behavior because it communicates a willingness to be wholly present and available; it promotes trust; and it sets an example that shapes clients' behavior. Ironically, the most important prerequisite for being reliable for clients in these ways involves setting limits around time and scheduling and maintaining boundaries around what you are willing to do for clients outside the sessions.

If your setting allows, it is advisable to have a working appointment schedule that involves each client having a specific time and day of the week in which he or she is seen. Each client's session should begin on time and end reliably at the same time, allowing time between sessions for documentation of chart notes. It is important to resist the urge to give a client more time during a session because he or she was late. The consequence of this seemingly benevolent behavior is that the therapist disappoints other clients by running late and makes work more difficult than it needs to be by missing the opportunity to write notes between clients. It is equally important to deny clients' requests to reschedule appointment times for nonessential matters because it often requires that the therapist change the established appointments of other clients.

Any effort you make to keep appointments timely and to maintain a set schedule establishes a precedent for clients to attend regularly, show up on time, and feel that your time allotment is fair and equivalent to that of other clients. Although it may occasionally involve denying gratification for clients who are more difficult or entitled, if you are firm with your limits around time and scheduling you will find that most of your clients show a greater level of respect for your time and efforts. In addition, you are likely to feel more centered and prepared before each session because you are not stressed by attempts to overextend to accommodate the unrealistic needs of your more difficult clients.

In addition to being predictable and consistent about appointments, it is vital to remember what you have offered to do for a client and to follow through on what you say you are going to do. This may be as simple as telling clients that arts and crafts is the activity planned for tomorrow and then ensure that this is what is done. In contrast, it may be as involved as telling a client that you will attempt to seek out a specialist with a certain type of expertise and inform the client of every effort made along the way to ensure that the appropriate professional is located. Failure to follow through on commitments decreases clients' faith in you and forces them to lower their expectations of therapy. In some cases, it may even have an effect on the client's view of the profession as a whole.

Confidentiality

Confidentiality is an ethical principle ensuring that any communication or behavior that occurs between a client and therapist is kept private by the therapist and is not divulged to anyone else. Confidentiality is vital to trust, and believing in it allows clients to feel comfortable sharing information with you that they may not feel comfortable sharing with anyone else. Confidentiality not only requires that you hold this personal information privately in your mind, but it also requires that you limit what you put in writing to only that which is essential for the documentation requirements of the setting and the insurer. Whatever is put into writing should be maintained in a locked cabinet with restricted access only by providers who have permission to view the file.

In most settings, there are a limited number of exceptions to confidentiality in which a therapist has permission to disclose certain information to another party. Depending on the area of the world and on the laws that govern licensure in that area, these exceptions to confidentiality often include circumstances in which:

- Using a document authorized by the setting and by local laws that govern practice, a client has given written permission to disclose specific information to a specific person for a specific purpose (e.g., for the purpose of receiving reimbursement from an insurance company)
- Clients pose a danger to themselves or others (i.e., a client has expressed an intention to commit suicide or to physically harm someone else)
- A child under a therapist's care is being physically abused, sexually abused, or neglected
- A client of any age, including an elderly individual, is experiencing any type of abuse or neglect

Throughout the world, various ethical guidelines, setting-specific policies, and laws have been put into place to protect clients' confidentiality and to preserve the privacy of their health-related information. You are responsible for familiarizing yourself with the policies and laws governing your local setting. Violating any of these policies or laws can cost you your employment and/or license and can put you at risk for legal actions.

Professional Boundaries

A *professional boundary* is a framework within which the client–therapist relationship occurs that protects both the client and the therapist from attempting to get certain emotional and psychological needs met that should not be met as a function of therapy. Boundaries help clients know what to expect (and what not to expect) from the therapeutic relationship, and they serve to reassure clients that you will not attempt to exploit, manipulate, or use the relationship as a means of getting your own needs met. Boundaries protect you by allowing you to structure and set limits on what you offer clients and when you offer it, so you are not pressured to overextend or accommodate clients with needs that are excessive or unrealistic. Boundaries allow you sufficient time and space outside your relationships with clients to pursue independent activities, personal responsibilities, relationships with others, and general self-care. When you set and maintain boundaries for a client, you do a favor for any health professional the client sees thereafter. This is because the client will already be familiar with what he or she can and cannot expect in a professional relationship. Thus, the client will be less likely to test limits and act out unexpressed emotional needs in treatment relationships.

Boundaries are important to establish at the beginning of the therapeutic relationship and to uphold throughout the course of the relationship. Establishing boundaries includes all of the following therapist behaviors.

- Setting a fee for services, even if it is nominal, just to define the relationship as a professional one
- Maintaining a consistent time at which each session begins and ends—not allowing clients to drop in at their leisure or attempt to manipulate their scheduled time as a means of gratifying emotional needs
- Limiting or restricting therapist self-disclosure of personal information
- Using touch judiciously (see Chapter 9)
- Being clear about your role and responsibilities as a therapist and any limits to that role
- Assuming a professional presence and conveying a take-charge attitude
- Freely setting limits on inappropriate language or behavior at the time in which it occurs
- Reminding clients of the exceptions to confidentiality (harm to self, harm to others, child abuse and neglect) and acting immediately to protect clients and others in situations of risk
- Ensuring that the therapy environment is appropriate and professional or creating a structure for therapy in an informal environment

Because of the inherent power differential in the therapeutic relationship, you as the therapist are always the person who is responsible for knowing and maintaining the boundaries. This is consistent with responsibility taking, which is an integral aspect of interpersonal self-discipline (see Chapter 3). Clients often initiate behaviors or make requests that blur or test the boundaries of the professional relationship. Typical circumstances where boundaries can be tested or blurred include:

- Asking the therapist personal questions or making requests that the therapist self-disclose personal information
- Giving the therapist gifts at inappropriate times or of inappropriate value or expense in an attempt to influence, impress, or treat the therapist as a close friend or family member
- Inviting the therapist to join in a dual relationship, such as going into business together or volunteering to fix a dent the client noticed in the therapist's car
- Ignoring the established structure or time frames of therapy

- Initiating physical touch with the therapist
- Calling the therapist by a nickname or other informal name that one might use with a close friend or family member (e.g., referring to the therapist as "Lu" when she chooses to present herself to clients as "Lu Ann")
- Inviting the therapist to lunch, dinner, or another social event with the goal of having a more personal relationship with the therapist

Occupational therapy is an intimate process that requires close interaction between client and therapist. This interaction may occur in a client's community, home, or other natural living environment, heightening the need for clarity and consistency regarding the limits and boundaries of the therapeutic relationship. There are times, however, when you may choose to relax one of the boundaries of therapy. In some cases, partially gratifying a client's request within limits, provided it is accompanied by an intentional discussion of the meaning of those limits, can be therapeutic for a client. This may take the form of giving a client a small transitional object that reminds him of therapy, receiving a greeting card or a small container of homemade cookies from a client, going out of your way to take a client to a more preferable location to swim, or responding to certain questions about certain aspects of your personal life to set a client at ease or allow the client to know you more as a person. An example of one therapist's intentional decision to respond to a client's request for the disclosure of highly personal information is provided in Box 14.1.

When deciding whether to relax a boundary of therapy, there are important questions to ask yourself.

- Would relaxing this boundary be consistent with the occupational therapy code of ethics?
- Would I be comfortable documenting this action in the client's file?
- Am I treating this client differently than I would treat other clients in this circumstance?
- How does it gratify my emotional and psychological needs?
- How does it gratify the emotional and psychological needs of the client?
- What are the long-term consequences of this action for the therapeutic relationship?
- Would I feel comfortable telling a colleague about this?
- Is this action in my client's ultimate best interest?
- Am I able and willing to sustain this behavior over time (e.g., possibly years)?

<hr />

Box 14.1   A Therapist's Response to Boundary Testing

Monsieur Boulanger[2] was a young adult with a diagnosis of schizophrenia who was referred to occupational therapy because of an increase in symptoms and suicidal ideation thought to be associated with recent separation from his girlfriend. At the beginning of therapy, he was emotionally shut down and completely unwilling to talk about himself. Each time I attempted to initiate a therapeutic discussion with him, he would begin to ask me personal questions. He would always protest by asking me why he was required to talk about his personal experiences and I was not. After several explanations, which included reframing the two different interpersonal contexts for him, clarifying my role as a therapist and his need to focus on himself, therapy sessions became less and less productive with time. Eventually, Monsieur Boulanger began to do things in order to avoid our individual sessions, and he refused to participate actively in setting collaborative therapeutic objectives.

One day, he asked me very directly if I had ever been divorced and alone. This question was personal and at the same time general enough for me to feel comfortable responding. Because I saw no other avenue for progress with Monsieur Boulanger outside of his need for me to self-disclose, I decided to tell him that I had experienced a kind of divorce and was alone for a year thereafter. I did not provide any other details, but at that point he began to express his fears of being alone and to reveal some of his feelings of rejection. At that point, I made an agreement with him. I told him that my response to his question about my divorce was, from that point

forward, the only personal information that I was willing to reveal. I told him that I had reached my limit and asked that he never try to pressure me into disclosing information again as a means of refusing to work on his own therapy goals. He agreed.

From this point forward, Monsieur Boulanger's behavior changed, and he became more emotionally available during our individual sessions. He also showed more of an investment in group therapy. He developed the ability to maintain a single continuous conversation about daily living challenges and other emotional difficulties in his life. Over time, he gained insight into his maladaptive behaviors and learned to apply different concrete strategies for affect management, and he learned to replace maladaptive interpersonal behaviors with more positive ones. Inevitably, his attempts to know more about my personal life continued during his entire course of therapy. However, he was able to accept the fact we had made an agreement before about the limits of the therapeutic relationship. Unlike before, he tolerated this limit without resistance, and he collaborated with me on therapy objectives. He still attends meetings on the unit with his psychiatrist, and from time to time I see him in the waiting room or in the hospital corridors. Every time he stops me and says, "Occupational therapy helped me a lot." Other colleagues, nurses, and social workers have told me about his positive comments regarding his occupational therapy sessions as well.

— **René Bélanger**

<hr />

[2] All client names and geographic information have been changed.

- Will this action invite more boundary testing?
- Will the client come to expect more from me than I am able and willing to give?
- Is there a chance that this action may cause the client confusion about the purpose of therapy or the limits of the relationship?

The Activities section of this chapter offers an exercise that allows reflection on various situations in which a therapist's boundaries may be tested. You are encouraged to reflect on these scenarios and share examples from your own practice.

Summary

This chapter reviewed the core values and ethics that provide the foundation for professional behavior in the field of occupational therapy. In addition, ways in which those core values are associated with the six interpersonal

modes were discussed. Specific aspects of professional behavior, including behavioral self-awareness, reliability, confidentiality, and professional boundaries were emphasized; and examples and exercises were provided to encourage reflection on these topics. At first glance, all of the professional behaviors covered in the chapter may seem straightforward. However, the purpose of the chapter was to reveal the hidden nuances and complexities associated with these behaviors. Experienced therapists know that sustaining these behaviors day after day and year after year with different clients and through all of the twists and turns in your personal and professional lives can be challenging at times. For this reason, the IRM principle of interpersonal self-discipline is particularly relevant to any discussion of professional behavior. When you are reflective and intentional about your application of occupational therapy core values and ethics, you benefit from added confidence in your decision-making when various dilemmas arise in practice.

References

American Occupational Therapy Association (1993). Core values and attitudes of occupational therapy practice. *American Journal of Occupational Therapy, 47,* 1085–1086.

American Occupational Therapy Association (2005). *AOTA: Occupational therapy code of ethics.* Bethesda, MD: AOTA. http://www.aota.org/.

ACTIVITIES FOR LEARNING AND REFLECTION

Resolving Ethical Dilemmas in Practice

This exercise describes a series of ethical dilemmas faced by occupational therapists in practice. Although these dilemmas reflect actual occurrences, the characters and details of the dilemmas have been fictionalized to protect the confidentiality of those involved. Please read each dilemma and respond to the corresponding questions. You may refer to Table 14-2 to guide your responses. You are then encouraged to share and discuss your responses with a partner or with a work group. At the end of the exercise, a question about your own experience is provided to allow for continued reflection and discussion.

Ethical Dilemma 1: Client with a Questionable Appearance

Terry is an occupational therapist with strong personal and political views about equality, discrimination, and racism. Her uncle, an Orthodox Jewish man, was once the victim of a hate crime committed by a so-called member of the white supremacy movement. Terry is the only occupational therapist working in a rural hospital on the spinal cord injury unit. The service recipient who has been referred to Terry is a White adolescent with his head shaved. He is wearing a jeans jacket that has a confederate flag sewn on the back, and he has an offensive tattoo on his arm. These characteristics remind Terry of images of white supremacy that she once saw on a television show. Terry begins to feel very uneasy about treating this person.

1a. What ethical principle(s) are at stake for Terry?

_____

1b. What steps should Terry take to resolve this situation?

_____

Ethical Dilemma 2: Different Worlds

Pat, a recently trained occupational therapist, just moved back home to rural Kansas from having completed her level II fieldwork training in a state-of-the-art hospital in California. Pat quickly realizes that her senior occupational therapy colleague is practicing outdated treatment techniques and using outdated equipment. Although it poses no safety hazard to the clients, Pat knows that they could be receiving better care. Because it is Pat's first job outside of school and she does not want to relocate, she is concerned that raising the issue might upset her colleague and cost her a job.

2a. What ethical principle(s) is Pat facing?

_____

2b. What ethical principles is Pat's colleague facing?

2c. What steps, if any, should Pat take to resolve this situation?

Ethical Dilemma 3: An Ambitious Doctoral Student

Marcy is a doctoral student who is only one step away from completing the degree requirements of her PhD program in occupational therapy. The only thing standing in her way is that she needs to have a sample of 50 research participants (adults with developmental disabilities). Marcy is on her 49th subject and just a week away from her deadline. She approaches the only adult in the last of three community homes who has not yet participated. He is known for refusing to participate in activities that are unfamiliar to him and is capable of choosing occupations he prefers. Marcy approaches him, and he declines to participate. However, she already has the signed consent of his guardian, who told her, "Just push him and he'll do it."

3a. What ethical principle(s) should Marcy bear in mind when facing this situation?

3b. What should Marcy do?

Ethical Dilemma 4: An Occupational Therapist in Need of Support

Ted, a long-time occupational therapist, is facing a difficult situation in his family. His daughter has cystic fibrosis, and her illness has worsened recently owing to a complicating episode of mononucleosis. Hospital visits and subsequent trips to the clinic have taken their toll on Ted. Because he spends after-school and evening hours with his daughter (his spouse takes the day shift), he has missed countless hours of sleep, has increased his alcohol intake, and has lost his appetite. However, Ted keeps on functioning and showing up to work day after day. His performance appears unaffected, but internally he is ready to vent to a colleague whom he can trust. Andrea is that colleague, and one day on the subway going home Andrea bears witness to Ted's painful story.

4a. What ethical principle(s) does Ted need to keep in mind as he faces this situation?

4b. What ethical principle(s) should Andrea keep in mind as she faces this situation?

4c. What steps, if any, should Ted take to resolve this situation?

4d. What steps, if any, should Andrea take to resolve this situation?

Ethical Dilemma 5: An Expert Facing a New Type of Client

Angie is a level I fieldwork student training at a prestigious rehabilitation center in New York City. Her supervisor, who is also the director of the clinic, is an experienced practitioner who is well known in the field for her expertise in assistive technologies. Angie is basically in awe of her as she has read her journal articles and attended her workshops at conferences. The first client to whom Angie is assigned is a child with an autistic spectrum disorder referred by his neurologist to work on sensory processing. Angie's supervisor starts to assemble supplies for sensory integration therapy and leads Angie into the gymnasium where sensory integration treatment takes place at the clinic. Chuckling, the supervisor confides that the only therapist with expertise in sensory integration is on maternity leave, so she will have to train Angie in sensory integration techniques. She then adds that she has never really practiced these techniques before but that she has watched her colleague practice from time to time and has read about them in various journal articles.

5a. What ethical principles is Angie facing as the therapist in training?

_____

5b. What ethical principles must the supervisor consider?

_____

5c. What should Angie do?

_____

5d. What should the supervisor do?

_____

Ethical Dilemma 6: A Concerned and Emotional Family Member

Ally is an occupational therapist practicing in an acute care inpatient unit in a hospital just outside of Los Angeles. When demonstrating transfer training with an elderly client in front of the client's adult daughter, the patient suddenly becomes faint and slips through Ally's hands and falls to the floor. At that point the patient's daughter becomes very distressed and threatens to sue both Ally and the hospital. Because the client only appears to have red marks on her elbow and hip and says she is ok, Ally is reluctant to file a report of the incident (as required by hospital procedures). Her reluctance is based on her hopes that the daughter was just being emotional and on her fear that, by putting the incident down on paper, she will make herself even more vulnerable to litigation.

6a. What ethical principles should Ally keep in mind?

_____

6b. What should Ally do?

_____

Ethical Dilemma 7: A Potentially Dangerous Liaison

Rachel is an occupational therapist living in Nebraska. Her former client, who has had severe bipolar disorder for most of her adult life, is now a user of occupational therapy services at a psychiatric day hospitalization facility in Wisconsin. Rachel's former client phones her at the clinic one day and confides that she has begun having an intimate relationship with a male occupational therapist who works in her day hospitalization program. She is overjoyed and tells Rachel that this is the best thing that has ever happened to her. She is even considering a return to work.

7a. What ethical principle(s) pertain to this situation for Rachel, the therapist in Nebraska?

_____

7b. What ethical principle(s) pertain to this situation for the therapist in Wisconsin?

_____

7c. If you were Rachel, what initial steps would you take to resolve this situation?

_____

7d. If those were not effective, what would you do next?

_____

Reflection Question

Have you ever witnessed or experienced one of these or some other ethical violation in a health care relationship? If so, briefly describe it here.

_____

_____

_____

To your knowledge, was the dilemma resolved? If so, how was it resolved, and what was the outcome?

_____

_____

_____

EXERCISE 14.2

Professional Boundaries

This exercise describes a series of situations where boundaries in the therapeutic relationship have the potential to be tested or blurred. Read and reflect on how you might manage each of these situations as the therapist. If possible, discuss your point of view with a partner or work group. Following the scenarios, you are encouraged to respond to some questions about your own practice experience.

• A client who you respect and like knows that you enjoy yoga. One day she invites you to come to her yoga center for a class together.
• A client's mother invites you to attend her daughter's graduation from grade school. She tells you she attributes much of her daughter's success in school to you. The pediatric client would be thrilled if you attended.

- Upon terminating your treatment relationship, a client, who is unemployed and receiving public aid, gives you a box of stationery as a sign of her appreciation of all that you did to help her reunite with her children.
- A client has mentioned before that he owns a condo in the Broadway district of Manhattan that he is trying to rent out. Your sister just moved to Manhattan and is looking to rent a condo immediately, as she has been burning through her money staying in hotels.
- During your treatment relationship, a client gives you a $200 gift certificate to your favorite four-star restaurant. She tells you that her uncle owns the restaurant and that it is a sign of her appreciation for all you have done for her.
- Following a severe fever, your husband has been fatigued and ill ever since returning from a trip to the Australian bush. He has seen his personal physician, who has reassured him it is probably a case of the flu. However, both you and he agree it seems much worse than that. One of your clients mentioned at the intake interview that his wife is one of the top infectious disease specialists in the United States.

In your own experience, have you ever encountered a situation in which a client or other service recipient did something or made a request that tested the boundaries of your relationship? If so, briefly describe the situation here.

_____

_____

_____

_____

What did you do to manage the situation?

_____

_____

In retrospect, is there anything you would have done differently a second time around?

_____

_____

CHAPTER 15

WORKING EFFECTIVELY WITH SUPERVISORS, EMPLOYERS, AND OTHER PROFESSIONALS

Whether you are a student, a therapist, an educator, an administrator, a fieldwork supervisor, or any combination of the above, you always stand to benefit from building relationships with other professionals. Many rehabilitation settings host multidisciplinary meetings, require periodic consultation or supervision, or incorporate co-therapy interventions that involve more than one professional. Depending on the needs of the population being served, occupational therapists may work collaboratively with a wide range of health care professionals. These may include, but are not limited to:

- Other occupational therapists
- Certified occupational therapy assistants
- Physicians from various specialties
- Physical therapists
- Physiotherapists
- Speech therapists
- Recreation therapists
- Art therapists
- Nursing professionals from various specialties
- Psychologists with various specializations
- Medical social workers
- Vocational rehabilitation specialists and rehabilitation counselors
- Aides of various kinds
- Other technicians
- Supervisors or employers from various disciplines
- Teachers/educators

Working collaboratively with another professional may be as simple as exchanging essential verbal information about a client or as complex as a long-term co-therapy relationship in which the collaborating professional joins the occupational therapist during treatment sessions over a period of weeks, months, or years. Irrespective of the complexity of the relationship, any time two professionals have contact concerning a client it presents an opportunity for a successful outcome (i.e., one that supports the best interests of the client) or an unsuccessful outcome (i.e., one that slows or interferes with the client's treatment).

Successful outcomes of any collaboration depend, at least in part, on whether the collaborators share similar goals for the client and similar opinions about how to approach treatment with the client (e.g., practice frameworks or theoretical orientations to treatment). The more similar the two professionals are in terms of the overarching values and techniques of their professional disciplines, their areas of specialization, and their training and practice experience, the more likely it is that their goals for the client and orientations toward treatment are complementary. However, even when two collaborators share common backgrounds and ideologies (e.g., both are pediatric occupational therapists who utilize sensory integration as a practice framework), it is inevitable that at some point the individuals will differ in opinion or in practice behavior. Ideally, if both individuals are open to learning about and incorporating the others' unique point of view, the collaboration will likely be successful and the client will likely benefit from what both professionals can offer. However, relying on chance for this to occur puts both the collaboration and the client at risk for failure. For this reason, it is important to approach any collaborative relationship with intentionality, no matter how straightforward it seems initially.

There are a number of ways in which you may approach a given collaboration with intentionality. They include:

• Asking the collaborator for education regarding the basic values, world views, and practice techniques used in his or her treatment approach. Alternatively, if this is not possible, educating yourself regarding these issues by drawing upon literary resources or other personal and professional relationships.
• Being able to describe your own orientation to practice and preferred practice techniques clearly and in a way that facilitates dialogue and further understanding. This begins by taking the initiative to provide such information as a means of introducing yourself to the collaborator.
• Being able to identify not only the strengths but also the weaknesses of your preferred orientation to practice. This requires knowledge of the pros and cons of any orientation to practice, and it demands that you exercise the Intentional Relationship Model (IRM) principle of critical self-awareness.
• Being able to describe your impressions of and goals for the client straightforwardly while at the same time demonstrating a willingness to learn and receive input from the collaborator.
• Continually monitoring the collaborative relationship for the potential occurrence of inevitable interpersonal events. The interpersonal events most likely to occur in collaborative relationships with other professionals include power dilemmas, empathic breaks that stem from differing perspectives and boundary issues, and events associated with the limitations of each professional's knowledge and scope of practice.
• Acting promptly to resolve any empathic breaks that do occur within the relationship.
• When significant differences in ideology or practice behavior disrupt the collaboration, using conflict resolution skills to prevent any negative long-term consequences.

Collaborative work with another professional may take place in the direct presence of the client or in the client's absence. The objectives and nature of the collaboration differ depending on whether the client is present. In addition, the rank or status of the other professional relative to your own rank or status may influence the course or eventual outcome of the collaboration. Each of these situations presents unique considerations for the collaborating professionals.

Collaborations in the Client's Absence

Contact with other professionals in a client's absence may be precipitated by a referral, a specific question about an existing client, a need for ongoing consultation regarding a client, or by an established norm for contact within a setting, such as an in-service meeting, a weekly staffing meeting, or a supervision meeting. Depending on the setting and the nature of the relationship between the involved professionals, collaborations that take place in the client's absence may assume any of the following forms.

• Spontaneous face-to-face discussion
• Spontaneous phone call
• Preplanned phone conference or face-to-face meeting
• Dialogue by e-mail

Each of these situations creates a different mood and a different expectation regarding how much information will be exchanged and the efficiency and style in which it will be exchanged. For example, a spontaneous discussion that occurs in the staff lounge may involve a more relaxed and candid exchange, or more blunt language may be used. A spontaneous phone call that interrupts the professional in the middle of his or her workday may result in a rushed conversation in which certain details are lost. With an e-mail exchange, there is a high risk that empathic breaks may occur because there is no means of assessing the affect and tone of voice of the other individual. When used as a means of addressing disagreements or handling conflicts, e-mail exchanges have the potential to lead to unresolved differences and permanent rifts in relationships. When applying the IRM, it is important to think about the context for interaction with another professional and to act thoughtfully when engaging in unplanned interactions.

Anytime contact with another professional takes place in a client's absence, issues of confidentiality are always a primary consideration. Whenever two individuals share information about a client, there remains a lingering possibility that the client may eventually become privy to that information. Clients may become privy to information by reading their own medical records (assuming the professional has documented the contact) or if one of the professionals involved chooses to share the content of the exchange with the client. Moreover, when clients are aware that two professionals have been in contact regarding their treatment, they often inquire about the nature and content of the conversation. In these instances, it is important that the two professionals be prepared for such questions and are able to present to the client (or others) a clear and consistent description of the conversation that took place.

In some instances, professionals may find the need to exchange information about a client that they do not wish the client to know. This kind of need arises most often in one of three circumstances.

• When two professionals disagree over an issue concerning the client
• When an empathic break or disagreement has occurred between one of the collaborating professionals and the client
• When the client's personal problems or psychological presentation affect the course of treatment and the collaborating professionals need to make an intentional plan about how to manage the interpersonal aspects of the situation together.

When two professionals disagree over an issue, they should make an intentional decision about whether to share their disagreement with the client. This involves weighing whether sharing the nature of the disagreement would support the client's best interests. In some instances, a disagreement between two professionals may be irrelevant to the quality of care a client receives. For example, revealing a personal conflict between two professionals to a client may confuse the client, lower his or her hopes about something one of the professionals had said or recommended, or damage his or her view of one of the professionals. An example of Jane Melton's decision not to inform a client about a conflict with the client's caseworkers (managers of his care team) is presented in Box 15.1.

In other situations, it is important for a client to know that a disagreement between two professionals has taken place. This is often the most ethical thing to do because it allows the client to weigh the perspectives of each professional and make an informed decision about the course of his or her own care. For example, if an occupational therapist and physical therapist disagree over the degree to which a young client with cerebral palsy should use powered mobility, it might be highly informative to the client's parents to hear the opposing perspectives on this issue so they can make an independent decision about what is best for their child.

Similarly, there will be occasions when a disagreement occurs between one of the collaborating professionals and the client. In this instance, the collaborator may con-

---

> **Box 15.1 Therapist's Choice Not to Inform a Client About a Conflict**
>
> Box 4.2 presented Jane Melton's conflict with the managers of Virgil's[1] care team, who were insisting that Jane provide a bath board for Virgil. Instead of providing the bath board, Jane felt obligated to inform the managers that the new housing situation for Virgil was unacceptable from an environmental design standpoint. When the managers resisted and attempted to remove Jane, she exerted her authority as an occupational therapist and informed the organization that was to fund Virgil's new housing that the environment was unsafe. In the section below, Jane provides her rationale for not informing Virgil about this conflict.
>
> > Virgil had been schooled in the notion that the accommodation was suitable to his needs. When I met him within his environment it was immediately evident to me that the setup of the house fundamentally did not facilitate his independence, maximize his dignity or provide a safe environment for staff to support him. I made the decision not to explain my position to Virgil at that point as his excitement of leaving the institution was evident and I did not want this situation to damage his delight. In time, the funding organization reviewed the situation and Virgil was moved to alternative accommodation where he was able to mobilize around his home and gain access to the bath, toilet, and other areas of the house. He was equally delighted with the alternative accommodation, so I felt that there was no need to inform him about all of the conflict that had occurred leading up to this point.
> >
> > — **Jane Melton**

[1] All client names and geographic information have been changed.

fide in other members of the team and provide them with certain details about the conflict in order to gather opinions about how to best manage the conflict. Approaching this interaction with intentionality would involve informing other team members that a conflict has occurred, disclosing any attempts to manage the conflict and deciding as a team whether and how to respond if the client should mention the conflict to another professional on the team. In most cases, it is best that other team members not become actively engaged in the conflict. Responding by suggesting that the client discuss the issue with his or her therapist and work to resolve the conflict privately is usually the best response a collaborating professional can give when approached by a disgruntled client. In many cases, clients would rather have another professional intervene to fix the situation instead of confronting the therapist on their own.

However, intervening in a conflict between a client and a colleague almost always infuses tension into the relationship between the two professionals and rarely results in an improved relationship between the client and the therapist originally involved in the conflict.

An alternative situation in which professionals may wish to keep the content of a conversation confidential is when a client's personal problems or psychological issues are affecting the course of treatment. For example, if an occupational therapist is working to intervene with a maladaptive dynamic within a family (e.g., parent and siblings laughing at a client when he fails at a task), the therapist may wish to provide a collaborating psychologist an update on the nature of this work. Sharing with the psychologist that the family becomes highly defensive when confronted about this dynamic and recommending that the psychologist try a less confrontational approach with the family if she should observe the same dynamic may be something that the occupational therapist does not wish for the family to know at that point in treatment.

In some settings, an organized meeting takes place with the purpose of exchanging information about a single client or about a group of clients within the setting. These meetings are sometimes referred to as in-service meetings, case conferences, grand rounds, or staffings. When such meetings occur in the absence of the client, it is equally important to establish group norms or guidelines for the exchange of information. Some questions to consider include:

- How will confidentiality be maintained within the group?
- What, if any information about the content or outcome of the meeting will be shared with clients (or their families)?
- What kind of information is relevant to the objectives of the meeting and acceptable to share with other professionals in this setting?

> Intervening in a conflict between a client and a colleague almost always infuses tension into the relationship between the two professionals and rarely results in an improved relationship between the client and the therapist originally involved in the conflict.

When norms such as these are introduced, some settings are better at adhering to them than others. Among the norms, confidentiality is the one that is the most important to uphold when information about clients is shared in a group context. Because it is always difficult to know how well any given individual in a group situation is going to remember guidelines surrounding confidentiality, prefacing comments about a client with a statement such as, "please keep this information confidential" may be a useful precautionary measure.

Collaborations in the Client's Presence

When collaborations take place in the presence of a client, they generally assume one of three forms.

- Co-therapy relationships
- Consultative relationships
- Meetings with the client (or primary caregivers) for the purpose of treatment planning, problem-solving, periodic reviews, or progress reports (e.g., staffings, in-service meetings, or meetings to review a child's individualized educational plan)

Collaborative interactions that occur in a client's presence need to include as much of an emphasis on intentionality as those that occur in a client's absence.

Co-therapy relationships are those in which two or more professionals get together to carry out an intervention with one or more clients/family members. Such interventions most commonly consist of group therapy sessions, family sessions, parent/caregiver education, or individualized sessions in which the professionals work together with the client toward a common treatment goal. Particularly when new or short-term, these relationships are most likely to be successful if the involved professionals make their collaboration intentional. Making a co-therapy relationship intentional involves the following actions.

- Spending a great deal of time planning the structural, logistical, and interpersonal aspects of the joint approach. For example, estimating the relative time each professional will spend with the client(s), determining specific role(s) or functions each professional will assume during the session, deciding on the content that each professional will introduce into the session, and predicting which interpersonal modes each professional is likely to use during the session and their anticipated effect on the client's relationship with the two professionals.
- Monitoring your own interpersonal behavior toward the collaborating professional in the client's presence, being careful to share power, to communicate clearly, and to assert yourself in a professional manner. Most importantly, you should always be careful not to undermine your collaborator by criticizing the collaborator in front of the client, by subtly joining the client if the client is unhappy with the collaborator's behavior, or by interrupting or contradicting the collaborator's approach. A helpful way to prevent these behaviors is to establish a planned time to share mutual feedback following the session.
- Monitoring your reactions to the interpersonal behavior of the other professional, taking mental note of what you would or would not change about the collaborator's approach, and deciding how to provide your collaborator with constructive feedback, if necessary. Typically, the most respectful time to provide a collaborator with feedback about his or her performance is in an isolated, confidential setting in the absence of the client. However, if the feedback is related to safety issues, it is best to bring it up immediately and in the presence of the client, if necessary.
- Following each session, processing each professional's impressions of the joint effort (e.g., deciding what about their approach worked and what did not work as well, sharing constructive feedback with each other about each other's approaches, and planning for the next session).
- Each professional being willing to make adjustments to his or her approach, or both being willing to adjust their joint approach together in anticipation of the next session.

Although they require extra time and effort, when these steps are followed before, during, and after each therapy session, co-therapy relationships tend to be more stable and successful over time. Most importantly, following these steps maximizes the likelihood that clients will experience the interpersonal aspects of the session positively and with the knowledge that the two professionals are working collaboratively to serve their best interests (Fig. 15.1).

Consultative relationships that involve contact with the client are similar to co-therapy relationships in that similar principles of intentionality apply. One distinction is that consultative relationships typically involve one of the professionals being in the position of "help-seeker" and the other being in the position of "help-giver." Thus, the collaboration is more overtly influenced by an undeniable power differential between the two professionals. The nature of the consultant's power is that he or she typically

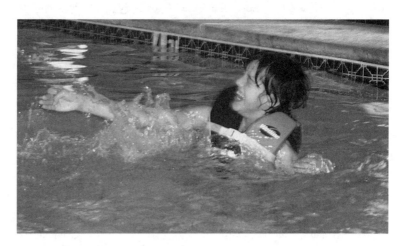

FIGURE 15.1 Being intentional about our work with other professionals inevitably serves the best interests of our clients

has a specialized type of knowledge that the help-seeker lacks. In addition, the help-giving professional may also be in a position to evaluate some aspect of the help-seeker's work or behavior. When the help-giver is not hired by the help-seeker but instead by the help-seeker's supervisor or boss, it intensifies the implications of the help-giver's evaluative role. Help-givers may misuse their power by:

- Assuming an inappropriate level of authority in front of the client and within the collaborative relationship
- Acting outside of the scope of their knowledge or acting in an overly confident manner about a given topic that is not an area of expertise.
- Evaluating or criticizing the help-seeking therapist in the presence of the client or in a way that is disrespectful or undermining.

Although the help-seeker is in a more vulnerable position than the help-giver, he or she typically wields a different kind of power—that which is related to his or her relationship with the client. Usually, the help-seeker has had contact with the client for a longer period of time than the help-giver and has likely formed some kind of a relationship with the client. In many cases, clients are likely to feel more comfortable with the professional who is more familiar to them. Some therapists may misuse their established relationship with a client to manipulate the client, turn the client against the help-giver, or undermine the help-giver's advice. This is most likely to occur if the help-seeker is feeling vulnerable, judged, or criticized by the help-giver. Although it is a common human instinct, this kind of behavior is maladaptive and ultimately harmful to both the client and the collaborative relationship.

Bearing these risks in mind, certain principles of the IRM may be applied to prevent the misuse of power by either professional. According to the IRM, help-giving professionals have the following responsibilities.

- To respect the help-seeker's existing relationship with the client and to recognize that the purpose of the consultation is not to exert authority but to support the help-seeker's efforts
- To recognize that your role in the relationship with the client is temporary and not to create a unique relationship with the client that is more intimate than the help-seeker's relationship with the client
- To refrain from evaluating or criticizing the help-seeking professional in a way that might undermine his or her power in the eyes of the client
- To be clear about the scope of and limitations to your knowledge and specific area of expertise

In return, the responsibilities of the help-seeking professional include:

- Being open and willing to consider the specialized knowledge or unique expertise offered by the help-giver
- Being willing to receive and consider the potential value or information or evaluative feedback in a nondefensive manner
- Being willing to change your approach in response to the feedback provided
- Being honest with the help-giver if you do not understand what is being offered or if you disagree with the feedback provided
- Refraining from using your relationship with the client as a means of retaliation against the help-giving professional

When both the help-seeking and the help-giving professionals adhere to these guidelines, it increases the likelihood that the outcome of the consultative relationship will be therapeutic for the client.

Supervisor/Employer and Student/Employee Relationships

Whether in the presence or the absence of the client, collaborations that involve a supervisor or employer carry risks that are similar to those accompanying consultative relationships. The same principles and power issues that apply to professionals in help-giving and help-seeking roles apply to those in supervisory/employer and student/employee roles. An additional element of the IRM that applies to these types of relationships involves familiarizing yourself with the power dynamics in a given treatment setting. To do this, you should consider the following questions.

- How is power organized within the setting?
- Are decisions made in a top–down manner (i.e., supervisor or employer controls decision-making and is not as receptive to feedback, suggestions, and input) or in a democratic manner (i.e., feedback, suggestions, and input from a student or employee are taken seriously and may be implemented by the supervisor or employer)?
- Which individuals in the setting are responsible for a given client's care?

- Which individuals in the setting are liable should an error occur during a client's treatment?
- What, if any, types of decisions may be delegated to students or employees?
- What decisions are students or employees prohibited from making independently?
- What are the expectations around seeking supervision or guidance at this setting? To what degree and in what capacities are students and employees expected to function independently in the setting? Under what circumstances is it mandatory that a student or employee seek assistance or supervision?
- In addition to clinical care and upholding the values and ethics of occupational therapy, what are your other responsibilities and obligations in this setting (e.g., how can I best become a team player in the setting)?

Many medical settings, such as hospitals or outpatient rehabilitation centers, have power structures that are similar to those of military operations. This means that there is a preestablished power hierarchy in which professionals have roles (or ranks) that designate how much of a decision-making role they are able to assume in the setting, to what degree they are responsible for the actions of other professionals, how much supervisory control they are able to exert over other professionals, and how much they are able to delegate certain tasks or duties to others in the setting. Regardless of what role or rank you occupy in a setting, you are more likely to have positive collaborative relationships if you approach power dynamics in an intentional manner. Those in supervisory or employer roles may benefit from considering the following issues when supervising students, managing employees, and/or assigning certain tasks.

- Identifying your own values concerning the use and delegation of power. This may require asking yourself: "What leadership qualities have I appreciated in teachers, employers, or supervisors I have known? What leadership qualities have I disliked in teachers, employers, or supervisors I have known?"
- Deciding what type of a leadership style you plan to use. This may require asking yourself: "What degree of decision-making will I allow my supervisees/employees?" "Will decision-making allowances depend on the rank or skill level of the employee?" "How much will I delegate tasks/assign cases to my supervisees/employees?" "What are the types of tasks/cases that I will delegate or assign and to whom?" "How much work will I do myself?" "What is the nature of the work I will do

myself?" "Under what circumstances will feedback from students/employees be solicited and incorporated into my decision-making"
- Being explicit in communicating to your students/employees your values and boundaries around use of power. This includes explaining your leadership style, being clear about the chain of command and about decision-making policies and expectations in the setting, and articulating the circumstances under which feedback from students and employees will be welcomed and considered.
- Making a special effort to ensure that you have been very clear in providing instruction or making your needs known regarding a requested task or assignment. Ensuring that you have left ample room for the student or employee to ask questions if he or she does not understand what is being requested.
- Being explicit about the kinds of tasks and activities you expect the student/employee to perform independently.
- Being explicit about the kinds of questions, dilemmas, decisions, or tasks, or activities that require the input or involvement of the supervisor or employer.
- Establishing formal (i.e., written evaluations) and informal (i.e., scheduled supervision sessions) mechanisms in place for evaluating the performance of those for whom you are responsible. Informing the student/employee of the criteria according to which he or she will be evaluated before beginning the relationship.
- Providing feedback to students/employees in a direct and prompt manner. If a supervisor or employer identifies an area of weakness or suspects that problems might develop, he or she should inform the student or employee as quickly as possible and schedule follow-up meetings until the behavior is corrected.
- Acting within the scope of your knowledge or expertise and seeking your own consultation if unsure of how to manage a specific issue.

Similarly, students and employees can approach supervisory relationships with intentionality by doing the following.

- Knowing your general reactions to, and opinions about, those who serve in roles of authority. To gain insight, you might ask yourself the following questions: "Who have been key authority figures in my past?" "How did they influence my life?" "What interpersonal qualities did I appreciate or admire about those authority figures?" "What interpersonal qualities did I not appreciate or find to be problematic?"

- Observing the supervisor's leadership style by watching what occurs with other students or employees. If uncertain, asking the supervisor or employer to explain his or her leadership style, including his or her expectations for performance, preferences regarding decision-making, and expectations involving independent functioning.
- Observing the supervisor to determine his or her level of openness to and preferred ways of receiving input and feedback from students and employees. If uncertain, erring on the side of being conservative and parsimonious about input and feedback until you are more comfortable.
- Introducing yourself to the supervisor and informing the supervisor of your strengths and areas of competence as well as any limitations or areas of weakness on which you would like to improve.
- Recognizing the supervisor's rank and authority and showing respect when receiving the supervisor's opinions, advice, and feedback
- Developing learning objectives or performance goals for yourself and sharing them with the supervisor to ensure that they are consistent with the supervisor's priorities and expectations.
- If they have not been made explicit, asking the supervisor about the criteria by which your performance will be evaluated.
- If a formalized structure for periodic supervision is not in place, occasionally checking in with the supervisor regarding your performance and when questions arise.
- Requesting that important issues be formalized in writing (e.g., contractual issues concerning the duration of employment/training period, salary, and benefits, expected number of hours per week, and any issues about performance)
- If you disagree with a supervisor about a request, raising the issue directly with the supervisor in a careful and respectful manner. The most conservative approach to doing this is by asking the supervisor for more of an explanation or a rationale for making the request. If you remain in disagreement, you might provide a rationale or explanation for an alternative point of view. In the long run, this is always more effective than acting

behind the supervisor's back in a way that is contradictory or even slightly different than what the supervisor has requested.
- Refrain from over-questioning, challenging, or contradicting a supervisor in front of a client or in front of other staff (unless it involves an urgent issue, such as a safety issue). Although it is often done in the interest of learning, this kind of behavior may be perceived as undermining by some supervisors.
- Under no circumstances allowing yourself to become a victim of or an accomplice to a supervisor's unethical or inappropriate behavior.

When both supervisors and their students or employees make an effort to make their relationship intentional in these ways, it increases the likelihood that both parties will be satisfied with the outcome. In the Activities section of this chapter, two worksheets are provided to allow you to rate your interpersonal behavior during supervisory interactions; one may be used by students or employees and the other by supervisors or employers. You are encouraged to utilize these worksheets to ensure that your relationships with others are as intentional as possible.

✳Summary

Occupational therapists witness and work with clients who are facing difficult and demanding life circumstances. Collaborating with other professionals in the midst of managing these challenges is often a requirement that only adds complexity to your role as a therapist. Remaining intentional about your collaborations with other professionals is an important aspect of the IRM, regardless of whether you are interacting with other professionals in the presence or absence of a client. When issues of pride and territoriality surface during collaborations, it has the potential to permanently affect relationships between professionals and to disrupt relationships between professionals and their clients. In this chapter, recommendations for maximizing the likelihood of successful relationships with supervisors, employers, and other professionals were provided.

ACTIVITIES FOR LEARNING AND REFLECTION

The worksheets provided in this section aim to allow you to feel more prepared to provide or receive supervision. Additionally, they are designed to encourage self-reflection about interpersonal behaviors while in the act of providing or receiving supervision. In responding to the various categories, you are encouraged to check all response options that apply or respond to the open-ended questions in the far right column. In the far right column, you are also encouraged to jot down any other reflections or goals for self-improvement in each area.

Intentionality Worksheet for Providers of Supervision		
Values Concerning Use of Power	I most admire leaders who are: · Authoritarian—they establish their own expectations for performance and do not deviate or waiver in response to individual differences or input from others · Collaborative—they establish their own expectations for performance and adjust them according to input from others or individual differences between those receiving supervision · Participatory—they look primarily to others to form their own expectations for performance and continue to adjust them according to the needs and individual differences of others. · Other (list and describe):	Reflections and goals · What life experiences have influenced my preferences? · What are the pros/cons of the leadership style I admire most? · What new interpersonal behaviors would I need to incorporate to replicate this style?
	I least admire leaders who are: · Unpredictable or chameleon-like—their style and moods vacillate, and one never knows what is expected or how the leader might respond. This results in disloyalty and dishonest or self-protective behavior among employees. · Eager to please—they are more concerned about being liked and accepted than about what people really need to do or learn in order to be effective. Because one can never please everyone, the leader risks becoming resentful, mistrustful, or competitive · Opportunistic—they have no loyalty to those who work harder or are more reliable. Instead, they put their energies into the person who is most convenient or most willing to do a job on a given day. This becomes a disincentive for more reliable or loyal employees. · Manipulative—they use guilt, lack of planning, sudden emergencies; or they emphasize their own plight in order to control others and encourage performance. · Abusive – they insult, humiliate, intimidate, make unreasonable demands, or unfairly punish in order to control others and encourage performance. · Weak or vulnerable – they are not competent in their role as leader and as a result the most dominant employees take control. · Other (list and describe):	Reflections and goals · What life experiences have influenced my aversion to the types of leaders I selected? · What new interpersonal behaviors would I need to avoid to ensure that I do not replicate this style?

(table continued on page 290)

Intentionality Worksheet for Providers of Supervision (continued)		
Leadership Style	Respond to the following open-ended questions: · What types of decisions will I allow my supervisees to make independently? · What types of decisions will supervisees be prohibited from making? · Am I more oriented toward allowing supervisees to make their own mistakes or do I have more of a tendency to watch my supervisees closely and intervene before mistakes occur? · With respect to supervisees' performance, am I more concerned with big picture issues, with getting the details right, or with a combination of the two? · How important is it to me that supervisees adhere to expected timelines or deadlines? · How will I reward supervisees for good performance? · How will I inform supervisees that their performance is not acceptable? · Will the types of rewards, punishments, or special allowances depend on the rank or skill level of the supervisee, on my relationship to the supervisee, or will they be applied uniformly across all supervisees based upon pre-established criteria? · How might different types of supervisees respond to my leadership style? · Which types of supervisees will respond best to my leadership style? · What kinds of supervisees might have difficulty with my style?	Respond here:
Communication of Leadership Style	Respond to the following questions · What aspects of my leadership style will I explicitly convey to supervisees? · What aspects of my style will I expect them to figure out for themselves? · When and how will I convey my leadership style to my supervisees? · What will I tell supervisees about the organization's chain of command and about decision-making policies and expectations in the setting?	Respond here:
Providing Instruction and Assigning Tasks	Respond to the following questions · What are the types of tasks/cases that I will assign to my supervisees? · What criteria will I employ in deciding to whom to assign which type of task? · How will I ensure that the supervisee understood my expectations or instructions? · How will I create an environment that encourages questions and communication if supervisees do not understand what is being requested. · When I expect a task or assignment to be completed independently, how will I communicate this to the supervisee? · How will I inform the supervisee of the kinds of questions, dilemmas, decisions, or tasks, or activities that require my input or involvement?	Respond here:

Orientation Toward Students and Supervisees	I work best with supervisees who are: · Exceptionally committed—working well beyond expected time frames and taking on larger than expected workloads · Exceptionally talented—learning quickly and excelling beyond their expected level of performance · Eager to please—orienting toward what I need most from them at any given time, frequently asking for feedback, and accepting of anything I ask · Driven to learn—asking several questions, requesting reading assignments, and expressing curiosity about a wide range of topics · Overcoming obstacles—facing barriers beyond their control, having good potential, and working hard to meet basic expectations. · Independent—easy to supervise and not demanding · Critical thinkers—challenging or questioning my approach or recommendations from time to time.	Reflections and goals · What about my own history, either as a supervisee or as a supervisor, has influenced my preferences toward certain types of supervisees? · What might I do to widen my appreciation of a greater variety of supervisee styles?
	I work least well with supervisees who are: · Challenging, questioning, or critical of my approach · Emotionally disengaged from the learning process · Doing only what is required and no more · Lacking in self-confidence about their own performance · Overconfident about their own performance · Reluctant to ask for help · So eager to please that I wonder if they are thinking critically or able to set boundaries for themselves · Lacking expected competence · Lacking in professionalism · Ignoring requests or feedback · Manipulative (using guilt or twisting rules to get out of certain tasks) · Lacking in maturity · Interpersonally difficult (emotionally labile or aggressive)	Reflections and goals · What about my own history, either as a supervisee or as a supervisor has influenced my aversion to certain types of supervisees? · Are there any new approaches that I would want to learn to better manage and communicate with these types of supervisees?
Evaluation and Feedback	Am I open to receiving unsolicited feedback from my supervisees? · Yes · No	Reflections and goals · What about receiving feedback from supervisees is difficult for me? · How can I better prepare myself to receive feedback?
	What are my limits and expectations regarding the nature or type of feedback I will consider? · I am comfortable receiving feedback from supervisees when I solicit it. · I am comfortable receiving unsolicited feedback from supervisees. · I am open to receiving any type of feedback provided it is delivered in an earnest and respectful manner. · I am comfortable receiving feedback from supervisees about workload issues. · I am comfortable receiving feedback from supervisees about my leadership style. · I am comfortable receiving feedback from supervisees about my technical approach to therapy. · I am comfortable receiving feedback from supervisees about my interpersonal approach to therapy. · I have a difficult time determining which types of feedback I should pay attention to and which types I should ignore.	Reflections and goals

(table continued on page 292)

Intentionality Worksheet for Providers of Supervision (continued)		
	How will the feedback I receive affect my decision-making and attitude toward the supervisee providing the feedback? · I will incorporate a supervisee's feedback into my decision-making or behaviors if I feel it is accurate or reasonable. · I do not typically change my decisions or behaviors significantly in response to feedback from supervisees. · My general attitude toward supervisees who provide feedback is one of admiration. · My general attitude toward supervisees who provide feedback is one of neutrality. · My general attitude toward supervisees who provide feedback is one of skepticism.	Reflections and goals
	Respond to the following questions · What formal (i.e., written) mechanisms have I put into place for evaluating the performance of supervisees and providing them with feedback? · How will I evaluate the performance of supervisees on an informal basis? · How and when will I inform the student/employee of the criteria according to which he or she will be evaluated? · Am I comfortable providing feedback early, directly, and clearly? · When I provide feedback do I offer a clear remediation plan, homework assignments, or other suggestions for ways to improve?	Respond here:
Self-Awareness of Limits	I would rate my self-awareness of limitations in the scope of my knowledge or expertise as follows: · I am comfortable informing supervisees about my area(s) of expertise. · I am comfortable informing a supervisee that I cannot answer a question or provide a service if it is beyond the scope of my knowledge or expertise. · I am comfortable extending beyond my scope of knowledge or expertise if I know enough about what I am doing and if it does not pose a safety risk to the client. · I regularly seek consultation or supervision if I have a question or if I am unsure about how to provide supervision on a specific issue.	Reflections and goals

Intentionality Worksheet for Recipients of Supervision		
Introduction to Supervisor	I would rate my ability to effectively introduce myself to a supervisor as follows: · I am comfortable volunteering information about my training and experiential background. · I am comfortable volunteering information about my perceived areas of strength and competence, including what I might offer a given setting. · I am comfortable volunteering information about any limitations or areas of weakness that I would like to improve upon.	Reflections and goals
Attitudes Toward Authority Figures	Respond to the following questions · Who are the most memorable authority figures in my past? · In which ways did these individuals influence my life? · What interpersonal qualities did I appreciate or admire about these individuals? · What interpersonal qualities did I not appreciate or find to be problematic? · What other life experiences have influenced my attitudes toward authority figures?	Respond here: When we are not intentional about our interactions, our attitudes toward authority figures have the potential to reveal themselves in our behaviors toward supervisors. Write down any additional reflections or goals for self-improvement in this area here.
Past Experience with Supervisors and Employers	What leadership and interpersonal qualities have I most appreciated about supervisors with whom I have worked in the past?	Respond here:
	What leadership and interpersonal qualities have I least appreciated about supervisors with whom I have worked in the past?	Respond here:
	Have I ever had difficulties with a supervisor? · Yes · No	If yes, please consider the following: In what ways did my own behavior toward the supervisor exacerbate or attenuate the supervisor's behavior? · *Exacerbating Behaviors*: · *Attenuating Behaviors*: If I should encounter a supervisor with similar qualities in the future, what steps can I take to ensure a reasonable or more positive outcome?

(table continued on page 294)

Intentionality Worksheet for Recipients of Supervision (continued)		
Orienting Toward the Supervisor's Leadership Style and Showing Respect	I would rate my ability to orient toward a supervisor as follows. · I make an effort to observe how my supervisor interacts with others so I can better know her/his expectations for performance, preferences regarding decision-making, and expectations involving independent functioning. · When necessary, I ask the supervisor about the criteria by which my performance will be evaluated. · I seek feedback independently by occasionally checking in with the supervisor regarding my performance.	Reflections and goals
	I would rate my ability to show respect or deference toward a supervisor as follows. · I observe the supervisor to determine the level of openness to and preferred ways of receiving input and feedback from supervisees. · I am able to acknowledge rank and show deference to my supervisor's opinions, advice, and feedback. · I ask when I need something (e.g., permission for time off) rather than tell my supervisor what my plans are. · I respect my supervisor's time by (avoiding canceling or no-showing for scheduled appointments, being consistently early or on time for appointments and asking to schedule times to talk rather than just dropping in). · When appropriate, I convey gratitude privately and/or publicly acknowledge the role my supervisor has had in my training and achievements. · I avoid behaviors that could be interpreted as undermining, inattentive, or disrespectful (e.g., I refrain from overquestioning a supervisor, directly challenging his or her opinion, asking for help and then rejecting what is offered, not attending fully to the supervisor's requests or instructions, or contradicting the supervisors in the presence of other people).	Reflections and goals
	When providing constructive feedback to a supervisor, I would rate my abilities as follows. · I provide feedback in a way that is straightforward but sensitive. Before making a criticism or suggestion, I consider its potential utility for students as a whole, rather than specifically for myself. · Before providing feedback, I think about why the status quo exists so I am able to validate the practical and theoretical sense behind it before making a recommendation for change. · If I am uncertain about how to provide feedback, I wait until I have established a positive relationship with the supervisor and until I have observed how the supervisor tends to respond to different approaches to providing feedback.	Reflections and goals

Being Clear and Assertive About Educational Needs and Learning Objectives	I would rate my ability to clarify my needs and objectives as follows. · I am comfortable sharing my educational or professional development needs and goals with my supervisor · I am able to develop learning objectives or performance goals independently · When asserting my needs, I am careful to be sure they are consistent with the priorities and expectations of the supervisor and setting.	Reflections and goals
Help-Seeking and Self-Awareness of Limits	I would rate my self-awareness of limitations in the scope of my knowledge or expertise as follows. · I am comfortable informing supervisors about my strengths or background as a therapist. · I am comfortable informing a supervisor of my weaknesses or areas in which I lack confidence. · I tend to push beyond the scope of my knowledge or experience if I know enough about what I am doing and if it does not pose a safety risk to the client. · I would rather seek supervision than risk making an error with a client. · I tend to lack confidence, seek approval, and overutilize supervision. · I seek supervision at an acceptable level—if I have a question or if I am unsure about how to handle a specific issue.	Reflections and goals
Awareness of One's Rights as a Supervisee	I am able to enforce my own rights as a supervisee in the following ways. · If employment guidelines, work hours, vacation times, and other administrative details and benefits information are not formalized in writing, I am comfortable asking for it to be put into writing. · If a supervisor raises an issue about my performance, I am comfortable asking for documentation of the issue in writing and for continued documentation of my performance until the issue is resolved. · I am able to avoid becoming a victim of or an accomplice to a supervisor's unethical or inappropriate behavior. · I am comfortable informing a supervisor verbally and in writing when I believe I am being mistreated or that my rights are being violated. · When necessary, I am comfortable going to a higher authority to report a supervisor's unethical behavior.	Reflections and goals

CHAPTER 16

ON BECOMING A BETTER THERAPIST:
Self-Care and Developing Your Therapeutic Use of Self

During the interviews with the 12 therapists introduced in Chapter 2, I asked them to share personal stories and inner thoughts about various situations and experiences that significantly influenced their professional development. They discussed critical life experiences that shaped their decisions to enter the field, explained what motivates them to continue to practice, and described various interpersonal lessons about practice that they learned the hard way. The therapists also explained how they actively reflect and manage themselves in light of certain types of clients, some of whom are interpersonally complementary to their personality styles and others of whom are interpersonally challenging. A consistent theme that ran through everyone's descriptions of how they cope with the demands of daily practice was self-care. The therapists emphasized that the ability to be both intentional and emotionally spontaneous with clients was directly correlated with the extent to which they made deliberate efforts to involve themselves with people and activities that were nurturing, relaxing, and enriching. The insights that emerged from these more personal discussions with the therapists led me to compose this last chapter about the roles of self-knowledge and self-care in developing your therapeutic use of self.

There is one thing the therapists agreed upon: Developing therapeutic use of self is a lifelong endeavor. You can continually work to improve it in endless ways. There is no fixed path or formula for becoming a better therapist. However, my own experiences and those shared with me

> Developing therapeutic use of self is a lifelong endeavor.

by the therapists suggest that embarking on this developmental process involves four important challenges, which are discussed in this final chapter.

The first challenge of developing a therapeutic use of self is cultivating critical self-awareness. It involves knowing those things about yourself that affect, for good or ill, your interactions with others in a therapeutic context. The second challenge is to cultivate the reflective use of your current strengths, weaknesses, limits, preferences, and world views. This is a critical component of the intentional use of self. It involves not only self-knowledge but active use of that knowledge to consistently behave interpersonally in ways designed to optimize the client's therapeutic process. The third challenge is to create and capitalize on opportunities for self-care that strengthen aspects of the self and allow you to develop new strengths for your therapeutic use of self. The final and fourth challenge is maintaining mindfulness of why you are an occupational therapist.

Self-Awareness and Reflective Use of Your Traits

Self-awareness and reflective use of your traits go hand in hand. The more you know about your personality, world view, strengths, weaknesses, limits, and values the more you can draw on that knowledge during the therapy process. Conversely, the more you cultivate an intentional use of self in therapy, the more self-aware you become. That is, by reflecting on what goes on in therapy and on how your communications or behaviors affect clients, the more self-aware you become. These two challenges of developing a therapeutic use of self are discussed in tandem.

Knowing and Responsibly Accepting Weaknesses and Limitations

As therapists, knowing our weaknesses and being aware of our limitations is as important as recognizing our strengths. Knowing which clients or situations are likely to be more challenging, draining, boring, or even threatening can help guide our clinical decision making, our efforts to seek guidance and support from colleagues, and ultimately our interpersonal efforts and behaviors in therapy.

It is important to recognize that even the strongest therapists have limitations and weaknesses and lessons they have had to learn. The key is recognizing these weaknesses, learning from them, and working with them rather than allowing them to become sources of embarrassment, self-disdain, or shame. The latter feelings tend to get in the way of self-awareness. Thus, self-acceptance is important to cultivate as well. Self-acceptance means knowing that you, like everyone else, have weaknesses and limits and that they are not personal failures but, rather, part of the human condition. Importantly, self-acceptance does not imply a take-me-as-I-am attitude. Rather, it means taking responsibility for how your weaknesses and limits may affect others by making decisions that minimize the possibilities of any ill effects.

For example, a therapist once told me that during a particularly difficult period in her personal life she found that she was more easily distracted and inattentive during her therapy sessions. Rather than focusing on her clients, her thoughts would often drift back to reflecting about her personal problems. This therapist was aware that her tendency to allow her mind to drift is a characteristic reaction for her when she is under stress. Most of the time, she could pull her attention back to the client without the client noticing. However, when she would find her thoughts drifting to such an extent that it became obvious to the client, she would admit and apologize to the client that she was mentally fatigued that day, reassure the client that it had nothing to do with him or her, and ask the client to restate whatever information she had missed. This strategy was important on several accounts. First, the therapist was

being honest and willing to admit her failures. This contributed to the building of trust within the relationship. In addition, by honestly admitting to the client that she had lost important information, it created an opportunity for the therapist to ensure that she could obtain the information she needed to contribute to the therapy process.

Recognizing and Cultivating Your Assets

Some of the traits that you bring into therapy involve natural qualities with which you are born, such as temperament, body size, tone of voice, or other aspects of your physical self. These more or less permanent qualities always have automatic implications for our therapeutic relationships. They are the first characteristics clients encounter as they are getting to know you. If used intentionally and appropriately, your natural qualities can be strengths and lead to more successful relationships with your clients. Using these qualities effectively means not only being aware of them but also actively cultivating an awareness of how they affect others, especially during therapy.

For example, René Bélanger discussed the virtues of being a man who is physically small. He is aware that his size means that his clients perceive him as less threatening. Because many of his clients have difficulty feeling safe in interpersonal relationships and can be easily threatened, this trait has become a real asset for René. His small physique also allows him more "room" to be authoritative with clients when he needs to be. That is, he can assert authority without coming across as threatening. Thus, when he perceives that clients need a firmer response, his physique allows him to take on an air of authority without his being perceived as controlling or threatening (Fig. 16.1).

Roland Meisel is an innately funny man. In everyday conversation he intersperses puns, jokes, and quips quite naturally. His practice can involve a fair amount of tension because it requires evaluation of whether clients merit continued benefits based on being unable to work. Roland consciously uses his natural humor to diffuse this tension and to come across as less authoritarian (Fig. 16.2).

Developing Aspects of the Self

Many of the positive traits that we have as therapists do not come naturally and may have been cultivated over time.

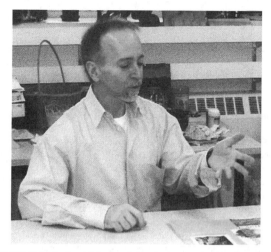

FIGURE 16.1 René Bélanger is frank about using his size as an asset during therapy

Many result from deliberate efforts toward personal development based on personal mistakes. Others come as the result of years of self-reflection on experiences in therapy. Some are the result of difficult experiences. The sections that follow examine these avenues of self-development.

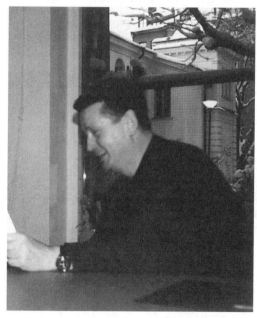

FIGURE 16.2 Roland Meisel uses humor effectively to build rapport and diffuse tension

Deliberately Cultivating Strengths from Mistakes, Problems, and Failures

Training to become a therapist invariably brings with it a desire to learn every skill possible so as to avoid making mistakes. However, it quickly becomes clear that the mistakes we make can serve as our best sources of learning and growth. One variable common to interpersonal excellence in clinical practice is the ability to recognize mistakes in relating and to strive continually to adjust your interpersonal skills to avoid making similar mistakes in the future (Box 16.1).

For example, as a young therapist I tended to become much more quiet and passive when in the presence of demanding, interpersonally aggressive, and critical clients. Over time and with sufficient feedback from these types of clients, I learned that this behavior only makes them feel rejected and abandoned. Now when I meet a demanding client, I force myself to become more engaged, firm, and frank about conveying my own impressions and feedback. What was once a weak area for me has now become a strength, and my new-found interpersonal strategy has proven effective on multiple occasions.

Receiving difficult feedback from clients, particularly when unsolicited, can be devastating, especially at the beginning of one's career. With time, however, experienced therapists learn to view client difficulties and feedback as opportunities for growth. Kim Eberhardt painted a definitive picture of how she uses unsolicited feedback from clients to improve on her interpersonal skills.

> It's the feisty clients who I enjoy.... They are the squeaky wheels ... very headstrong and very motivated, energetic people. Many of them can be difficult, critical and demanding, but I find this very challenging.... I enjoy these people because they really care about the quality of the therapy they are receiving and about the relationship they have with me, even if they have negative things to say at times. They inspire my creativity and get me thinking about what else they might need at an interpersonal level.... I keep in touch with people over time, and it helps me work with others like them. They give me confidence that if I was able to do something that they found helpful then I know I'll be able to benefit the people I am currently seeing.

Kim's continual striving to learn from clients and build on her own skills reflects a consummate focus on the task-oriented aspects of the relationship rather than on her own personal emotional injuries or reactions. Kim places her own feelings and pride aside and focuses on building a

Box 16.1   Mistakes Therapists Make

Any discussion of interpersonal lessons learned the "hard way" would be incomplete if it did not include examples of some of the more basic mistakes students and therapists tend to make. Because many of the therapists featured in this book also serve as fieldwork supervisors or employers, I asked some of them to share their perspectives on the types of mistake they most commonly witness when supervising students or observing other therapists. Collectively, they described the following.

- *Self-disclosure.* "Some therapists tend to self-disclose in ways that make them vulnerable to empathic breaks and don't reflect good judgment or foresight. For example, one student disclosed to a client that she and her intimate partner were living together. This went against that particular client's religious views, and it introduced an unnecessary level of complexity into the student's relationship with that client."
- *Inappropriate emotion or tone of voice.* "Some are just too perky for the clinical situation at hand…. They introduce themselves to a client in a way that says "My life is going just great, and the world couldn't be better." It shows a level of disrespect for the client's emotional state and a lack of empathy. Others talk to children as if they are infants—in a patronizing, sing-song tone of voice. Parents often attribute this to inexperience."
- *Unrealistic expectations.* "Some people new to the field expect miracles from their clients. They repeatedly expect too much out of treatment and then become disillusioned quickly if it doesn't happen. Some lack an understanding that, even when clients share the same impairment, different people progress at different rates and reach different levels of outcome. The clients can feel the therapist's disappointment because it is often reflected in the way they ask questions, phrase things, or in their tone of voice."
- *Presumptuousness.* "Some behave too much like an expert with their clients, and they do not take the time to listen to and value the client's perspective. Some give off subtle signals that they consider themselves to be the idyllic parent that the child never had by providing too much education and instruction and by taking too much control. Parents often respond to this type of behavior defensively by acting in ways that say 'Don't tell me how to parent or what to expect from my child.' Others insist on using first names with clients without asking them first how they would like to be addressed."

- *Lacking confidence.* "In contrast, it is clear that some students or newer therapists are nervous about their own performance, and they do not convey an appropriate level of confidence and professionalism…. They may speak too softly, mumble, chuckle nervously, make too many jokes, or fiddle with things. Some are so anxious about their own performance that they cannot center their attention adequately on their clients. As a result, they overlook key communications and details about the interaction. By being anxious or lacking an appropriate level of leadership they also convey to their clients that they are not up to the task of serving in the role of therapist. Some clients tend to question these therapists more frequently, which only serves to make the therapists more anxious."
- *Forgetting about use of self.* "Some therapists tend to focus too much on one aspect of the person (i.e., motor control) and often the wrong aspect (e.g., the client's need for hope or encouragement might be the most pressing issue during that particular session)."
- *Too much information.* "Often in their desire to show clients or parents how much they know about a given topic, therapists go into long descriptions or have repeated technical discussions with parents about the impairment. This can be harmful to the relationship (and to the child) if the information is unsolicited, poorly timed, or excessive."
- *Lack of empathy.* "Some therapists judge clients for being difficult to work with, failing to show up, or not following through—rather than strive to understand why. Often you see a great lack of empathy for the parents of disabled children if the parent does not meet the therapist's expectations."
- *Being ego-involved.* "Many students and new therapists have great difficulty coping with client criticism or negative feedback. Some become easily defensive or too domineering with clients if clients question them or disagree with their approach. Others have a hard time tolerating it if clients don't establish a good connection or rapport with them. They feel personally wounded if a client doesn't respond to them in the way they had hoped they would. These therapists are the ones who, if they do not change their perspective, are the most vulnerable to becoming burned out from performing therapy. We have to understand that it's a given in OT that some of our clients reject and become disappointed with us at times."

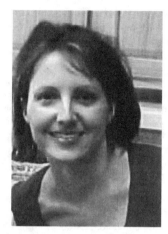

FIGURE 16.3 Kim Eberhardt enjoys working with clients who might be viewed by others as interpersonally challenging

growing database of how to gain maximal interpersonal effectiveness in therapy (Fig. 16.3).

Sometimes a given trait can be a source of both strength and weakness, depending on the client or the therapy situation. One such challenge, which several therapists talked about, was the tendency to show emotion. Kathryn Loukas, Belinda Anderson, and Carmen-Gloria de Las Heras all talked about both the strengths and the potential vulnerabilities involved in reacting spontaneously or showing their feelings to their clients. Kathryn (Fig. 16.4) explained how, when she is moved by something during therapy, she has a tendency to show what she is feeling.

My weakness is my emotionality but it is also my strength.... I can be overly emotional ... when I laugh with clients I laugh hard.... I cry easily ... and when I am hurt or disappointed I show my irritation or frustration openly.... I can find things hard to let go of.... This both hurts and helps me in my relationships in life and in OT.

Similarly, Belinda (Fig. 16.5) described the challenge of differentiating between clients with whom it is appropriate to show emotion and those with whom it is not.

Sometimes I might be too empathetic and sometimes you have to not be so empathetic.... On occasion I might find myself crying with somebody about their child's situation.... I recognize I must control my tendency to become too emotional because I realize that some people get the wrong message and may want to take advantage of it.... When they see that you are that soft they begin to think

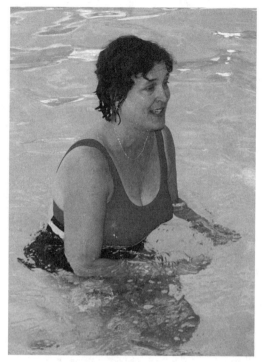

FIGURE 16.4 When interacting in the pool, Kathryn Loukas does not hide her reactions

you are their friend rather than their therapist.... They attempt to call you up and invite you places, and they get confused about the boundaries.

For Carmen, it is natural to show her emotional reactions spontaneously and openly as they unfold. This tendency to be emotionally transparent is something that Carmen describes as part of her essential nature. It is also something that is not always well accepted by clients. Consequently, Carmen explained that she must be highly judicious about showing emotion with clients whom she does not know well or with those who themselves lack emotional control. Similarly, Kathryn and Belinda recognize that they have to be critically aware of their own emotions and when it is appropriate or inappropriate to make them transparent.

In addition to experiencing and revealing strong emotions, another challenge that many therapists identified is a tendency to have an overly optimistic view of their clients coupled with a tendency to go out of their way to accom-

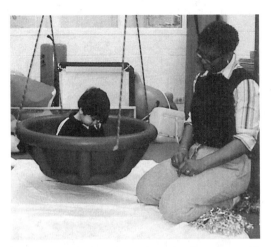

FIGURE 16.5 Belinda Anderson's emotional resonance with a young client is palpable

modate, or provide, for a client. As a consequence, therapists are sometimes misled or come to be seen as a boundless source of unending time and resources. Realizing the limitations of some of their clients and maintaining their own limits and time for themselves is a difficult lesson to learn.

Belinda Anderson provided the most poignant description of this common tendency to overfunction for clients only to be disappointed later.

I'm too optimistic, and I can be gullible sometimes.... I miss seeing the downsides of it.... For example, I sometimes overextend for people, especially if I see that a family is in great need. However, I can't predict when a certain family won't show up for the session to benefit from all the work and planning I have done.... Having limits and boundaries and time for myself is my greatest weakness.

Belinda shared one particularly revealing story that described the emotional risks and disappointments that many therapists experience when they overfunction for clients.

When I teach parents how to follow through with certain sensory integration treatments at home, I usually give them my pager number in case they have any questions. I have usually left it open, and it hasn't been a problem.... But this one parent of a little girl who was visually impaired and sensory defensive was different. The child was challenging to work with, and the parent required a lot of extra time on the phone. After a long period of treatment and a lot of tears and nervousness, the treatment was ultimately

successful. At the end of our treatment, the parent invited me to a wedding and in the same phone call she also mentioned that she wanted the ability to continue to call me at home. I gently told her I could not go to the wedding and that she could not continue to call me at home because the treatment period had ended. She then became very angry with me and did not treat me in a respectful way.... Now, I tell clients up front the limits around what they can and cannot expect from me. I encourage them to make decisions for themselves,... I don't overfunction and call doctors for them.... I don't get materials for them.... I learned that if you start that they expect more and more from you. This is something I had to learn on my own.

Therapists tend to encounter people at their most vulnerable moments and in the midst of personal crises. Clients need and can demand a lot from therapists. There is a duty to meet those demands when reasonable. However, therapists are human too and do not deserve to be taken advantage of or mistreated. Locating and maintaining a comfort zone that reflects your personal limits and boundaries is an essential and ongoing process in the journey to professional development.

Limits and boundaries go hand in hand with other self-care efforts that allow therapists to cope with the day-to-day demands of practice. Box 16.2 contains a series of examples of ways in which therapists assume the responsibility of taking care of their minds and bodies as means of preserving their ability to be wholly present and effective in their interactions with clients (Box 16.2).

Transforming Personal Difficulties and Challenges into Gifts

While seeking to understand how good therapists develop, another unanticipated and striking discovery emerged from my conversations with the therapists. It involved the fact that many of them have found ways to transform significant personal difficulties and challenges into gifts used in practice. Many of these therapists view themselves as more empathic, sensitive, thoughtful, caring, passionate, or scrupulous because of the problems they have endured. The next section describes some of the ways in which the therapists built on losses and hardships to become stronger, more empathic, or more motivated in their work to support others.

Michele Shapiro was the first therapist who piqued my interest in the idea that therapists who are more emotionally and interpersonally present during their interactions with clients are those who have found means of transforming significant life challenges into interpersonal gifts.

Box 16.2 Examples of Therapist Self-Care Efforts

Work in the field of occupational therapy has enlightened me to the numerous nurturing, relaxing, and enriching occupations that therapists choose as means of self-care. One of the most effective ways to ensure that you are being intentional and deliberate about self-care is to set aside regular and specific times in your schedule for these occupations. Another approach to self-care involves seizing in-the-moment opportunities to gain support, connection, and nurturance through contact with others and engagement in occupation. Although the possibilities for occupations that can be considered as promoting self-care are as numerous and unique as the therapists who engage in them, the following is a list of some of the more interesting stories I have recorded from both students and therapists over the past few years.

- "I cook my favorite meal."
- "I complain about my day to my boyfriend."
- "I exercise more."
- "I bounce ideas off of one of my peers, or I talk to a supervisor about it."
- "I actively use psychotherapy when I feel I need to. I love therapy."
- "I seek support from my family members."
- "I have a hobby that I never do with clients."
- "I read fiction."
- "I see a movie."
- "I watch my favorite TV show."
- "I play with my dog."

At one time I thought that my sensory processing difficulties would greatly impede my ability to serve as an occupational therapist. It was only many years after working in the field of OT that I understood that I am a good OT *because* of my own hypersensitivity. Because I am more sensitive to sensory stimuli as well as to psychological stimuli, I am better able to understand the complexity of the problems my clients face. I think this understanding is different and more nuanced than what nondisabled therapists can only learn from theory.

The sensitivities Michele is referring involve a sensory processing disorder that she has had since childhood. Michele is overly sensitive to tactile, vestibular, and auditory stimuli.

In June of 2001, Michele began a sensory diet in an effort to treat these difficulties. She believes that this very difficult and challenging process changed her life and influenced her ability to empathize with her clients. Michele describes this empathy as not only psychological but also somatic. Kielhofner (1992) coined the term "somatic empathy" and first described its nature and importance.

> The therapist must deeply empathize with how such a patient is attempting to accomplish movement to do a task. This special "somatic empathy" is necessary for a therapist to be able to work with a patient in an activity and know something of the experience of struggling with a particular body to move in order to accomplish an intention. This is complicated by the fact that the patient's body cannot move in the way the therapist's body does. Therapists must be able to project themselves vicariously into patients' bodies in order to comprehend what is going on and to direct it in the therapeutic encounter. (p. 228)

I was curious to learn more about Michele's interpretation. She described her somatic empathy as follows.

> It's being able to imagine in your own body the experiences that your client is undergoing in his or her own body.… It's attempting to feel those experiences within your own nervous system.

Michele's example epitomizes the transformation of a situation of great pain and suffering into one from which tremendous will and strength emerged (Fig. 16.6).

Another example of a therapist who has been able to transform difficulties into strengths is Kim Eberhardt. Kim's unique ability to center herself in another person—to distinguish between what her clients really need for themselves and what she thinks might be best for them—also suggested to me that a significant personal life experience might have influenced her outlook about her relationships with clients.

> Being in the position of some of my patients has influenced my view of what people really need when they are hospitalized for long periods of time. As a young child I was hospitalized for two years with kidney problems. Later on in my mid-twenties my mother was hospitalized with cancer and I served as her caretaker. I vicariously experienced some of the challenges that hospital environments bring from a caregiver perspective, which is something I never experienced before. It shed light on some of the concerns that family and friends have. When you have personal experiences I think you develop a kind of empathy that can be helpful.… I think every health care provider should spend time in a hospital once in their lives.

Jane Melton is another therapist whose work is characterized by a high value for empathy and for promoting client's individuality and autonomy. The perspective-

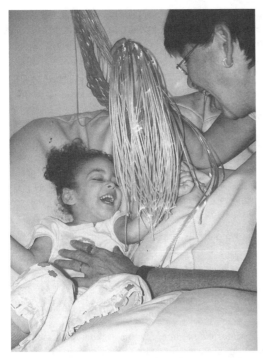

FIGURE 16.6 Michele Shapiro draws on her own experience when using touch with a vulnerable client

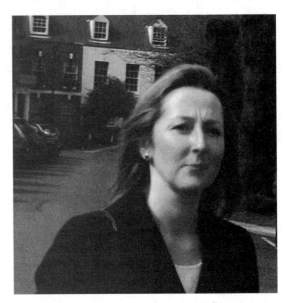

FIGURE 16.7 When encountering aggressive clients, Jane Melton draws on lessons from the past

changing experience that Jane Melton (Fig. 16.7) described occurred to her when she was very new to the field.

As a junior therapist I was seriously injured by a client at work. The situation was badly handled by the organization for the client and me. Though it was a very hard at the time, this difficult situation made me more determined to work to affect positive change in this field. I still do not feel at ease working with aggressive people displaying violent behavior, but I have learned that most acts of aggression have a reason.... When I do have to work with people who are hostile, I have learned to now focus on the positive aspects of their situation—for example by discovering ways to enable them to take more control of their lives and to engage in something meaningful and fulfilling. This helps me manage and put into perspective my own human response of apprehension about my own well-being.

René Bélanger is known for his high level of personal investment and passion about his work. When I asked him to reflect on significant aspects of his life that have influenced his work, he spoke of the complexities that accompany his sexual orientation.

The fact I am openly gay gives me the ability to recognize when clients try to avoid reality or adopt a false identity. I am familiar with the perils of trying to conform to an unrealistic idea of what some consider a 'normal life situation.' Because of this, I am able to confront and support clients who endure pain because they have an unrealistic view of themselves or they are hanging on to impossible, false, or idyllic ideas about what life should be like.... The fact that I'm a sexual minority also allows me to respect human diversity and people with very different values and world views. However, respecting this diversity does not mean that I would ignore the necessity for change when it is clear that conflicts of roles or habits are causing significant problems for a client.

Carmen-Gloria de Las Heras described the following difficulties and how she has managed to endure them.

Since my late adolescence I have had severe, chronic depression, which gave me the experience of the deepest feelings of helplessness, hopelessness, emptiness, no personal meaning, and feeling so different than who I was... I felt the terror of the symptoms.... For a long time, medications were not available to me in my country. I continued life and I now receive medications and psychotherapy. I accept it as part of myself now.... About five years ago I also had a brain tumor and underwent brain surgery. I have rheumatoid arthritis and I had a difficult marriage that involved overcoming domestic violence, the experience of a separation, and witnessing the pain that my children had to endure.

All of this somehow has influenced my practice in a good way. I think that I learned to be very sensitive, warm, and empathic towards others. I have an open mind, flexible approach, a deep sense of the other, I can be empathetic, and people can feel that I feel with them. My children and my work, music, nature, and cooking are my best allies and friends for facing and overcoming these difficulties.

Maintaining Mindfulness of Why You are an Occupational Therapist

A final feature that contributes to the ongoing journey of becoming a better therapist, I refer to as *mindfulness*. It refers to keeping in the forefront of your mind the meaning of your work. Mindfulness can involve recalling why you entered the field in the first place. It can be a reflection on a particular client or event that had meaning. It can involve drawing on some other aspect of yourself such as spiritual, cultural, or political beliefs. There is no real formula for mindfulness. Perhaps the best way to discuss it is to provide some examples.

I begin with Carmen-Gloria de Las Heras. Her description of what drew her into the field leans toward the suggestion that she was fated for this profession. Indeed, much of Carmen's mindfulness about being an occupational therapist reflects a personal conviction that it was destiny. Carmen describes a situation that illustrates how she first discovered occupational therapy as a child, long before she knew there was such a profession.

I met occupational therapy when I was so little (10 years old), and I never stopped living its values. My mother was a volunteer for an OT who worked with children who had terminal cancer. At that late stage and at that time in history (1970), there were not many ways of helping these children cope with their illness. But we introduced play, activities, clay, and other resources into the hospital.... From our efforts we could see the children smiling and laughing. One day we did a big project with clay in which the children made figures.... The children waited until nightfall when the lights were off and began to play war with the clay figures... The next day, the entire room was littered with clay.... I knew the children had been happy.... The next week two of the children had died. At that moment, as a child, I felt that I wanted to be able to do things that made people happy—even if they knew they were going to die. Thanks to the smiles of those children, I became and will never regret becoming an OT!

The mindfulness of some of the therapists I interviewed was influenced profoundly by spiritual experiences

or religious beliefs. For other therapists, spiritual or religious beliefs have brought new meaning into their practice or have reminded them of the significance of the work they do for others. Certainly, spiritual belief or experience is not a prerequisite for becoming a good therapist, but for some it is part of the path.

For example, I asked Michele Shapiro about being an occupational therapist. Her answer was consistent with what I would consider a spiritual perspective.

Today at the age of 55, when I look at my life in retrospect, I think that God led me to be an occupational therapist. I liked the idea of helping people, but I thought that I was too sensitive a person and that I wouldn't be able to cope because witnessing other people's pain would make me too sad. A wise person then said "It is *because* you are so sensitive that you will be able to help others." Little did I realize then how important that statement was. My understanding comes from my life's experience. But I became an OT before I understood all this, so I can only thank God for leading me down the right pathway."

Michele's beliefs are fueled by a powerful personal experience. Following major surgery in 1993, Michele experienced a life-threatening bilateral pulmonary embolism. For a brief period, she was declared clinically dead. Michele recalled that experience and explained how, during the period in which she was declared dead, she thought God gave her a choice of whether to live or to let go. According to Michele, choosing to live and surviving this near-death experience has had an endless and powerful influence on her value for life. Michele described her outlook as follows.

Years ago I remember saying to myself—If I were an OT just to help this one particular child, then my life has been worthwhile. Now I have said that so many times, but each time it feels wonderful all over again!

Like Michele, Belinda Anderson also mentioned her belief in God as motivating her to become an occupational therapist. She described the following life-changing incident.

The thing that really changed my mind was something that happened when I was 19 years old. On New Year's day my sister and I were going to go to a party. My mother gave us keys to the car, and we tried to start it, but something was wrong. I got out of the car to see what was wrong and my sister was still in there. I remember seeing the smoke and as I yelled "get out" the fire came up all around the perimeter of the car. Thanks to God, neither of us was hurt. But from then on I said to myself that I must be here for a reason and felt that the Lord wanted me to work with children. I felt that my duty to God was to be influential in a lot of people's lives.

When I asked Belinda what allows her to continue to practice, even during rough periods in her life, she relayed the following.

My mother, with whom I was very close, passed away a few years ago. I never thought that I would be able to do without her. But I felt that God gave me a kind of strength—kind of like a message that I was ready to continue practicing and that I was not alone. Plus my mother had always prepared me to be on my own.

Kathryn Loukas is another therapist who brought up issues of spirituality during our discussions of her work as a therapist. She relayed the following story as being highly influential in her motivation to continue to practice.

On one occasion I felt like it was a calling to work with a client. Matthew[1] is a very bright and a very likable young man. When he was 11 he experienced a catastrophic open head injury as a result of a car accident. His mother's car was struck by a drunk driver. His mother was killed, and his brother suffered extensive internal injuries. At that time, a woman, who would later become Matthew's home health care nurse, heard the accident and ran outside of her home to the scene to help.

After undergoing seven weeks of inpatient therapy at a local medical center, Matt continued to work with me for three solid years, three times per week, from fifth to eighth grade. During that time, we developed a strong therapeutic relationship, and Matt felt comfortable talking about a range of topics. We would talk about losing a parent, we would talk about the changes in his brain, the changes in his family situation at home, the changes in his left side, the visual-perceptual problems, the things he could not do with his left hand....

During this process, Matt and I became very close. I think he considered me as serving in a kind of maternal role for him, and I also felt very maternal toward him. However, his father had fallen in love with the home health nurse—the woman who had been at the scene of Matt's accident and worked a long time with Matt's brother. Toward the end of our work together I realized that I needed to step back and let this new woman in Matt's life move into his world. His father had become emotionally dead since the accident, and for the first time he came alive after initiating a relationship with this woman.

Stepping away from the family and from Matt in particular was very difficult for me. However, under the circumstances I felt it was vital to Matt's relationship with his new stepmother that I do this. The outcome of Matt's therapy had been unusually successful. Matt became a consistent honor roll student and the recipient of an award as an outstanding science student. There was no longer a pressing need for me to serve as his therapist. Letting go of our time together was not an easy process for me.

Later that year, I came across a book on handwriting in the library that was dedicated to Matt's mother. It was on the shelf next to another book I was looking at. I opened it up out of curiosity, and it just happened to open to the dedication page. Even though I have stopped working with Matt and his family, I still feel a strong sense of spirituality about Matt. I believe that, for the time I worked with him, God, and maybe even Matt's mother, wanted me to have a special place in his life.

The stories above illustrate ways in which spirituality can infuse meaning into occupational therapy work. Sociopolitical circumstances that affect our world views can also be strong influences on the meaning ascribed to practice. For example, Vardit Kindler, an occupational therapist who practices in Jerusalem, Israel noted:

I live in a highly tense part of the world where during specific periods of time difficult events envelop me. There is no doubt that they influence who I am and how I deal with life. I believe that all people in this country and region should be treated equally with recognition of cultural and religious differences. The variety of people whom I encounter and interact with in my work as an OT reflects my world view. In the therapeutic process my focus is on health and the child's functional needs within the context of the family and participation in daily activities. I believe that it can only be done via a dynamic reciprocal and interactive relationship with the child.

Vardit provides occupational therapy to children from both Israeli and Palestinian families. Given the ongoing threats, risks, and violence, Vardit and many of the other therapists I met in the Middle East (regardless of their ethnic and religious orientations) had a surprisingly optimistic and humanistic approach to therapy with the wide range of clients they see. It is a region of the world where difference abounds. Contrasting religious outlooks and political viewpoints create deep and painful divisions. For some therapists, the daily political, religious, and cultural tensions had a paradoxical effect of influencing their view of their work with a passion for respect of all people. For them, providing occupational therapy was one means of healing the wounds that divide so many.

---

[1] All client names and geographic information have been changed.

Summary

This final chapter explored four challenges involved in a therapist's ongoing journey toward professional development. As we saw, some therapists began the journey at an early age. For others, the journey peaked when they achieved a unique level of wisdom from having to confront an uncommon, difficult, or deeply spiritual human experience or circumstance.

The core aspects of your temperament, personality, personal values, and world view coupled with ongoing experiences, inside and outside of therapy, shape who you become as a therapist. In the end, you have to rely on your unique combination of natural interpersonal strengths, cultivated interpersonal abilities, and areas of challenge. The key to intentional practice is not to strive to be someone else but to gain awareness of your own therapeutic qualities and to build on and refine those qualities. Three exercises located in the Activities section of this chapter are provided to help you begin this endeavor.

This book featured the stories of a dozen exceptional therapists. They were recommended to me by their peers as people with well developed interpersonal skills who infuse their practice of occupational therapy with a high level of judgment, care, and empathy. In writing this book it is my hope that these individuals will serve as very human and approachable role models of intentional interpersonal practice. I am convinced that with time I might have found many more therapists who could serve as equally stellar role models. As a final note, I encourage you to find those nearby who can best serve as peer advisors, models, and mentors for yourself and to use the guidelines in this book to shape your mutual learning endeavors.

ACTIVITIES FOR LEARNING AND REFLECTION

Cultivating Self-Awareness in the Face of Challenges

Cultivating self-awareness involves knowing those things about yourself that may have positive or negative effects during therapy, particularly when you are confronted with a situation that is interpersonally challenging. In some cases, your interpersonal behavior in response to a challenge is more likely to have positive effects on the relationship. For example, being empathic is a positive trait provided it is not overused to the extent that it enables a client's negative behavior to continue. In other cases, a behavior is mainly a liability in that it produces negative effects. For example, being impatient with a client or sidestepping an issue when it should be confronted are almost always liabilities. In still other instances, an interpersonal behavior may be a proverbial double-edged sword. In this chapter, we saw that a tendency to be emotionally transparent was such a behavior. There are times when, and clients for whom, it can be very positive and others when and for whom it can lead to unanticipated complexities.

Although developing an ability to be critical of your own behavior does not require you to write down your interpersonal reactions and behaviors, it can be helpful as a means of reflecting on your personality style. One way of performing this self-reflection is to record, on copies of the form below, traits you notice about yourself and ways in which others may react to this trait when you encounter challenging interpersonal situations (both positively and negatively, if this is the case). You may use experiences from both inside and outside of therapy to complete the form. It is helpful to write down either a general description of what you notice about how others react to this trait and/or to write specific examples. Keeping a copy of the form(s) you complete and updating it (them) from time to time based on experience can be a useful way to maintain critical self-reflection.

Developing Critical Self-Awareness in Response to Challenges		
Interpersonal behavior exhibited when feeling a challenge, stress, or tension	**Negative impact of this behavior in interactions (describe or give examples)**	**Positive impact of this behavior during interactions (describe or give examples—you may write "none" if you see no potential benefit of this behavior)**

EXERCISE 16.2

Cultivating Reflective Use of Your Current Strengths, Weaknesses, Limits, Preferences, and World Views

Reflective use of your traits in therapy involves three aspects: (1) anticipating how you might use or curtail a particular personal tendency in therapy; (2) noticing the impact of a particular personal behavior during therapy and then continuing, discontinuing, or modifying it strategically to achieve a better outcome; and (3) reflecting on something that happened as a result of your behavior during therapy and clarifying the lesson for the future.

The following are some ways to increase habitual awareness.

- Anticipate how you might use or curtail a particular personal tendency during therapy. Before each session with a given client take just a moment to reflect on:
  - What this client needs from you on an interpersonal level
- Process the effects of your behavior after stressful encounters. After a particularly challenging client or group session, take a moment to reflect on:
  - Your emotional reactions during and after the session
  - What interpersonal behaviors you exhibited and their consequences for the relationship
- Keep a journal of reflections on particularly salient moments during therapy.
- Identify someone (supervisor, colleague) who can serve as a mentor when you have questions about your therapeutic use of self.
- Set specific goals for yourself to eliminate or reduce a behavior that you know is not therapeutically effective and monitor your progress using a tally sheet, calendar, or other concrete way of documenting the behavior.
- Set a specific goal to use a new interpersonal style or strategy during therapy. Document your progress, and note its consequences.

These are just a few strategies for developing aspects of your therapeutic use of self. Whether you use one particular strategy is not as important as finding what works for you and consistently using it in a self-reflective manner.

EXERCISE 16.3

Mindfulness

It is a good idea to periodically think about the meaning of your role as a therapist. One means some people find helpful is to take some time to write and reflect on it. This reflection can take on many forms, for example:

- Write down what it means to you to be a therapist and keep what you wrote in a designated place. Periodically go back to read it and add other thoughts.
- Identify some specific times you can set aside to reflect on being a therapist (e.g., the anniversary of your becoming a therapist; whenever you finish with a particularly challenging client).
- Find an individual or a group open to discussing the topic of your life work in a mutually supportive way and have occasional conversations about it.

GLOSSARY

Activity focusing Strategies for responding to interpersonal events that emphasize doing issues over feeling or relating issues.

Boundary testing Client behavior that violates or that asks the therapist to act in ways that are outside the defined therapeutic relationship.

Conflict Disagreement, argument, or dispute between a client and a therapist.

Contextual inconsistencies Any aspect of a client's interpersonal or physical environments that changes during the course of therapy.

Crisis points Unanticipated, stressful events that cause clients to become distracted and/or that temporarily interfere with clients' ability for occupational engagement.

Critical self-awareness Having a working knowledge of one's interpersonal tendencies while interacting with clients of different personality styles and under different conditions and circumstances.

Cultural competence Incorporates a therapist's knowledge of, respect for, and ability to incorporate the customs, behaviors, belief systems, world views, and health care practices of individuals with backgrounds other than their own.

Denial A way of coping with a painful or uncomfortable event that involves denying its existence, minimizing its impact, or rejecting one's personal connection to the event.

Desired occupation Task or activity that the therapist and the client have selected for therapy.

Difficult interpersonal behavior Any recurring, enduring, or high-intensity communication or other behavior that prompts one or more negative emotional reactions in another individual.

Difficulty with rapport Evident when a client is unfriendly or unresponsive to any attempts to make casual conversation or to find a common ground for communication.

Difficulty with trust Becomes apparent over time as a client expresses various forms of skepticism and uneasiness about the process of therapy.

Doorknob comments Occur when clients allude to something important in a vague way or time what they say inappropriately so as to leave the therapist with a choice of whether to pick up on the hint or ignore it.

Emotional buoy Therapist who continually orients and guides clients through the interview by highlighting shifts in major topic areas, marking how much has been accomplished and how much is left to do, and describing the questions to come. Therapists occasionally provide positive feedback to clients about their behavior during the interview.

Emotional climate Refers to the nature and intensity of affect and the style in which affect is expressed by both the client and the therapist during an interaction.

Emotional disengagement Occurs when a client is not experiencing spontaneous and authentic emotional reactions to the interpersonal events of therapy.

Emotional resonance Defined as feeling the same type of emotion as the client and allowing one's feelings to show through one's affect or in what one says.

Emotionally charged therapy tasks and situations Activities and circumstances in therapy that can lead clients to become overwhelmed or experience uncomfortable emotional reactions such as embarrassment, humiliation, or shame.

Empathic break Situation in which a therapist fails to notice or understand a communication from a client or initiates a communication or behavior that is perceived by the client as hurtful or insensitive.

Enduring characteristic Stable and consistent interpersonal aspects of the client that comprise an interpersonal profile idiosyncratic to the client.

Excessive dependence Occurs when a client is resistant to any attempts by the therapist to promote independent thinking and/or functioning.

Expressions of strong emotion External displays of internal feelings that are shown with a level of intensity beyond usual cultural norms for interaction.

Hostility Multifaceted verbal or behavioral expression of anger or rage.

Human diversity Defines differences between individuals or groups of individuals in any number of characteristics, including sex, age, race, ethnicity, language, and religious orientation.

Hyperverbal When clients talk to the point that they are unaware of the natural rhythm, shifts, pauses, and boundaries of conversation.

Impression management Consists of intentional statements and behaviors that allow the client to begin to trust in the therapist's personal and professional integrity.

Interpersonal event A naturally occurring communication, reaction, process, task, or general circumstance that occurs during therapy that has the potential to detract from or strengthen the therapeutic relationship.

Interpersonal event cascade When more than one interpersonal event follows the therapist's initial response to a single interpersonal event.

Interpersonal focusing Strategies that emphasize feeling and relating issues over doing issues.

Interpersonal reasoning Process by which a therapist consciously and reflectively monitors both the therapeutic relationship and the interpersonal events of therapy in order to decide on and enact appropriate interpersonal strategies.

Interpersonal self-discipline Ability to anticipate, measure, and respond to the effects of ongoing communications with a client.

Interpersonal skill base Interpersonal skills that are judiciously applied by the therapist to build a functional working relationship with the client.

Interpersonal style Therapeutic mode or set of modes that characterize a therapist's general approach to interacting with clients.

Intervening Refers to saying or doing something deliberately aimed to modify (rather than validate) the client's emotional expression.

Intimate self-disclosures Statements or stories that reveal something unobservable, private, or sensitive about the person making the disclosure.

Judicious use of touch Refers to knowing how to use touch that is intended to have interpersonal effects in a way that respects clients' boundaries and meets their needs for closeness or distance.

Labeling Involves describing what one observes in a client's affect or behavior in order to highlight, clarify, or validate it.

Limitations of therapy Restrictions on the available or possible services, time, resources, or therapist actions.

Managing emotional intensity Entails knowing what to do when clients exhibit pronounced feelings of sadness, anger, or anxiety.

Manipulative behavior Refers to underhanded efforts to maintain control or have one's own way when interacting with others.

Mindful empathy An objective state of observation in which the therapist comes to feel and understand a client's underlying emotions, needs, and motives, while at the same time maintaining an objective viewpoint.

Mode matching and versatility Refers to the therapist's ability to anticipate which interpersonal mode is best suited for a client at any given time and to flexibly apply modes as needed using mode shifts.

Mode shift A therapist's intentional decision to change the way he or she is currently interacting with a client by discontinuing use of one mode and initiating use of another mode.

Multimodal Describes a therapist who is able to utilize any of the six interpersonal modes with equal accuracy, comfort, and effectiveness and is able to select the appropriate mode according to the needs of the client and the situation at hand.

No cross-talk rule Guideline for listening during conflict resolution. It means that the other individual must listen fully and never interrupt the person who is explaining his or her point of view.

Nonverbal cues Communications that do not involve the use of formal language.

No retribution rule Guideline for listening during conflict resolution. It means that each participant must not blame the other for having raised an issue or disclosed a perspective.

Ongoing critical awareness Constant mindfulness of what one is communicating verbally, nonverbally, and emotionally along with what one is withholding, limiting, or otherwise not communicating and the implications of these noncommunications for the therapeutic interaction.

Phenomenological perspective Understands problematic behavior as based in something a person is experiencing, thinking, or feeling about the situation at hand.

Power dilemmas Tensions that arise in the therapeutic relationship because of clients' innate feelings about issues of power, the inherent situation of therapy, the therapist's behavior, and/or other circumstances that underscore clients' lack or loss of power over aspects of their lives.

Rapport building Involves making deliberate efforts to make a client feel comfortable in the therapist's presence and to establish a common ground for communication.

Reluctance Disinclination toward some aspect of therapy for reasons outside the therapeutic relationship.

Resistance Client's passive or active refusal to participate in some or all aspects of therapy for reasons linked to the therapeutic relationship.

Response mode Concrete action or communication that reflects the therapist's use of a given mode.

Response mode sequence Series of mode shifts in which the therapist draws on more than one category of response mode to address one or more interpersonal events that occur sequentially, or a cascade of interpersonal events.

Situational characteristics Characteristics that are inconsistent with the way an individual typically behaves when interacting with others. In practice settings, they are usually linked to stressful circumstances.

Strategic questioning Asking clients questions in a way that intends to influence their perspective, convey a certain message, or cause them to reflect on and evaluate their thinking about a given topic.

Symptom focusing Specific approach to managing an impairment that involves spending a great deal of mental energy, time, and/or physical effort giving in to one's symptoms (or impairment) and spending considerably less time attempting to ignore, implicitly endure, or adjust to symptoms in order to engage in occupations.

Tangential When clients digress onto related topics or have difficulty getting to the point when responding to a question.

Therapeutic mode One of six specific ways of relating to a client.

Therapeutic relationship Socially defined and personally interpreted interactive process between the therapist and a client.

Twinship need Defined as an individual's deep psychological need to connect with others who are perceived as similar in fundamental ways, such as their world view, religious orientation, or cultural background.

Witnessing Refers to being present in the room with the client but not necessarily saying or doing anything to intervene in the expression of emotion.

INDEX

Note: Page numbers followed by f refer to figures; those followed by t refer to tables.